Contents

CRIPPING INTERSEX

DISABILITY CULTURE AND POLITICS

**Series Editors: Christine Kelly (University of Manitoba)
and Michael Orsini (University of Ottawa)**

This series highlights the works of emerging and established authors who are challenging us to think anew about the politics and cultures of disability. Reconceiving disability politics means dismantling the strict divides among culture, art, and politics. It also means appreciating how disability art and culture inform and transform disability politics in Canada and, conversely, how politics shape what counts as art in the name of disability. Drawing from diverse scholarship in feminist and gender studies, political science, social work, sociology, and law, among others, works in this series bring to the fore the implicitly and explicitly political dimensions of disability.

This is the fifth volume in the series. The previous volumes are:

Mobilizing Metaphor: Art, Culture, and Disability Activism in Canada, edited by Christine Kelly and Michael Orsini

Disabling Barriers: Social Movements, Disability History, and the Law, edited by Ravi Malhotra and Benjamin Isitt

The Aging–Disability Nexus, edited by Katie Aubrecht, Christine Kelly, and Carla Rice

Disability Injustice: Confronting Criminalization in Canada, edited by Kelly Fritsch, Jeffrey Monaghan, and Emily van der Meulen

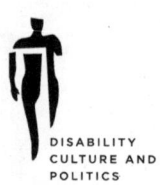

DISABILITY
CULTURE AND
POLITICS

CRIPPING INTERSEX

CELESTE E. ORR

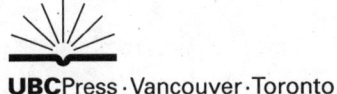
UBCPress · Vancouver · Toronto

31 30 29 28 27 26 25 24 23 22   5 4 3 2 1

Printed in Canada on FSC-certified ancient-forest-free paper (100% post-consumer recycled) that is processed chlorine- and acid-free.

Library and Archives Canada Cataloguing in Publication

Title: Cripping intersex / Celeste E. Orr.
Names: Orr, Celeste E., author.
Series: Disability culture and politics.
Description: Series statement: Disability culture & politics | Includes bibliographical
    references and index.
Identifiers: Canadiana (print) 20220281572 | Canadiana (ebook) 2022028203X |
    ISBN 9780774865531 (hardcover) | ISBN 9780774865548 (paperback) |
    ISBN 9780774868549 (PDF) | ISBN 9780774865654 (EPUB)
Subjects: LCSH: Intersex people. | LCSH: Intersex people—Health and hygiene. |
    LCSH: Intersex people—Psychology. | LCSH: Intersex people—Medical care. |
    LCSH: Intersex people—Social conditions. | LCSH: Intersex people—Identity. |
    LCSH: Discrimination against intersex people. | LCSH: Discrimination against
    people with disabilities.
Classification: LCC HQ78 .O77 2022 | DDC 306.76/85—dc23

Canadä

UBC Press gratefully acknowledges the financial support for our publishing program of the Government of Canada (through the Canada Book Fund), the Canada Council for the Arts, and the British Columbia Arts Council.

This book has been published with the help of a grant from the Canadian Federation for the Humanities and Social Sciences, through the Awards to Scholarly Publications Program, using funds provided by the Social Sciences and Humanities Research Council of Canada.

Printed and bound in Canada by Friesens
Set in Futura Condensed and Warnock by Artegraphica Design Co.
Copy editor: Robert Lewis
Proofreader: Jesse Marchand
Indexer: Matthew MacLellan
Cover designer: David Drummond

UBC Press
The University of British Columbia
2029 West Mall
Vancouver, BC V6T 1Z2
www.ubcpress.ca

Acknowledgments

To the scholars, activists, advocates, friends, chosen family, and others who struggle against and seek to dismantle compulsory modes of being: thank you for sharing your work, knowledges, and insights with me in direct and indirect ways. The formation of this book would not have been possible without so many astute, thoughtful, and deliberate intellectual giants educating me along the way.

Thank you to my publisher, UBC Press, specifically my editor, James MacNevin, who kindly helped guide me through this process. James's insights and supervision have been instrumental. Thank you to the Disability Culture and Politics series editors at UBC Press, Michael Orsini and Christine Kelly, for offering invaluable support. I am forever indebted to Michael, who saw this work as a book project long before I knew that such an undertaking was even possible. I extend my deepest gratitude to my peer reviewers for taking the time to engage with my manuscript and for offering their enthusiastic support and thoughtful commentary. I am also grateful to the production editor, Meagan Dyer, copy editor, Robert Lewis, and the book cover designer, David Drummond. Additionally, thanks to the Social Sciences and Humanities Research Council of Canada for aiding in this book's publication.[1]

Corrie Scott and Shoshana Magnet, who were my PhD supervisor and co-supervisor respectively, have helped me with this project since its earliest conception. I feel incredibly fortunate that I had such clever, generous, rigorous, and caring supervisors. Without their support, encouragement, and innumerable lessons, this book would not have been possible. To this day, I consistently remind myself of Corrie's lesson to think creatively and of Shoshana's lesson that it is alright to sit with bad feelings and not to be okay all the time.

For epitomizing feminist academes and teaching me so much, thank you to Alexandre Baril and Kathryn Trevenen, whose kindness and wisdom continue to influence and inspire my work and way of be(com)ing in the world. Additionally, I am grateful to Jennifer Blair, Alison Kafer, and Denise Spitzer for supporting this project in its earlier form.

Thank you to my friends and (chosen) family for always offering care, support, patience, and love. I extend my deep gratitude to Hayley Crooks, Keelan Harkin, Nicholas Hrynyk, Alessia Iani, and Meg Peters for being intellectual visionaries and the best of friends throughout much of my graduate and professional life. Additionally, El Yazid Alaoui, Lucy Ellis, Moneca Lu, Sarah MacKenzie, Meghan Martel, Lisa Nazarenko, Lucy Ngo, Dylan Spicker, and Melissa Van Bussel have been indispensable, loving supports. All of these shrewd feminist killjoys continue to restore, energize, feed, and hydrate me. Thank you to my family, especially my gram, June Orr, and my parents, Margee Duffield and John Orr. In their own unique ways, they have provided me with encouragement during my academic pursuits. I am also grateful for the invaluable support of my partner's family. A special thank you to Quinn Cassady, Guy Cassady, Lee-Ann VanWees, and Truus VanWees.

Lastly, I extend my heartfelt appreciation to my partner, Dana Cassady, whose incredible love sustains me and whose propensity to make trouble motivates and emboldens me. Dana, my love for you is immeasurable; never stop being a magnificent, gorgeous troublemaker.

CRIPPING INTERSEX

Introduction
Intersex and/as/is/with Disability

Intersex activist and co-founder of Organisation Intersex International, Vincent Guillot (in Lohr 2016), recounts that after his mother gave birth, she was told that "she had given birth to a monster." She had given birth to a supposedly aberrant, shameful, disordered baby with intersex traits that defied the sacrosanct male-female sex dyad. Or, in more medicalizing terminology, Guillot was born with a disorder of sex development (DSD) that demanded a medical "cure." Rather than being given the truth about his diagnosis, Guillot was lied to. At the age of seven, told that he had appendicitis warranting surgery, Guillot underwent the first of several surgeries to exorcise his body of the "monstrous" intersex characteristics. "They wanted to make a boy out of me," Guillot explains, "so they simply cut away whatever they didn't like ... After all, I was a monstrosity." Guillot's undeniably tragic, painful experiences of pathologization, shame, and deceit are unfortunately not unique. Given that most medical professionals across the globe insist that intersex variations are medical emergencies – innate pathologies, disorders, diseases, or disabilities – that require curative interventions, countless people with intersex characteristics are routinely subjected to, to borrow from disability studies scholar Eunjung Kim (2017, 10), "curative violence":[1] gratuitous cosmetic surgeries, hormone replacement therapies (HRT), medical surveillance, and so on. Given the violent nature of these procedures, they typically result in myriad short- and/or long-term disabilities such as depression, anxiety, suicidal ideation, loss of genital sensation or ability to orgasm, incontinence, anesthetic neurotoxicity, chronic infection, and genital pain.

Guillot's and other intersex people's stories have largely remained outside of popular cultural consciousness due, in part, to medical professionals' insistence that intersex traits, diagnoses, and medical interventions must remain secret. In some cases, medical professionals have explained to parents/proxies that their intersex infants or children must never know of the diagnosis. Knowing about their "monstrous" difference would be too traumatic. Others have instructed parents/proxies to tell their children that they must never speak of their differences and diagnoses, why they were in the hospital, or why medical interventions took place. This approach has prevented intersex people from knowing their own bodies and medical histories, as well as from taking pride in their bodies, connecting with other intersex individuals, and developing trusting bonds with their parents/proxies and doctors. Additionally, these secrets and these instances of routine curative violence that aim to exorcise intersex have resolidified the sacred cultural belief and investment in the idea that there are only two sexes, "female" and "male." However, many intersex people have learned the truth and spoken the truth. After fighting to get hold of their medical records, they were finally told the truth, and they shared their stories and formed invaluable bonds and alliances with other intersex people. The Intersex Rights Movement was born, along with intersex studies, a field that radically challenges interphobic curative violence and all forms of interphobia.

Due to the tireless and successful labour performed by intersex activists like Guillot as well as intersex advocates and intersex studies scholars, intersex human rights issues are entering mainstream conversations like never before. The ostensible intersex monsters are coming "out of the shadows" (Caplan-Bricker 2017). The "I" is apparently "no longer silent" in "LGBTIQ" (S. Richards 2018). The "I" is "speaking" about the harms of pathologization, lies, and curative violence, and many people are ready and willing to listen and ready to question medical professionals' exalted cultural reputation and supposed investment in "first do no harm." In an effort to resist curative violence, many intersex activists, advocates, and intersex studies scholars counter medical professionals' claims that intersex traits are pathological, maintaining that intersex variations are not a disability, disorder, or disease.

That is, according to medical professionals, intersex characteristics are innate disabilities, disorders, or diseases that must be cured – eradicated. On the contrary, many intersex activists, advocates, and intersex studies scholars posit that intersex traits are *not* disabled, disordered, or diseased.

They insist that intersex characteristics are normal, natural, or simply atypical human variations that do not require a cure. Rather than nonconsensually and irreversibly altering intersex people's biological traits to make them "fit" the sex dyad, medical professionals must do away with the sex dyad. There must be radical shifts in how biological sex is understood and in how medical practitioners approach, interpret, and "treat" intersex variations. If, for instance, intersex traits were not construed as disabilities, disorders, or diseases – if they were not deemed heretics of the female-male sex binary that demand exorcisms – Guillot and countless other folks with intersex traits would not have been understood as monstrous; they would not have been subjected to disabling curative violence.

There is evidently a warranted debate over what intersex is and how medical professionals respond to intersex characteristics. And this debate over what intersex means clearly hinges on what disability, disorder, and disease mean. As this debate continues and as conversations about intersex, the consequences of intersex medical management, and intersex human rights issues become more mainstream, it is vital to reflect on how intersex is understood and what specific understandings accomplish. If pathologization calls for curative violence, does insisting that intersex traits are not pathological disabilities, disorders, or diseases successfully combat said violence? Are intersex characteristics really or really not disabilities? Does claiming that intersex variations are not disabilities, disorders, or diseases help to undermine the sex dyad? To answer these questions, this book explores the political, discursive, and embodied connection between intersex and disability. To investigate this connection, I place intersex studies in conversation with disability studies to see if, how, when, and why intersex and interphobia intersect with, collapse into, or become indistinguishable from disability and ableism. In doing so, I propose and demonstrate the need for a new field of study, crip intersex studies, as well as a crip approach to intersex activism.

Integrating disability studies into intersex studies and effectively transforming it into crip intersex studies offers the tools required to break down the traditional sex binary and what I term "compulsory dyadism": the instituted cultural mandate that people cannot undermine the sex dyad by possessing intersex traits or housing "the spectre of intersex" (Sparrow 2013, 29). The spectre, according to this mandate, must be exorcised. Distancing intersex from disability by insisting that intersex is "not that" reproduces ableist discourses and prevents intersex studies scholars, activists, and advocates from using the necessary tools offered by feminist disability and crip studies to successfully combat the ableism that underpins compulsory dyadism. Effectively undermining compulsory dyadism is impossible without also resisting ableism and undermining "compulsory able-bodiedness" (McRuer 2013, 369). Given that people with intersex traits who "fail" the sex dyad are deemed disabled, disordered, or diseased and are often subjected to medically unnecessary interventions to "cure" that which is supposedly out of order, studies and activism regarding intersex and disability must be actively politically linked.

One may consider analyzing intersex issues through disability frameworks to be inappropriate or odd given that intersex traits are not immediately legible or understood as disabilities outside of medical contexts. Given that intersex variations concern one's biological sex, intersex is typically presumed to be under the jurisdiction of gender, queer, and sexuality studies. As a result, a crip intersex project or field of study may seem out of place. Nevertheless, as noted by Emi Koyama (2006), a multi-issue social justice activist and the founder of the advocacy organization Intersex Initiative (IPDX), "gender and sexual frontlines are not distinct from the battleground of disability politics." Sex, gender, sexuality, and disability – indeed, any part of one's embodiment, experiences, or identities – do not exist in isolation.

Moreover, it is important to keep in mind that socio-medical "body-mind" (Clare 2017, xvi) categories and diagnoses are constantly in flux and contested. As a result, there is very little reason to debate whether intersex variations are "really" or "really like" disabilities. How intersex and/as/is/with disability are understood is a discursive process, not an objective assessment. Actively resisting association with disability – or attempting to demonstrate that intersex is not "really like that" – is counterproductive given that ableist ideologies are exploited to justify compulsory dyadism and interphobic curative violence. Intersex traits that breach compulsory dyadism are understood as simultaneously violating compulsory able-bodiedness.

Disability studies scholars Anna Mollow and Robert McRuer (2012, 13) write that "what is interpretable as disability" – or a disability issue – "need not be tethered to a disability identity." Likewise, drawing connections between intersex and disability does not require that intersex people understand themselves as disabled or claim disability or crip as identities. This anti-essentialist and post-identity-politics approach "enables sitings of disability," as well as intersex and/as/is/with disability, "in multiple, often unexpected, locations, rather than solely in the bodies and minds of a few individuals" (Mollow and McRuer 2012, 13).[2] Ultimately, intersex is a disability issue because intersex characteristics are increasingly being integrated into conventional, ableist notions of disability, disorder, and disease to justify curative violence and other forms of cultural violence, erasure, and exclusion.

In the 1990s, many people in Deaf communities attempted to resist pathologization and to celebrate Deaf culture by claiming that Deaf people are not disabled but a linguistic subgroup. Disability studies scholar Lennard J. Davis (1995, xix–xx), however, endeavoured to draw a political link between Deafness and disability at this time:

> There has been too little examination of the connection between Deafness and disability. Because many Deaf activists have strongly defined themselves as a linguistic minority and not disabled, political bonds and political activity have been discouraged between the Deaf and people with disabilities ... I want to move through issues of Deafness to general statements about disability. While I understand that such a move will displease some in the Deaf community, I ask that they forbear in order to see what benefits, if any, may accrue from such a method.

Critical projects like Davis's have outlined overlaps between Deafness and disability and have shown the advantages of these camps forming political bonds. In response, many (but not all) Deaf people have productively and positively engaged with disability. Rather than espousing "stigmaphobic distancing" from disability, many Deaf people have gotten involved in reinventing disability not only by resisting the ableist, medical model of disability – the idea that a person's disabilities or impairments are an innate problem and, therefore, must be cured and avoided at all costs – but also by celebrating Deaf culture and disability (McRuer 2006, 85). The idea of being a valuable linguistic minority and the idea of being disabled were no longer understood as mutually exclusive within Deaf communities.

Similar to Davis's (1995) acknowledgment that there was too little examination of the relationship between Deafness and disability, *Cripping Intersex* remedies the lack of examination of the fraught relationship between intersex and disability. At this particular moment, when the Intersex Rights Movement has been deemed the "next civil rights frontier" (Andrews 2017) and when there is evident distancing from disability, this analysis of the connection between intersex and disability will perhaps result in some discontentment. Analyzing said connection may trouble some people who view intersex characteristics as entirely normal or who conceptualize intersex people as a sex/ual minority, queer, or the third sex, not as disabled, disordered, or diseased. Nevertheless, like Davis's bold request, I ask possible discontented readers to forbear in order to see what benefits emerge from cripping intersex studies.

Dis/association with Disability

Amid the cultural battle over what intersex means, Morgan Holmes (2009b, 5–6) claims in the introduction to her edited collection *Critical Intersex*, "Intersex studies draws as much from the impulses, theoretical frameworks and critical lens of *disability studies* as from the development of queer theory/studies and gender studies informed by feminist theory" (emphasis added). In addition to Holmes, a handful of other intersex studies scholars, activists, and advocates enthusiastically and liberally draw from disability studies.[3] Yet, to the detriment of their work, many do not implicitly or explicitly engage with disability scholarship. For instance, although Tiffany Jones and colleagues (2016) suggest in their book, *Intersex: Stories and Statistics from Australia*, that intersex issues could be folded into disability studies and activism, they note that there are disputes about whether that should actually happen.

One of the main points of contention concerns dissociation with or "stigmaphobic distancing" from disability, disorder, or disease (McRuer 2006, 85). Queer and disability studies scholar Abby L. Wilkerson (2012, 185) notes that given dominant ableist ideas about what it means to be disabled, be diagnosed as disabled, or live with a disability, some intersex activists "vehemently refuse any association with it." Due to these ableist perceptions, and in the attempt to resist pathologization, some intersex individuals do not align or identify with disability. Perhaps their perceptions of disability or diagnosis do not align with their lived realities. This resistance is evidenced by some intersex people's disidentification with intersex medical nomenclature that emphasizes disability or disorder, specifically the diagnostic term "disorder of sex development" (DSD).

When DSD terminology was introduced, it caused considerable, warranted anger. In October 2005, fifty experts from various fields, including urology, genetics, endocrinology, gender studies, and activism, gathered to revise the medical treatment guidelines for people with intersex traits (G. Davis 2015; Greenberg 2012; Karkazis 2008). This meeting was the first (but not the last) of its kind. The results of the meeting were published in *Archives of Disease in Childhood* and titled "Consensus Statement on Management of Intersex Disorders" (I.A. Hughes et al. 2006). In re/medicalizing fashion, "intersex" was replaced with DSD terminology; the idea that intersex is a disorder was effectively solidified. Even though the statement claims that having intersex anatomy is not shameful, the practice of "normalizing" surgery, particularly for children assigned female, is still endorsed. Despite the misleading use of the word "consensus" in the article's title, the meeting participants were not all in agreement, and the article was not met with general accord. Many intersex activists and intersex studies scholars rightly note that the statement does not do enough to prevent nonconsensual and irreversible medical procedures. Others, such as intersex studies scholar and activist Georgiann Davis (2015, 54), argue that introducing DSD terminology enabled medical professionals "to reclaim their jurisdiction over intersex" just as the Intersex Rights Movement was gaining considerable ground and attention (also see Holmes 2011).

Since the advent of DSD nomenclature, there has been significant conflict concerning the discursive relationship between intersex, disability, disorder, and disease. For example, a participant in Davis's (2014, 19) study argues, "DSD is not ... something a lot of people want to identify with ... nobody wants to be a disorder ... Who wants to be a fucking disorder? ... I don't." Likewise, summarizing an interview with Marissa Adams, an intersex person, Nora Caplan-Bricker (2017) writes in the *Washington Post,* "The Intersex Rights Movement has a message for the world: We aren't disordered and we aren't ashamed." Susannah Cornwall (2013, 373), quoting Intersex Human Rights Australia (IHRA) (then known as Organisation Intersex International Australia), similarly draws readers' attention to the fact that some intersex activists reject disability: "INTERSEX is *not* a medical condition or a disorder or a disability or a pathology or a condition of any sort."[4] These kinds of declarations are intended to combat pathologization and curative violence. One may assume that an association with disability will fuel medical interventions and stoke stigma. Nevertheless, perhaps unwittingly, such declarations reproduce the cultural perception that disabilities or disorders are inherently inferior or undesirable. Even if one does not personally maintain that disability is innately wrong or degenerate, such assertions distance intersex from disability because of the belief that "such an association" may "worsen" intersex people's position (Cornwall 2013, 373). However, fuelling medical interventions and stoking stigma are not the inevitable or logical conclusions of aligning with disability or cripping intersex. Rather, doing so reproduces ableism and does not effectively undermine the ableist intersex-as/is-disability medical model. A crip intersex approach ensures that ableist ideologies do not underpin intersex human rights claims and proves that disability ought to be important to intersex studies and to intersex human rights projects.

The critiques about DSD terminology and curative violence are unquestionably valid and needed. The institutionalization of DSD terminology and the "Consensus Statement on Management of Intersex Disorders" ultimately highlight the medical community's resistance to conceptualizing intersex traits as anything other than disordered pathologies that require a cure. DSD terminology and the "Consensus Statement" also clearly illustrate the discursive solidification of intersex-as/is-disability – the interconnectedness of compulsory dyadism and able-bodiedness. As a result, an approach rooted in crip intersex studies is required both to productively address this connection and to ensure that an anti-ableist framework is mobilized. Resisting pathologization and critiquing DSD language need not involve rejecting disability or entail stigmaphobic distancing from disability, disorder, or disease.

Cripping intersex also grants intersex studies scholars and intersex activists and advocates access to disability and crip knowledges, philosophies, and methods that can effectively dismantle compulsory dyadism. The sophisticated theorizations of, for example, "normality," the deployments of ableist discourses and metaphors in medical and nonmedical contexts, interdependency, and self-determination that have emerged from disability studies and activism can only bolster intersex projects as intersex studies scholars and activists grapple with the ableist intersex-as/is-disability medical model. Moreover, forging an alliance with disability groups may provide many intersex people with more much-needed space to share their experiences of medicalization and living with various traumatic – indeed, disabling – outcomes created by medical interventions (Cornwall 2009). Ultimately, without wielding the unique tools that disability studies provide, projects that combat compulsory dyadism and interphobic curative violence will fall short in some respects.

That being said, in addition to emerging intersex studies literature that integrates disability studies, there are some promising steps being made and alliances being formed between intersex and disability activist communities. For example, Koyama (2006) has for some time now recognized that disability politics must be important to intersex human rights projects. Further, IHRA's statement – "INTERSEX is *not* a medical condition or a disorder or a disability or a pathology or a condition of any sort" – is no longer featured on the organization's website. In line with this removal,

Morgan Carpenter (2012), intersex activist and president of IHRA, writes that "the intersex experience, and the intersex movement, has many intersectionalities with experiences of disability ... Intersex people are medicalised, stigmatised and suffer discrimination due to our distinctive biological characteristics."

This consideration of disability gestures to a productive and much-needed collaborative relationship between intersex and disability activism and studies. Given the dominant ableist intersex-as/is-disability medical model, the interphobic violence that intersex people experience is inextricably tied to and supported by ableism. The fact that interphobia and ableism are fundamentally intertwined systems of oppression must be underscored and centralized. Without full acknowledgment that interphobia and ableism are interwoven – and not, for example, merely tangential – a crucial and detrimental distance between intersex and disability is maintained. By unequivocally stating that disability is an intersex issue, scholars, activists, and advocates alike can better address and resist the ableist intersex-as/is-disability medical model and, in turn, can conceptualize an intersex-with-disability politics – a crip intersex politics.

Interestingly, some disability studies scholars, typically without explanation, narrate intersex as a disability or a disability matter. For instance, Rosemarie Garland-Thomson (2005, 1558) asserts, "Feminist disabilities studies acknowledges communities of all people based on shared disability experiences, and it recognizes the differences among the wide variety of stigmatized forms of embodiments that constitute disability in its broadest conceptualization – from blindness to *intersex* to dyslexia" (emphasis added).[5] This sort of inclusion of intersex in disability studies literature signals an openness and commitment to the porousness of disability experiences as well as to disability as a cultural concept, discourse, creation, identity, and embodiment. The inclusion of intersex in some disability literature – even if a brief mention – is a promising acknowledgment of the ableist oppression that intersex people face, a form of oppression that goes largely unrecognized. Such inclusion also calls other scholars, from a variety of fields, to regard intersex and disability as intertwined.

Cripping Intersex Studies

In stark contrast to the many biomedical and bioethics professionals who take essentialist, pathologizing approaches, intersex studies scholars from across disciplines often root their studies in feminist and queer theories, aptly underscoring the fact that sex and gender binaries are a farce.[6] "Male," "female," and "disordered" sex are not essential characteristics or essences; and there are no stable or objective positions from which to make assertions about biology, sex, gender, or sexuality. As Suzanne J. Kessler (1998, 44–45) explains in *Lessons from the Intersexed*, "how hard one 'looks' at genitals and what one 'sees,'" or does not see, "is not constrained by the optic nerve but by ideology." Rather than comprising innate attributes, sex is culturally, discursively, and literally re/constructed and performed. Intersex studies scholars use these sorts of theories to illustrate how and why dominant discourses, practices, and institutions "administer" (Ezie 2011, 141) or prescribe sex in order to uphold the epistemological myth of sex, sexuality, and gender dimorphism. Given that the sex binary is an untenable myth, intersex studies scholars demonstrate that medical interventions that are aimed at fitting intersex people's body-minds into the fiction that is dyadic sex are violent human rights violations.

Cripping intersex by integrating disability studies, specifically feminist disability and crip theories, pushes these intersex analyses further. Feminist disability studies, Kim Q. Hall (2011, 1) explains, is not "simply a combination of feminism and disability"; rather, "it transforms both fields" by denaturalizing and reimagining disability, sex, and gender. A crip intersex approach, therefore, brings into focus precisely how compulsory dyadism and able-bodiedness are intertwined as well as how pathologization and curative violence can be resisted alongside the reimagination of the relationship between inter/sex, gender, sexuality, and disability. A feminist disability lens prompts one to interrogate the ableist, intersex-as/is-disability medical model – how disability is deployed by medical professionals to maintain compulsory dyadism. Such a lens identifies and opposes the ableism used to justify curative violence. A crip intersex approach, therefore, advocates for an intersex-with-disability approach and pushes analyses about intersex characteristics further than feminist and queer theory alone.

Given intersex studies' commitment to queer theory and the contemporary articulation of intersex-as/is-disability, cripping intersex is only logical. Crip theory (McRuer 2006) emerges from disability studies and uses queer theory to nuance and develop new analyses. It recognizes that queer and disability activism and theory have overlapping and collective interests, such as challenging pathologization and medical "expertise." Crip theory explores the ways that queer and/or disabled embodiments are conceptualized – how we make meanings of queerness and disability – under neoliberal capitalism. Rather than focusing on identity politics – indeed, crip theorists are critical of said politics – crip theory is attuned to the ways that compulsory heterosexuality and able-bodiedness are institutionalized in intersecting and mutually constitutive ways. Additionally, crip theorists aim "to crip or destabilize categories of meaning" (Rinaldi and halifax 2016, 245). In understanding the critical edge of crip theory and remaining vigilant to the ways that all compulsory modes of being intersect with compulsory dyadism, cripping intersex can effectively consider how intersex figures into the political project of cripping and subverting hegemonic, heteronormative, queerphobic, ableist, and racist discourses and categories.

Feminist disability and crip studies enable radical new articulations of the profound problems with and effects/affects of compulsory dyadism. The analytical capacity of cripping intersex is, for example, demonstrated when one considers queer social justice movements and how some movements reproduce ableist discourses, collude with violent institutions, and come at the expense of people with disabilities, including intersex people. Consider the push for same-sex marriage. Same-sex marriage has been framed as fundamentally liberatory and liberal, but the project colluded with historically violent institutions: marriage, capitalism, heteronormativity, and neoliberalism (Duggan 2002; Van Eeden-Moorefield et al. 2011). Moreover, some arguments for institutionalizing same-sex marriage reproduce homonormative, queerphobic, and ableist narratives. As McRuer (2006) notes, same-sex marriage was sometimes justified on the grounds that instituting it would be an adequate remedy to the spread of HIV/AIDS, a highly stigmatized disabling chronic illness. Conflating queerness with the supposed horrific spread of disability, disease, and degeneracy, queer folks and (queer) people with HIV/AIDS are unnecessarily re/stigmatized. Justifying same-sex marriage need not include re/stigmatizing already marginalized groups. A crip intersex approach sharpens the critical edge of this analysis even further: the often-celebrated institutionalization of same-sex marriage ignores and erases the fact that "disabled" intersex people's body-minds are literally cut up to fit into the dyadic same-sex/different-sex marriage model.

A crip intersex lens also nuances, for example, Iain Morland's (2009, 296) claim that queer theory demonstrates and underscores the value of pleasure and, therefore, "lets us argue that desensitization is not an acceptable side effect of normalizing surgery, because genitalia are for touching." Genitalia are for touching, exploring, licking, urinating, and so on; they are not for performing nonconsensual surgeries on. Cripping this intersex analysis brings into focus the ableist ideologies that fuel this violent, curative model. Moreover, a crip intersex approach highlights the tragic irony of this situation: in the attempt to "fix" or "enable" apparently disabled intersex people, medical professionals perform procedures that typically result in various short- and/or long-term body-mind disabilities. Medical professionals gratuitously and violently create disabled subjects.

Gesturing to the social model of disability – the idea that one is disabled by literal, legal, and ideological barriers in society, not by one's impairments or disabilities themselves – Koyama (2006) implicitly reveals some of the benefits of cripping intersex projects:

> To a disability theorist, disability is not simply a characteristic of one's body, but the product of social institutions that divide human bodies into normal and abnormal, privileging certain bodies over others. In this view, the physical condition that necessitates the use of a wheelchair in order to move about is not itself a disability; social and architectural structures that deprives [sic] a wheelchair user of full participation in the society is what disables her. Similarly, intersex activist Esther Morris's observation that "not having a vagina was not my problem; having to get one was," can be paraphrased to say: not having a vagina was not a disability; the social expectation that she needed to get one in order to live a happy and productive life marked her body disabled.

Koyama claims that, rather than body-minds themselves, society disables people; this is essentially the social model of disability. The social model of disability can help intersex scholars and activists to better articulate that assessments of sex "ambiguity" or "disorder" are ideological allegations, not objective facts. By situating intersex activism alongside disability, Koyama implies that cripping intersex ought to be centralized; an effective, radical intersex politics requires an intimate relationship with disability politics and theories.

However, more nuanced disability theories strengthen this analysis and better reflect many intersex people's lived realities of living with impairments and desiring medical interventions, as well as the disabling consequences of curative violence. Feminist disability and crip theorists have been thinking beyond the social model of disability as well as the binary social-medical model of disability. Alison Kafer's (2013, 4) "political/relational model" (P/R model) of disability is particularly well suited to leaving room for such complexities and lived realities. Kafer, like so many other disability studies scholars, is suspicious of the medical model of disability as well as the social model of disability. The former places the entire presumed problem of disability in people's body-minds, frames disabilities as entirely negative and undesirable, and therefore seeks to eradicate disabilities entirely. The latter, although it productively challenges the medical model and advocates for literal, legal, and ideological changes, can ignore how impairment and pain structure many people's lives and how some people with disabilities, disorders, and diseases require or want medical interventions.[7] As a result, Kafer (2013, 4) proposes a "hybrid" model, the P/R model. There is much to appreciate in Kafer's (2013, 8, 7) model: as "a direct refusal of the widespread depoliticization of disability," it posits that disability and impairment should not be conceptualized as separate from "social meanings and understandings."

There are a number of ways that integrating the P/R model into intersex studies and effectively cripping intersex can bolster and nuance analyses and rights claims. To illustrate, I will outline three ways. First, the P/R model underlines that anti-essentialist arguments about sexual "ambiguity" and disorder are socially and relationally constructed. Second, the P/R model reframes and politicizes conversations about the disabling and impairing effects of curative violence that many intersex people live with. For instance, reconsider Morris's observation that "not having a vagina was not my problem; having to get one was." Although the effects of "having to get one" are not explicitly outlined, extending this line of reasoning is judicious given that so many intersex people testify to the disabling consequences of curative violence. The "problem" of having to get a vagina (or penis) too often involves then living with various short- and/or long-term impairments, pain, or disabilities. Third, using the P/R model to acknowledge impairments can recalibrate one's relationship with intersex people who want medical intervention because, for instance, their intersex traits, in and of themselves, cause impairments, disabilities, distress, or dysphoria. The fact that intersex traits in and of themselves rarely cause pain, impairments, or health issues is often stressed and used as evidence that medical interventions are unnecessary. Rather than minimizing, ignoring, or possibly shaming intersex people with these experiences that stem from their anatomical characteristics, cripping intersex via the P/R model allows intersex studies scholars and activists to openly and unashamedly acknowledge that some intersex people may desire medical interventions in order to comfortably live in and move through the world. Arguing against nonconsensual interventions need not involve distancing from disability or ignoring impairments, pain, distress, or dysphoria, even if uncommon. Cripping intersex via the P/R model enriches and offers up more nuanced theorizations about exactly how intersex people are rendered disabled as well as how they experience and live with disabilities.

A few intersex studies scholars and activists pose compelling and clever analyses that intersex and disability ought to be considered in tandem. Or, as Holmes (2008b, 169) explains, approaching intersex with disability in mind is crucial given that "the medical presupposition that intersex characteristics are inherently disabling to social viability remains the taken-for-granted truth from which clinical practice proceeds." Without feminist disability and crip studies, compulsory dyadism will not wholly or successfully be challenged. The critical edge of intersex projects, theories, and rights claims will not be fully realized without cripping intersex.

The Language of Disability and the Consequences of Curative Violence

Whereas this book strategically employs the language of disability – actively iterating that the discursive and literal consequences of pathologization and curative violence are disabling – intersex studies scholars and activists typically employ other terms and discourses. For instance, the language of mutilation, including the expression "intersex genital mutilation" (IGM), is often used to emphasize the damaging consequences of various medical procedures (see Chase 2002, 2006; Ehrenreich and Barr 2005; and Pagonis 2017b). IGM underlines the fact that these interventions are similar to, the same thing as, or sometimes more harmful than female genital mutilation/cutting (FGM/C). That is to say, like FGM/C, IGM is a cultural practice, not "objective" medicine. Medical projects and their consequences have also been referred to as "medical rape," sexual assault, torture, and queering by scholars, activists, advocates, nongovernmental organizations (e.g., StopIGM.org), and intergovernmental organizations (e.g., United Nations) (Monro, Crocetti, and Yeadon-Lee 2019, 789).[8] Although the disabling consequences of curative violence are evidently implied by these narratives, I maintain that explicitly naming the outcomes as disabilities is an important and useful means to illustrate the connection between intersex and disability as well as to capture the lived realities of so many intersex people who have been subjected to curative violence.

I have come across one case that explicitly frames the effects of curative violence in disability terms. This case involves M.C. (pseud.), an intersex child. In 2017, Pamela and John Mark Crawford, on behalf of their adopted son, M.C., filed a ground-breaking lawsuit against the Medical University of South Carolina, South Carolina Department of Social Services, and Greenville Hospital System for facilitating and/or performing medically unnecessary genital surgery on M.C.[9] The language of disability, specifically impairment, was used to defend M.C. and to explain the effects of said surgery. "The Order Approving Settlement on Behalf of a Minor," signed by the presiding judge, DeAndre Gist Benjamin, states that "plaintiffs in this case allege that Petitioner M.C. has incurred medical bills, pain and suffering, psychological damages, and permanent impairment." That is, M.C. incurred body-mind disabilities. Although the defendants denied all claims, M.C. was awarded US$440,000. This may be just one instance, but it is clear that framing the consequences of medical intervention as disabling or impairing is not only representative of the injuries incurred but also a pragmatic rhetorical strategy. This case indicates that using the political power of disability discourses can aid in legal battles and can help articulate the violence of the current medical protocol.[10]

Narrating the consequences of curative violence as disabling is not a rejection of the other narratives used to understand and combat compulsory dyadism. Rather, conceptualizing the effects as disabling is a constructive discursive tool that can be used to hold medical professionals accountable and that can help to alter policies about intersex medical protocol. Additionally, referring to the effects as disabling illustrates the connection between intersex and disability and, in many circumstances, accurately reflects intersex people's experiences of living with body-mind disabilities caused by medical protocols and procedures.

That being said, one cannot ignore the potential political dangers of referring to the consequences of unnecessary medical interventions as body-mind disabilities or impairments. Doing so could be misinterpreted as or twisted into what disability studies scholar Eli Clare (2017, 129) refers to as "cautionary tales." In such tales, disabilities become symbols and are used as justification for advocating against unjust, violent practices and against oppressive circumstances. Noting that medical violence enacted on intersex people produces body-mind disabilities could be misread as or repurposed into a cautionary tale. Such a tale would read something like this: medical interventions need to be stopped because they produce disabilities; disabilities are inherently inferior, bad, and undesirable; therefore, they ought to be avoided at all costs. One could even argue that ableism and disability were used in this symbolic manner during M.C.'s legal battle or is reflected in Morland's (2009, 296) observation, "desensitization is not an acceptable side effect of normalizing surgery." Rather than focusing on the fact that these medical practices are unjustly violent, violate the Hippocratic oath (Ford 2001; Pagonis 2017b), and are rooted in the unsubstantiated and indefensible ideologies of compulsory dyadism and able-bodiedness, a cautionary retelling of this narrative relies on ableist ideologies to oppose violent practices.

Nevertheless, we must also ask how we might ethically account for and "bear witness to body-mind loss," a loss that is often profoundly felt and embodied (Clare 2017, 60). Clare suggests that, although critiquing and avoiding ableist cautionary tales is crucial, we also need to bear witness to, acknowledge, and ethically foreground body-mind loss created by oppressive systems. Indeed, many intersex people describe in detail these painful, disabled aspects of their body-minds, note that they are resentful of having to live with these consequences, and use them as reasons for why unnecessary medical interventions need to be outlawed. Hence, not only do intersex testimonies of body-mind loss need to be respected and centralized, but rejecting oppressive systems and ideologies must also be centralized to avoid reproducing ableist cautionary tales.

Kim's (2017, 10) expression "curative violence" allows me to hold both of these threads together. As Kim (2017, 27) states, "I use 'curative violence' to describe the exercise of force to erase differences for the putative betterment of the Other. Curative violence occurs when cure is what actually frames the presence of disability as a problem and ends up destroying the subject in the curative process." Applying Kim's (2017, 14) terms to intersex medical management, we can say that the curative violence to which many intersex people are subjected involves body-mind and discursive violence that often destroys the subject. Hence, "cure and disability coexist as a process" (Kim 2017, 9).[11] Rather than reproducing cautionary tales, Kim's expression "curative violence" emphasizes the instituted, violent nature of "cure" and simultaneously leaves room to bear witness to intersex people's acquired body-mind disabilities and profound sense of loss. The "violence" in "curative violence" captures the visceral nature and consequences of medical intervention. The "curative" in "curative violence" foregrounds a tragic paradox: in an effort to "cure" or "enable" apparently disabled intersex people, medical professionals subject people with intersex traits to disabling violence that often leads to short- and/or long-term disabilities. Importantly, the term "curative violence" does not use disability as a symbol but instead emphasizes where blame lies by showing that many intersex people experience body-mind loss due to policies and practices that institutionalize compulsory dyadism and able-bodiedness.

Moreover, the expression "curative violence" does not foreclose on the fact that intersex individuals can and/or do take pride in their body-mind disabilities, even though they were created in brutal circumstances. Although violently acquired body-mind disabilities cause many intersex people to experience loss and suffering, their disabilities and intersex characteristics themselves are not innately wrong. Indeed, intersex pride as well as community cohesion and self-love, despite or perhaps because of violence, are evidently palpable within intersex activist communities. "Bodily and/or psychic ... scars," to quote disability and queer theorist Karen Hammer (2014, 160), "become not only evidence of wounding but also a new surface on which to form community," self-love, and identity. Although difficult at times, it is possible to acknowledge and "balance loss and pride" (Clare 2017, 131).

What follows from negotiating this balance and from centralizing disability and the violence of cure is restoration, justice, or restorative justice.[12] Restoration includes instituting an "age of ethics," as posited in the title of Alice Domurat Dreger's (1999b) edited collection *Intersex in the Age of Ethics.* Such an age would involve, for instance, deinstitutionalizing compulsory dyadism and able-bodiedness; outlawing violent, coercive medical practices; ensuring that intersex people who have undergone curative violence receive the body-mind care that they need; attending to the wounds and scars that haunt many intersex people; listening to intersex individuals and bearing witness to their stories on their terms; granting intersex people body-mind autonomy and full civil and citizenship rights; holding medical professionals and institutions legally accountable; compensating intersex people who have undergone such procedures; and creating diverse, positive, and destigmatizing representations of intersex people in medical and popular cultural contexts. Cripping intersex studies is an effective way to achieve this goal. Doing so offers the means to undermine the ableism that underpins compulsory dyadism, strengthen human rights claims, bear witness to intersex people's trauma and disabilities, and advocate for restorative justice.

Compulsory Dyadism

I propose the expression "compulsory dyadism" to describe the instituted cultural mandate that people cannot violate the sex dyad, have intersex traits, or house "the spectre of intersex" (Sparrow 2013, 29). Said spectre must be, according to the mandate, exorcised. However, trying to definitively cast out the spectre via curative violence always fails. The spectre always returns: a new intersex baby is born; one learns that they have intersex traits in adulthood; and/or medical procedures cannot cast out the spectre fully, as evidenced by life-long medical interventions, routines, or patienthood status. And the effects of compulsory dyadism haunt in the form of disabilities, scars, memories, trauma, and medical regimens (e.g., HRT routines). Compulsory dyadism, therefore, is not simply an event or a set of instituted policies but is an ongoing exorcising process and structure of pathologization, curative violence, erasure, trauma, and oppression.

Why this expression? "Dyad" – meaning two – is often employed in gender and sexuality studies to name the two (contested) sexes and genders. Some intersex activists and organizations also employ dyad nomenclature to describe, as intersex and trans activist and scholar Cary Gabriel Costello (2009) aptly puts it, the "myth of dyadic sex."[13] Further, "compulsory dyadism" draws inspiration from many other scholars' use of the term "compulsory" to underline the ways that modes of being – able-bodiedness, heterosexuality, motherhood, reproduction – are culturally mandated and instituted.[14] The phrase "compulsory dyadism" is a useful theoretical tool with which to name and identify the myriad ways that the epistemological fiction of sex dimorphism is institutionalized as well as to resist the cultural demand that people must not have intersex traits.

Dyad terminology, however, is contested within intersex communities, where some intersex people use "dyad" and "dyadic" as synonyms for non-intersex people. Intersex activist Karin Plattner (2011) explains, "'Dyad' is a noun used by some intersex people to refer to non-intersex people ... 'Dyadic' is the adjective used in reference to non-intersex people." Put simply, dyad is to intersex as cisgender is to transgender, enabled is to disabled, and heterosexual is to homosexual. Although there are benefits to having a name for non-intersex people, some fear that its usage could reinforce problematic male-female and dyad-intersex binaries. These contested grounds must be attended to in order to fully define and contextualize the use of "compulsory dyadism."

Intersex activist and biological anthropologist Claudia Astorino describes some of the benefits of dyad nomenclature. The benefits accrued mirror those of the academic and mainstream proliferation of "cisgender" or "cis" terminology. Astorino (2012) elucidates,

> Having a term like "intersex" without an opposite serves to identify an individual as intersex, but doesn't really help you understand what a not-intersex person is. The implication is that non-intersex people are just "normal," and because they're "normal," they don't need to have an extra word applied to them. The extra-word burden is on those people that are

different. But having an opposite-word can be really important, because instead of having the "normal" state of being and the weirdo one with the funny name, having two words means that for this state of being, there's more than one way to be. There's no value judgment implicit in having multiple terms for different states of being like there is in having a term only for the less-typical one.

For Astorino, "dyad" and "dyadic" help to abate the "extra-word burden" that renders intersex people pathological deviants and upholds the male-female sex binary. These terms resist defining intersex individuals as Other and defining "dyadic" people as normal, and they productively identify compulsory dyadism and interphobia.

In addition to Astorino's (2012) point, having a word for non-intersex to pair with intersex positively complicates cis-trans rhetoric, effectively resisting the linguistic erasure that "cisgender rhetoric facilitates" (Viloria 2014). As explained by queer, intersex, and Latinx activist, writer, and consultant Hida Viloria (2014), who acknowledges the benefits of cis nomenclature,

> if you are born intersex, this [cis-trans discourse] doesn't actually apply to you because there *are* no gender norms attributed to your biological sex as society doesn't even acknowledge that it exists. Indeed, as "cis" means "on this side of," and "trans" means, "on the other side of," those of us who are not on *either* side of this binary framework of sex are inherently excluded from cisgender rhetoric. And note, we [intersex people] didn't used to be, back when people simply said "trans*" or "non-trans*."

In an effort to prevent the intersex erasure that the promotion and adoption of cis rhetoric unwittingly produces, Costello (2014a, 2014b, 2015) proposes adding the expression "ipso gender" to trans and cis discourses. "Ipso" simply means "self"; and to clarify, "inter" means "between." "A cis gender intersex person would be one with an intermediate gender identity, since that 'matches' their birth sex," Costello (2014b) posits; "an ipso gender intersex person would identify with the binary sex they were medically assigned ... And a trans gender intersex person would be one who identifies with the binary sex other than the one they were assigned by doctors." Explaining Costello's proposed term in *LGBT Weekly*, Autumn Sandeen (2014) writes, "In chemistry, which gives us the language of cis and trans isomers, there are chemicals based upon a ring structure, called arene rings. When a chemical substitution is made in the same place on the rings, this is referred to as 'ipso' substitution."[15] According to Costello's suggested terminology, ipso gender intersex people identify with the male or female sex that they were socio-medically assigned; their gender identity remained "in the same place," so to speak. Although there are disadvantages to "ipso gender," insofar as it "does not resolve the challenges that intersex people pose to successfully discussing 'cisgender privilege'" (Viloria 2014), these linguistic devices and conversations are vital in combatting intersex erasure and are integral to intersex people's self-determination and narration.

Returning specifically to dyad nomenclature, there are concerns that it will reinforce binary thinking (Marquez 2019a). Astorino (2012) outlines these worries:

> I don't think that dyadic is the greatest choice. The term dyadic means "two" – a dyad, a pair. By calling a non-intersex person a dyadic male or female, you're basically saying that everyone who's not intersex fits nicely into that binary of male, female. But the fact that intersex people exist at all means that there is, and never was, dyadic sex ... By using the term dyadic to refer to non-intersex people, it totally glosses over the implications of intersex people existing: that binary sex is actually real.
>
> If biological sex isn't binary, then using a term like "dyadic" to describe non-intersex makes about as much sense as saying we've got a binary color wheel that's composed of red and blue, when we know full well that there's purple and orange and magenta out there, being awesome.

The colour wheel, spectrum, or kaleidoscope of body-mind and identification differences is not fully represented by the male-female or intersex-dyad binaries. "Dyad" could problematically reinforce binary thinking.

As a result, although some people still use dyad terminology, other terms have been proposed, debated, and used. For example, "perisex" ("peri" meaning "about" or "around") has been used to name non-intersex people. On the online Tumblr discussion board "Fuck Yeah Sex Education," the term "perisex" is endorsed by one of the forum's contributors, Mod H, who writes that "it does not imply a sex binary nor does it imply non intersex people strictly fit a binary system, rather it suggests that there are people who are closer to" – they are about or around – "what has been constructed (in western culture) to be 'male' and 'female' and those people do not fall into the intersex umbrella." The term "perisex" avoids reproducing the idea that sex is dichotomous. Nevertheless, another contributor, Mod C, rejects "perisex" and prefers "dyad" on Tumblr's "Actually Intersex" forum:

I don't remember who exactly coined it ... but it happened after a certain intersex blogger made a post (intended for the intersex community only!) criticizing the word "dyadic" and while I didn't necessarily agree with their opinions, I understood their point of view. However, dyadics took the opportunity to coin their own phrase that was less othering of them (as if they haven't been othering us since forever). It's kinda like Mod D said a while back; if dyadics really had their way, they'd just be called "normal."

In a similar vein, an anonymous individual on the same forum writes, "What is perisex and why do dyadics keep telling me to call them that instead? Honestly, until they all stop calling me the H-slur [hermaphrodite] I literally DGAF [don't give a fuck] about what they'd like to be called." Mod C responds, "My feelings exactly. It's the same as when cis people flip out over being called 'cis' and demand a label of their own invention. We won't do it. Perisex is a silly word and was invented by dyadics to restore their power imbalance, and I'm not having it." I cannot confirm who coined "perisex," and there is a lot of debate and uncertainty about who did. For instance, on Tumblr's "Ace Eyes" forum, an anonymous person asks who coined "perisex" and notes that "whenever I google it I don't get anything back." In response, a contributor identified as vergess writes, "I'm not sure who did. Perisex definitely originated in the tumblr intersex community." Nevertheless, given that intersex people have historically and systematically been denied the power to name and define their body-minds, rejecting language that may not have been created by and for intersex people in the attempt to name and combat compulsory dyadism is a meaningful repudiation – a means to re/claim power and re/define ab/normality. That being said, "perisex" has not garnered a lot of use in more mainstream intersex activist communities or literature.

In contrast, the term "endosex" ("endo" meaning "within") has garnered considerable attention, usage, and acceptance in recent years. Although some scholars define endosex people as "assigned and conforming to the assignment as only male or female" (Sumerau and Mathers 2019, 54), many intersex activists prefer "endosex" precisely because it does not reinforce the male-female dichotomy in the way that dyad nomenclature does. Endosex people are recognized within medical definitions of male and female biology, but endosex does not demand that one conform to or accept a male or female gender assignment. Endosex people can identify as any gender, not just as cis men or women (Marquez 2019a). As gender and sexuality scholar and activist Surya Monro (2019, 131) explains, "endosex" describes people "born with sex characteristics that are seen as typically male or female at birth" and are "therefore not medicalized as intersex."[16] "Endosex" appears to be the mostly widely accepted and used term in academic and activist literature, perhaps mainly because it offers up more flexibility than "dyad."[17]

There are, however, some detractors. For example, vergess claims on the "Ace Eyes" forum that "endosex," like "dyadic," is problematic because it reinforces the sex binary. Yet the ways that "endosex" is being deployed and defined does not support vergess's claim. Alternatively, on the online forum "Actually Intersex," Mod C claims that "endosex," like "perisex," is problematic because "it was invented by a dyadic person, so ... ew." Mod D writes of "endosex," "It's gross ... It sounds a lot like intersex and is kind of a subliminal way of minimizing privilege." As with "perisex," I cannot confirm who coined "endosex." However, as noted above, I recognize the importance of rejecting language that may not have been created by and for intersex people. Nevertheless, I will continue using "endosex" at this juncture. Having a word for non-intersex is incredibly useful, and "endosex" is both widely supported by intersex activists and sidesteps some of the problems that "dyadic" poses. However, I want to underscore that conversations about nomenclature pertaining to endosex people and embodiments will continue within and between activists, scholars, transnational communities, cultures, and languages. Indeed, language is alive – always in process. I remain open to these conversations and to prospective rhetorical shifts that better explain people's embodiments, challenge compulsory dyadism, and support intersex people's self-determination.

Given the proliferation of "endosex" in many intersex activist circles, organizations like Egale Canada Human Rights Trust understandably feel the need to justify not using "endosex" to describe non-intersex people, instead sticking with "dyad." Egale Canada Human Rights Trust's (2019, 4) publication *Supporting Your Intersex Child* reads,

> Some activists are pushing for the use of the term "endosex," which simply means not intersex. This push is to avoid endorsing any binary ideals that the term dyadic linguistically suggests. While it is important to recognize that the binary is limiting and harmful, we will still be using the term dyadic in this resource because the medical system, healthcare system, and society at large that you and your child must navigate within still operates between the confines of the binary.

My proposed term, "compulsory dyadism," sidesteps the problem with naming endosex people dyadic and underscores the fact that intersex people and their parents/proxies must navigate a system deeply rooted in the sex dyad. Rather than using "dyad" to name endosex people, I use dyad nomenclature – the sex dyad – to describe both systemic oppression and an ideology. Using "dyad" in this context is not contested. "Dyad" is befitting. Accordingly, I use "dyad" in "compulsory dyadism" to highlight, describe, and resist the instituted cultural demand that people must embody the myth of dyadic sex and therefore not have intersex traits. I do not use this expression to describe a definitive biological state or to reinscribe any binaries. People's body-minds are not dyadic; they are more various, beautiful, and defiant than instituted ideologies and systems expect and allow them to be. To quote Astorino (2012) again, "There's purple and orange and magenta out there, being awesome." Yet compulsory dyadism is real and has profound material consequences.

Ghosts of Compulsory Dyadism

Using hauntology as a linchpin to examine compulsory dyadism and its connection with compulsory able-bodiedness reveals that these mandates are not simply an event or a set of instituted policies but are also ongoing processes of pathologization, curative violence, trauma, and marginalization. Attending to the ghosts of compulsory dyadism – the ways that the socio-medical erasure of intersex traits and curative violence haunt – is imperative.

The language of haunting is not a fanciful, stylistic flare intended to sensationalize the violent circumstances in question or people's experiences; haunting is a site of theoretical inquiry. Hauntology, which was first introduced by philosopher Jacques Derrida (1994), provides a critical lens for exploring history, memory, trauma, and temporality. Hauntology provides a framework with which to investigate and give language to the liminal: things that cannot be classified as either being or nonbeing, traumatic consequences that are not constrained by linear time, and the relationship between absence and presence. By taking stock of the in-between, the not-quite-there, the being/nonbeing, and the things that haunt and linger, one gains a unique perspective on the continuing, deferred, or denied outcomes of systemic, inequitable power relations. Reflecting on her pivotal book *Ghostly Matters: Haunting and the Sociological Imagination* (2008), sociologist Avery Gordon (2011, 2) explains that "haunting is one way in which abusive systems of power make themselves known and their impacts felt in everyday life, especially when they are supposedly over and done with." Put differently, attending to that which haunts reveals the "complex rhetorical relationship between memory, ghosts, and justice" (Hoag 2014, 3) – between body-mind dis/abilities, being, becoming, and in/equity.

"A scar is more than a wound"; a scar is "more than just the body's method of remembering a wound" (Hammer 2014, 159). Body-mind scars and disabilities created by curative violence are evidence of, and are ghosts of, abusive systems and compulsory modes of being. Perhaps unsurprisingly, then, haunting imagery is peppered throughout both intersex and disability studies scholarship that contends with systemic violence. "The spectre of disability" (Belser and Betcher 2013, 344), or "the disability to come" (McRuer 2006, 5), "haunt[s] us all" (Garland-Thomson 1997, 9). The shifting "phantasm" (Holmes 2002, 175) or "the spectre of intersex" (Sparrow 2013, 29) haunts intersex people even if they have been surgically or hormonally "cured."[18] In other words, the disabling outcomes of curative violence exist "in between the past and the future," occupying "in-between spaces" (Kim 2017, 9). Likewise, Michael O'Rourke and Noreen Giffney (2009, x) write in Holmes's edited collection, *Critical Intersex*, that intersex "is not ontological, but rather hauntological." Although metaphors that are ghostly, for lack of a better word, haunt some disability and intersex studies literature, I liberally draw from hauntology because doing so captures the ongoing, nonlinear consequences of curative violence, compulsory dyadism, and compulsory able-bodiedness while underlining the need for restorative justice.

Although being haunted by trauma is not unique to intersex and disabled people,[19] attending to how intersex people are haunted by the disabling effects of compulsory dyadism demonstrates the need to crip intersex analyses in order to fully comprehend the body-mind loss that many intersex people experience. Many intersex individuals are haunted by, for instance, traumatic memories, acquired body-mind disabilities, an ability that was taken, or a "paradoxical nostalgia ... for all the futures that were lost" (Fisher 2013, 45). Tiger Devore (in Lahood 2012), a clinical psychologist, sex therapist, and intersex activist, speaks about the futures lost or stolen due to curative violence: "I'm very angry at the genitals that were taken away from me, very angry at how much good sensation was taken away from me. I would like to have had a whole lot more say over the body I would have had, the life I would have had, the identity I would have had." Testimonies like Devore's illustrate that the effects and affects of being denied body-mind autonomy and self-determination do not disappear once medical instruments are put away and sutures dissolve.

As noted above, "haunting is one way in which abusive systems of power make themselves known and their impacts felt in everyday life, especially when they are supposedly over and done with" (Gordon 2011, 2). The traumatic body-mind consequences of curative violence haunt intersex people even when imposed medical management, surveillance, surgery, and HRT are supposedly over and done with. Traumatic memories, a sense of shame, the knowledge of possible future curative violence, and/or acquired body-mind disabilities are never over and done with. They haunt. Ultimately, attending to that which haunts reveals the nonlinear, fragmented "relationship between memory, ghosts, and justice" (Hoag 2014, 3), the complex relationship between intersex and disability, and the need to crip intersex.

Intersex, as an idea, diagnosis, or discourse, is also elusive and ghostly. Intersex, Holmes (2002, 175) confirms, is "a perpetually shifting phantasm in the collective psyche of medicine and culture." Intersex is a morphic, mysterious spectre constantly under revision. Who is or is not labelled intersex, sexually "ambiguous," or sex "disordered" has always been and continues to be contested. Who is imagined to house "the spectre of intersex" serves a political purpose and depends on the ideological context, not on the "optic nerve" (Kessler 1998, 45). Attending to this shifting discursive phantasm is not simply an abstract endeavour to draw attention to the fact that categories are socially constructed and in constant flux. Analyzing who has been and who currently is labelled intersex, sexually "ambiguous," or disordered is about tracing and combatting compulsory dyadism and about recognizing that intersex is currently being integrated into conventional notions of disability. And it therefore proves that we must crip intersex to combat the insidious, complex nature of compulsory dyadism and able-bodiedness.

Chapter Summaries

The following chapters begin the formation of a crip intersex studies and archive. They focus on three seemingly distinct, but intimately intertwined, sites of compulsory dyadism: nonconsensual medical intervention, sport sex-testing policies as well as sport sex and dis/ability segregation, and the promotion and employment of preimplantation genetic diagnosis (PGD), a reproductive technology, to select against intersex variations. Although ostensibly separate, these three sites demonstrate the diffuse, but interconnected, nature of all forms of compulsory dyadism. At the crux of all iterations of contemporary compulsory dyadism are pathologization, able-ism, and subsequently, the call for curative violence to exorcise the spectre. Moreover, these sites of compulsory dyadism illustrate that compulsory dyadism profoundly impacts not only living intersex people with medical diagnoses but also, for example, suspect intersex people (e.g., athletes) and (potentially) pregnant people who may house and gestate the apparently unviable, disabled, queer, crip intersex phantasm. Whether the intersex spectre is detected in an infant, an adult during a routine medical exam, an athlete, an embryo, a fetus, or a pregnant person's uterus, the pathologizing and exorcising response is consistently rooted in ableist logics. To cast out the intersex spectre is to simultaneously cast out the disability spectre. In other words, although the three sites of compulsory dyadism that I analyze may, at first blush, seem unconnected, it is clear that no matter the site of compulsory dyadism, if intersex analyses are not cripped, one cannot fully understand or successfully undermine any form of compulsory dyadism.

Part 1, "Exorcising Intersex: Mutilation and Medical Malpractice," attends to the medical management of people with intersex characteristics. The first chapter, "The Question of Health Risks and Intersex Variations," unpacks the disputed medical claim that intersex traits pose a threat to one's health. Although doctors' intentions are benevolent, the health risks associated with intersex variations are at best contested and at worst exaggerated. Despite this debate, medical professionals employ ableist narratives to justify medical intervention, insisting that surgery will be no big deal because an infant will not even recall the event. Such procedures, however, are not isolated incidents. In addition to the fact that surgeries often prompt subsequent operations, rendering intersex people life-long patients, the body-mind loss or acquired body-mind disability is inevitably enveloped into one's be(com)ing.

The second chapter, "Medical Interventions and Acquired Body-Mind Disabilities," reframes conversations about four commonplace medical protocols: HRT, surgery, genital examinations, and withholding information or explicitly lying to intersex patients and to the parents/proxies of patients. Typically, the language of mutilation, torture, or assault is used to describe the consequences of these medical interventions. Centring intersex people's testimonies about curative violence presented in various mediums, I argue that it is also prudent and representative to narrate the consequences as body-mind disabilities. Doing so emphasizes the irony that, in the attempt to "enable" intersex people – in the attempt to enforce compulsory dyadism via compulsory able-bodiedness – intersex folks are actively disabled by medical interventions. Acknowledging the trauma as incurred disabilities unequivocally demonstrates the productive potential of an approach rooted in crip intersex studies that conceptualizes intersex as a disability issue, and it identifies a locus where intersex and disability issues align.

Chapter 3, "Is There Medical Recognition of the Disabilities Created?," asks whether medical professionals realize or recognize that their medical practices disable intersex individuals' body-minds? Many doctors typically do not explicitly acknowledge – indeed, they often deny – the harm caused and body-mind disabilities created by various interventions. Yet the clinical term "hypospadias cripple" signals otherwise. Doctors reserve the expression "hypospadias cripple" for intersex people with hypospadias who have undergone failed "corrective" surgeries, experience short- and/or long-term body-mind disabilities, and "require" further surgical revision. Hence, even though medical professionals often refuse to explicitly and publicly recognize the disabilities created, this descriptor is an unequivocal admission. As a result, we must construe the current medical management of intersex people as medical *mal*practice.

Part 2, "The Racialized Intersex Spectre," considers the seemingly unending mainstream, medical, and academic fascination and concern with the un/fairness of sport (inter)sex testing policies and procedures. First, however, Chapter 4, "Temporarily Endosex," reworks the disability adage that able-bodied people are only ever *"temporarily* able-bodied" (Clare 2009, 82) and argues that endosex people are only every temporarily endosex. The intersex spectre haunts all people. One can learn that they have intersex characteristics at any point in their life and, subsequently, be at the mercy of curative violence. Hence, this chapter attends to the debate over who is intersex and who is endosex? If intersex haunts all people, it apparently does not haunt all people equally. Historical and current representations of intersex are racialized. We see this fact in the ongoing institutional and mainstream media focus on and fascination with alleged intersex athletes. The phantom is currently represented as haunting women track athletes of colour in colonized nations of the Global South. Race, gender, and nation are central to the construction of sexual "ambiguity," intersex, and DSD.

Chapter 5, "Cripping Sport Sex Testing," tackles sport sex testing. By tracing past and present sport sex-testing practices, I determine that sex testing is and always has been not only anti-science but also a complex discriminatory multi-tool that aids in projects of war, colonialism, imperialism, sexism, racism, interphobia, and ableism. This chapter also crips sport sex testing and uncovers a troubling discrepancy: intersex is pathologized, defined as a disorder, disability, or disease, and represented as an inherent, degenerate, and disabling lack by medical professionals in and outside of sport contexts, but in the context of sport, intersex traits are represented as (unfair) advantages. Cripping this site of compulsory dyadism provides us with the tools to identify the discriminatory and anti-scientific il/logics that sport governing bodies employ to uphold sex testing and, in turn, sport sex segregation. Since these beliefs are the scaffolding that upholds this practice, sport must be cripped and decolonized. A means to this end is exploring the desegregation of sport.

Moving forward with the discrepancy noted above, I ask whether intersex athletes should (not) be relegated to "special" sporting events like the Paralympics if intersex characteristics are construed as a disorder, disability, or disease. Chapter 6, "Sport Sex and Dis/ability De/segregation," considers this query and contests the supposed need to police "disordered" intersex athletes and to segregate sport by (perceived) sex and dis/ability binaries. Sport is not as sex- *or* dis/ability-segregated as it is presumed to be; in fact, sport never could be successfully sex- or dis/ability-segregated. Theorizing intersex and disability sport segregation together provides us with the opportunity to reimagine sport policies and the organization of sport by complicating the relationship between disability and intersex and by blurring the line between Olympian and Paralympian. Hence, I offer up pragmatic ways to change sport culture and sport organization for the better.

Part 3, "New Eugenics: Preimplantation Genetic Diagnosis and Compulsory Dyadism," turns its attention to preimplantation genetic diagnosis (PGD), a reproductive technology that can accompany in vitro fertilization. PGD is used to detect and select against culturally devalued traits, including some intersex variations. Hence, PGD can enact a prenatal exorcism of sorts to ensure that the potentially pregnant person does not house and gestate an unviable disabled intersex spectre. Chapter 7, "Intersex, PGD, and the Eugenics Agenda," argues that intersex has always been on the eugenics agenda and remains on the agenda. The relationship between intersex, PGD, and eugenics deserves immediate attention despite the fact that PGD usage is still relatively uncommon because of its high cost; one cannot underestimate the possible future ubiquitous use of PGD, its broader eugenic implications, and its impact on the intersex population.

Chapter 8, "A Crip Intersex Approach to PGD," analyzes the ableism, queerphobia, and racism integral to eugenic anti-intersex selection via PGD. Whereas racism and queerphobia fuel eugenic anti-intersex selection, claims that intersex traits are inherently unhealthy, diseased, disabled,

disordered, unnatural, and deformed dominate bioethics articles that endorse anti-intersex selection, fertility clinic documents and guidelines, and
governmental policies concerning access to and regulation of PGD and reproductive technologies more generally. Ableist narratives figure prominently in discriminatory literature and in conversations about PGD because
harnessing ableist logics is more culturally admissible than explicitly employing queerphobic or racist rhetoric. Ableism is typically undetected or
perceived to be natural and a matter of common sense. As a result, ableism is liberally mobilized. Since ableism is so central to promoting this new
eugenic application of PGD, I suggest that anti-ableist discourses and disability analyses of reproduction, choice, and eugenics are vital as intersex
studies scholars and activists continue to critique and combat this eugenic
practice.

The concluding chapter, "Eradicating Exorcisms," underscores that intersex futures will be enriched by disability and that disabled futures will be
enriched by intersex. Cripping intersex will benefit scholars and activists in
the ongoing battle against compulsory dyadism, which is intertwined with
(or an iteration of) compulsory able-bodiedness. As a result, I suggest four
possible projects that demand crip intersex analyses: same-sex/different-
sex marriage laws; bathroom gender segregation; the seemingly innocuous
but dangerous gender-reveal parties, where (prospective) parents "reveal" a
fetus's gender to family and friends; and the ways that sex is taught at all
levels of education. If – as intersex activist, writer, and artist Pidgeon Pagonis
(2015c) declares in their art – "the future is intersex," then as this future takes
shape, everyone will encounter intersex and/as/is/with disability in complex,
intersectional, unexpected, multiple, phantasmal, and intersexy ways.

PART 1

EXORCISING INTERSEX:
MUTILATION AND MEDICAL MALPRACTICE

The Question of Health Risks and Intersex Variations

Benevolent Intentions

Medical professionals and scholars who endorse, prescribe, or perform curative or "normalizing" interventions, such as surgery or hormone replacement therapy (HRT), on people with intersex traits do so with benevolent intentions (G. Davis 2017; Karkazis 2008). They were taught and believe – or at least communicate to intersex patients and/or their parents/proxies – that these procedures reorder the innately disabled, diseased, or disordered intersex body-mind. Medical interventions may or will "save" the intersex child from a life of medical problems. For example, given that intersex traits are presumed to increase one's risk of cancer, doctors "save" the child from an impending cancer diagnosis by performing a gonadectomy. They may also believe that they are being kind – preventing a child from enduring stigmatization, teasing, a sexless adult life, infertility, or bullying for "[living] with and through difference" (Holmes 2008b, 175) – and they may insist that the infant or child will not remember the medical procedures anyway (Roen 2009).[1] They do not conceptualize these procedures as a means to restabilize compulsory dyadism, able-bodiedness, heterosexuality, and reproduction.

That said, do intersex traits really pose a threat to one's health, well-being, life, and longevity? Are these medical interventions warranted given the assumed health risks? Intersex activists and advocates, medical professionals, and scholars from a wide variety of disciplines argue over these questions. Evidence suggests that the health risks associated with intersex characteristics are at best contested and at worst exaggerated (G. Davis 2013). Not only do medical professionals overstate claims of future medical problems (e.g., cancer), but they also employ fear-mongering ableist rhetoric as well as discourses of "care," "consent," and "gender affirmation" to justify the current "curative" medical model. In turn, scholars, activists, and advocates as well as parents/proxies of intersex children who challenge "curative" procedures are implicitly framed as unreasonable or illogical for supposedly trying to deny a child the chance to live a fulfilling life free of medical and health problems. Moreover, given that infants will apparently forget the procedures because they are so young, the procedures are presumably "no big deal" – and critics might even be framed as absurd for trying to prevent infants from undergoing "curative" medical intervention.

Are medical interventions really no big deal because infants and children will likely forget? Many intersex people's accounts contradict this claim and "paint a disturbing image of half-crazed doctors running down hospital corridors wielding knives" (Karkazis 2008, 2). Intersex people remember; the trauma of curative violence haunts. In addition, surgeries often prompt subsequent operations, and intersex people are rendered life-long patients. The body-mind loss or acquired body-mind disabilities are inevitably enveloped into one's be(com)ing. Good intentions do not necessarily result in good, ethical care. As intersex activist Karen A. Walsh (2015, 120) reminds us, "The Road to Hell is Paved with Good Intentions." Benevolent intentions and curative violence are not mutually exclusive.

"The Unremembered Past": Challenging the Assumption That Intersex Infants Will Forget

Even though surgical interventions are often understood as traumatic events, many medical professionals assume that the violence of surgery will be forgotten by intersex infants and children because the procedures take place (or supposedly ought to take place) when they are too young to remember. However, surgical procedures can and do take place throughout one's infancy, childhood, and adolescent life, largely because intersex children typically undergo more than one operation. Not only that, but the "human autobiographical memory" – the ability to cultivate clear memories of events in one's past – "emerges gradually across the preschool years," when children are two to four years old (K. Nelson and Fivush 2004, 486). Children remember; these procedures are not and cannot be wholly forgotten by the body-mind.

According to sociologist Katrina Roen (2009, 21), medical professionals are misguided when they presume that procedures, if performed early enough, will be forgotten – an assumption that regards infant flesh as

> malleable enough that such delicate surgery might be "successful" and might be forgotten such that no loss might be experienced. This is the body as an object. Here, the act of surgery is understood to exist in the unremembered past of the self: the infant has not yet *become* a subject to whom the body is an important marker of selfhood.

The body-mind is not an object. The body-mind is an ongoing "event," "a continual, life-long *becoming* in which any early surgery will be ever-present. The scarring, the aesthetic difference, the changes to sensation, are lived continuously. They are not discrete events ... They are necessarily imbricated in the process of the emerging self" (Roen 2009, 21). Nonconsensual procedures are not isolated incidents; the body-mind loss, memories, scars, or acquired body-mind disabilities are inevitably enveloped into one's construction of the self.

As noted in the Introduction, the experience of intersex activist Tiger Devore (in Lahood 2012) illustrates this fact: "I'm very angry at the genitals that were taken away from me, very angry at how much good sensation was taken away from me. I would like to have had a whole lot more say over the body I would have had, the life I would have had, the identity I would have had." Not only do many intersex people experience numerous interventions throughout their lives, but such interventions also literally de/reconstruct these people's body-minds, lives, and identity formations. They continue to shape and comprise one's cultivation of (a medicalized) self. As intersex activist Hida Viloria (2017, 82) writes, "Genitals that were removed can't be brought back. It's a wound that can't be healed." These unhealable wounds haunt, shape, and continue to shape one's memories, embodiment, experiences, possibilities, life, and identities.

Health Risks (or Lack Thereof) Associated with Intersex Variations

Intersex people do not forget. Scars, disabilities, memories, and stolen futures linger and comprise the ever-emerging self. So one may be compelled to ask whether the health risks that intersex traits pose are threatening enough to justify this profound body-mind loss and trauma.

Intersex studies scholars, intersex activists, and many nongovernmental organizations claim that intersex variations themselves do not typically pose health risks; rather, the socio-medical responses are what cause harm. That said, there is no unanimity about the health issues, risks, or impairments that stem directly from intersex traits. Synthesizing literature regarding the supposed medical issues associated with intersex traits themselves (not with medical responses to said traits), Georgiann Davis (2013, 52) observes that "the risks ... vary substantially from study to study, leaving us to act on (what might be misguided) predictions about health factors." In addition, one of the co-founders of Organisation Intersex International Europe, Dan Christian Ghattas, rightly noted at the "Public Consultation on Protection against Violence and Discrimination Based on Sexual Orientation and Gender Identity" (United Nations Human Rights 2017) that there is a "frightening lack of follow up studies that would prove the actual benefits of non-lifesaving cosmetic genital surgeries and other medical interventions." Even though there are limited (and contested) health risks associated with intersex variations themselves, interventions intended to erase intersex traits occur all over the world and are strategically masked as necessary forms of cure and care.

Some of the most noted supposed medical problems that stem from intersex traits include urinary issues, hormone imbalances, cancer, "blind pouch vaginas," and infertility. I address each presumed problem in turn.

Urinary Issues

Some medical professionals justify surgically altering intersex people with variant genitals to prevent (upper) urinary tract infections (UTIs) and their symptoms (e.g., pain in back and sides, fever, nausea, burning sensation when urinating, frequent or intense urge to pee, and kidney damage) as well as lower urinary tract symptoms (LUTS) (e.g., poor/intermittent stream, straining to urinate, incontinence, feeling of bladder not emptying, and drippling). Although advocating against surgery performed on unconsenting intersex infants and children, biology and gender studies scholar Anne Fausto-Sterling (2000, 58) notes that "some intersex babies [with variant genitalia] might have problems with urinary tract infection, which, if very severe, can lead to kidney damage." However, there is not enough evidence to conclusively claim that intersex people with variant genitals are more prone to UTIs or LUTS. In fact, as I note elsewhere (Orr 2019), surgery can cause urinary problems (e.g., UTIs), as well as a whole host of other body-mind disabilities.

Moreover, intersex people's urinary issues are "sporadically reported" (Cools et al. 2018, 422), the effects of surgery "on urinary function and the pelvic floor (including safe urine storage and drainage, urinary continence and risk of infection) are often insufficiently addressed" (Cools et al. 2018, 421), the long-term impacts on kidney function are "largely unknown" (Cools et al. 2018, 422), and studies concerning intersex genital surgeries typically "neglect urinary functioning" – instead focusing on appearance – which "can lead to inappropriate conclusions" about how successful surgery is (Cools et al. 2018, 426). The fact that studies concerning the outcomes of surgery usually neglect to mention urinary function indicates that preventing urinary issues is not the main aim of surgery in the first place. Rather, appearance – the ability to conform to the sex dyad – is the main aim.

Studies that do address urinary function contradict the claim that variant genitals are disproportionally prone to urinary problems. In turn, they suggest that immediate surgical intervention is unnecessary. For example, according to Zeina M. Nabhan, Richard C. Rink, and Erica A. Eugster (2006, 815), the children with intersex variations whom they observed had UTI incidences similar to those of the endosex population. They posit that there is no correlation between an increased risk of UTIs if surgical intervention is delayed. Likewise, Riitta Fagerholm, Risto Rintala, and Seppe Taskinen (2013) report that they have not seen severe LUTS in their patients diagnosed with a disorder of sex development (DSD). Comparing intersex patients who have undergone surgery with intersex patients who have not, they determined that LUTS were just as common in each group. In other words, surgery did not effectively reduce LUTS. The claim that surgery is required to prevent urinary issues is unsubstantiated.

Surgical interventions should not be performed on these grounds. Rather than subjecting unconsenting infants and children to traumatizing, potentially disabling, and life-changing surgery to treat (potential) urinary problems, medical professionals should opt for means to solve urinary issues, if or when they arise, that are not surgically invasive. Surgery is an unduly radical response to (potential) urinary problems. Medical practitioners risk intersex infants' and children's genital sensation and ability to orgasm based on unsubstantiated and contested claims of (potential) urinary issues. It is clear that these interventions are not medically necessary but are instead cosmetic procedures. Yet these cosmetic procedures occur because they are narrated as a preventative measure and necessary cure for a "disorder."

All that being said, I acknowledge that some people with intersex traits may or do experience health problems or body-mind impairments because of their intersex anatomy (e.g., UTIs, dissociation, and dysphoria). Rather than minimizing or ignoring these people's experiences, we ought to fight to ensure that these people can readily practise their autonomy and access the care (e.g., surgery, HRT, and therapy) that they require. Opposing non-consensual or coercive interventions and fighting for the right for people to consent to interventions are not mutually exclusive.

Hormone Imbalances

Congenital adrenal hyperplasia (CAH), a chronic adrenal condition attributed to and sometimes conflated with intersex, is one variation that causes medical concern. People with CAH have adrenal glands that do not make enough vital hormones. They have problems making enough cortisone, a hormone that aids the body in responding to stress or trauma (e.g., viruses and broken bones). Mineralocorticoids, hormones that maintain one's salt balance, and androgens, steroid hormones, may also be affected. As a result, people with CAH typically need to take a variety of hormone replacements (e.g., hydrocortisone, prednisone, and fludrocortisone) throughout their entire lives to ensure hormonal and metabolic balance. Cosmetic, genital surgery is not needed to manage CAH, but when intersex traits are identifiable, such surgery typically occurs.

To clarify, CAH is attributed to and sometimes conflated with intersex because some people with CAH have variant genitals. Not all individuals with CAH have variant genitals. CAH rarely causes intersex characteristics in people with XY ("male") chromosomes. Alternatively, CAH can cause intersex variations in XX ("female") individuals. Hence, intersex traits could be a sort of symptom of or signal that there may be an underlying health issue (i.e., CAH). The difference between XY and XX individuals is due to the fact that CAH is associated with higher levels of prenatal testosterone and, therefore, may "virilize" or "masculinize" an assigned female fetus. That is, an assigned male's "masculine" traits (i.e., phallus) are not deemed intersex because such traits are expected and deemed normal. Assigned females are deemed incongruous, intersex, and disordered.

The supposed disordered masculinization of assigned females with CAH is, apparently, both physical and psychological. The pathologization of assigned females who apparently will physically and psychologically masculinize highlights the fact that hegemonic femininity as well as compulsory heterosexuality, dyadism, and able-bodiedness underpin "normalization" practices. Supposed physical masculinization is identified as genital "ambiguity" or variance (e.g., an "enlarged" clitoris). Psychological virilization is looking or behaving in an "unfeminine" manner and "developing" lesbianism or bisexuality. The idea of psychological masculinization was developed by John Money in his book *Sex Errors of the Body and Related Syndromes: A Guide to Counseling Children, Adolescents and Their Families* (1968). Lena Eckert (2009, 64–65) explains,

> Money's assertion that CAH females show increased intelligence and a propensity toward lesbianism as a consequence of virilization is proving of this patriarchal implication in the process of intersexualization. Money reports that 'it is possible that the genetic factor responsible for CAH is linked to another genetic factor responsible for intellectual superiority' (Money 1968, 40). Virilization as biological process based on hormones and genetic dispositions is thought to be responsible for intellectual achievement – a rather commonsense assertion that reveals deeply patriarchal reasoning.

The evidently reductionist, biological-essentialist, sexist, and queerphobic proposal that assigned females with CAH pathologically, physically, and psychologically masculinize has been and continues to be used to justify nonconsensual and unnecessary genital surgeries, such as clitorectomies/clitoroplasties. This idea has also fuelled the development and prescription of dexamethasone, a drug that can be prescribed to a pregnant person with an assigned female fetus with CAH (Dreger, Feder, and Tamar-Mattis 2012; Sytsma 2006). Even at the risk of the pregnant person's and fetus's safety and health, dexamethasone is prescribed to prevent the development of supposed physical and psychological virilization. That is, according to this logic, medical intervention is necessary to avoid the health "risks" of pathological queerness. Ultimately, surgical interventions are not at all needed to manage CAH.

Although HRT is necessary for many people with CAH, many individuals with intersex variations are coerced into taking medically unnecessary "female" or "male" hormones so that their embodiments "coincide" with or emphasize their socio-medically assigned sex/gender. Borrowing from philosopher Paul B. Preciado (2013, 191, 387), I argue that imposed HRT is "biodrag," an internalized "[technology] of gender" that aims to reorder or "cure" the queerly disordered or crip intersex subject on the molecular level. Moreover, HRT is presumably necessary because "normal" sex hormone levels are essential for "normal" (i.e., heteronormative) gender and sexual-identity formation. Intersex people's deviation away from compulsory dyadism renders them queerly disordered, disabled, or diseased – deviants from compulsory heterosexuality and able-bodiedness. Given the "ideology of cure" (Clare 2017, 5), disorder, disability, or disease demands curative intervention. As a result, many intersex people are literally re/produced and de/reconstructed by HRT as well as by a variety of other "curative" interventions. Ultimately, even though HRT is often medically unnecessary, it is employed to straighten out and reorder the body-mind given that intersex people are perceived as developing queerly or abnormally – or, to use Kathryn Bond Stockton's (2009, 1) term, "sideways."

In other circumstances, the medical need for hormones is created by medical professionals. For example, Walsh (2015, 122) had to begin a life-long HRT regimen because of an unnecessary surgical intervention:

> I know now that it was not necessary to remove my gonads – my only source of endogenous hormones. [Because of the unnecessary gonadal removal,] I am at extraordinary risk for osteoporosis, as well as problems with libido. Additionally, I had problems feminizing during my "puberty," since the Premarin was not well absorbed. It is a myth in the treatment of intersex that exogenous hormones work as well as endogenous ones. This is a lifelong problem for me ... I wish I had been given the choice to keep my testes with regular monitoring instead of rushing to surgery. Hormone replacement therapy is a poor substitute for the real thing – especially at age 15 with a long life ahead.[2]

Due to the needless rush to remove Walsh's testes, Walsh must remain on HRT and must anticipate or confront various disabilities. Rather than imposing or creating a need for HRT, medical professionals must listen to individuals' needs and "put people in the hormonal environment where they feel comfortable" (Anne Tamar-Mattis, quoted in Wall 2015b, 119). Depending on the person, HRT intervention may or may not be required or desired. When people are not (put) in the hormonal environment that enables them to live the life that they are comfortable living, they do not simply feel uncomfortable. Forcing people to embody an ideology, a sex, or a gender that is not their own can cause them to experience profound body-mind disabilities, such as anxiety, depression, dysphoria, and dissociation, as well as unnecessary (prospective) disabling illnesses like osteoporosis and cancer.

Cancer

In addition to the above scientifically unsubstantiated justifications for intersex medical interventions, intersex traits are compared to and regarded as though they were life-threatening diseases (see Christensen 2011; Holmes

2000; and Mitra 2014a). Georgiann Davis (2015, 69) verifies that some medical professionals "compare intersex traits to dangerous diseases, despite the fact that most intersex traits have minimal, if any, health risks. Dr. C., for instance, viewed DSD terminology as 'an analogy. It's like talking about skin cancer and brain cancer.'"[3] The analogy is distinctly misrepresentative when one takes into account, for example, that the five-year survival rate of children diagnosed with brain cancer varies from 40 to 80 percent and that, if they survive, they will deal with an array of long-term consequences (e.g., cardiac problems, depression, and post-traumatic stress disorder).[4] Children with intersex traits cannot potentially die from their intersex traits themselves. Rather than being diseased or "sick," Morgan Holmes (2000, 97) posits, "it is the culture around the child which is *dis-eased,* as it were, made uneasy by the child's intersex characteristics." Regarding intersex variations as diseases or as (potentially) cancerous or comparing intersex to diseases enables medical professionals to more readily justify gratuitous exorcising technologies. Borrowing from Phil Smith's (2004) analyses of disease metaphors, I argue that "the disease metaphor" is a useful means to create body-mind disability categories and to justify eliminating what is culturally disruptive or perceived to be "repulsive and revolting."

Moreover, many medical professionals claim that intersex people are at a greater risk of developing cancer in their gonads (i.e., testes, ovaries, and ovotestes) – which, as a result, must be preventatively removed by a gonadectomy. Yet the risk of developing cancer "is often hard to predict" (Cools et al. 2006, 468), and claims of cancer development are contested and regularly inflated. Once children's gonads are removed, they no longer have the option to biologically reproduce, and they are dependent on HRT for the rest of their lives. Morgan Carpenter (2013) writes,

> Sterilisations [i.e., gonadectomies] are typically carried out on adolescents, on the basis of inflated claims of cancer risk with Australian studies quoting upper bound rates of 30% to 50%. Overseas studies quote risks from 0.8 to 5% in the case of AIS [androgen insensitivity syndrome]. The lifetime risk of breast cancer in women is 12.2% according to the US National Cancer Institute – but we don't routinely remove women's breasts on the basis of that cancer risk. Sterilisation turns us [intersex people] into lifelong patients, even if it's the only intervention carried out: we need HRT.

The logic of increased cancer risk is used selectively to justify curative violence, effectively removing both anatomical attributes and possible life paths from children without their proper consent. Furthermore, the apparent risks of cancer are inconsistent and ought to be considered alongside the fact that everyone is at risk of developing certain types of cancer, depending on, for example, anatomical characteristics, family history, life choices, geographical location, and age. If cancer is truly a risk, rather than literally removing one's possible life paths and disabling them, medical professionals can employ routine cancer screenings, similar to routine mammograms and Papanicolaou tests. Indeed, Ulla Döhnert, Lutz Wünsch, and Olaf Hiort (2017) suggest that doctors should perform biannual screens for cancerous tumours in at-risk intersex people.

In fact, one's risk of developing cancer (e.g., breast/chest cancer and gastric cancer) markedly *increases* because of long-term HRT (Pizot et al. 2016). HRT with one hormone (as opposed to two or more) can increase breast/chest cancer risk by up to 10 percent for each five years of use, and after fifteen years of HRT, the risk is typically increased by 36 percent (Ross et al. 2000). Linda K. Weiss and colleagues (2002) report a pronounced increased risk of breast/chest cancer in people who are on HRT and explain that this risk decreases once HRT use is stopped. Many intersex individuals, however, do not have the choice to discontinue HRT because nonconsensual gonadectomies have literally removed that choice. Their health both depends on and may dissipate because of these hormones. The almost indistinguishable spectre of intersex and disability will forever linger. Ultimately, the effort to reorder the supposedly disordered intersex body-mind – as a means to ostensibly prevent cancer – increases one's risk of cancer due to the required HRT.

Nevertheless, some parents/proxies of intersex children have been told that their children *will* develop cancer and that, in order to prevent such a calamity, surgery is necessary. Some parents/proxies, having been blatantly lied to or told only partial truths, are advised to perpetuate lies by telling their children that they had to undergo surgery because they had cancer. For example, Pidgeon Pagonis and their family were told such lies. As a child, Pagonis (2015a) was told that they were born with cancer, whereas their parents were told that their child would develop cancer:

One of the first lies my mother told me was that I was born with *cancerous ovaries* and that they were removed in a life-saving post-birth operation. You [i.e., doctors] instructed my parents to tell me this made-up story, and it became a root in my development. When I began asking questions about why I couldn't get a period or have biological children, you told my mother to *just stick to the cancer story* – and she did. Sad I wouldn't be able to have kids, confused about the reason why, and scared the cancer would return, I began to retreat inward to a world of shameful silence. You didn't tell my parents the same lie. Instead of telling them I was *born* with cancer, you hyped the risk that my "underdeveloped ovaries," which you decisively referred to as "gonads" – and really were my undescended testes – would likely develop cancer if left intact. You noted in the records after my gonadectomy that the tissue samples came back negative and "no term other than gonad was used." This manipulative tactic meant to induce willingness in scared parents is a byproduct of a culture that insists, sometimes by force, that humans only come in two polar opposite varieties. Instead of removing my undescended testes and causing a life-long dependency on hormone replacement therapy (HRT), you could have instead been honest with us and offered to monitor them annually for signs of cancer. I know other Androgen Insensitive (AIS) intersex folks who still have their testes, and they wouldn't trade them for the world. These types of decisions about our bodies belong to us and never to you.

As Pagonis aptly alerts readers, these lies are manipulative means to gain "consent" from parents/proxies for doctors to perform interventions that work to re-enforce and restabilize compulsory dyadism. Doctors lie and exploit parents'/proxies' fear of illness, disability, and death so that culturally mandated ways of being can be upheld. And, ironically, because of the attempt to enforce the intersecting logics of dyadism, heterosexuality, and able-bodiedness through lying, intersex people live with body-mind disabilities, hormone dependencies, and futures that were stolen.[5]

Regarding intersex as or the same as a type of cancer creates a "state of exception," which then "lay[s] the groundwork for justifying medically unnecessary interventions" (G. Davis 2015, 23). This state, which is cultivated by medical professionals, exploits parents' anxieties about chronic ill health, disabilities, and death to justify curative violence. Parents/proxies are understandably profoundly distressed and believe that they are acting in the best interests of the child. Synthetizing the literature about the supposed benefits of surgical interventions, Human Rights Watch and interACT: Advocates for Intersex Youth (2017) conclude, "The results are often catastrophic, the supposed benefits are largely unproven, and there are generally no urgent health considerations at stake. Procedures that could be delayed until intersex children are old enough to decide whether they want them are instead performed on infants who then have to live with the consequences for a lifetime." This is the type of information that doctors should be sharing with parents/proxies of intersex children.

Blind Pouch Vaginas

Similar to the cancer metaphor, the ableist metaphor "blind pouch vagina" is employed by medical professionals to justify invasive curative violence.[6] These vaginas are apparently "blind" because they are too short. In addition, a person with a blind pouch vagina may not have a ("properly" formed) uterus or cervix and may be infertile. To make the vagina "see," vaginoplasties are often performed. Vaginoplasties "can cause infertility; ... the constructed vagina can smell like a bowel; it can necessitate constant use of sanitary napkins; it frequently requires repeated surgical revisions" (Arana and Human Rights Commission Staff 2005, 12). In addition to vaginoplasties, dilators – hard dildo-like instruments – are often used to maintain or "improve" vaginas surgically constructed by vaginoplasties in order to make sure that the vagina does not "go blind" again. Or, if surgery was not performed, dilators are often used to nonsurgically deepen the vagina so that it can "see" better. Unsurprisingly, dilation "is often painful and humiliating" (Arana and Human Rights Commission Staff 2005, 21).

The metaphor "blind" provides us with quite a bit of insight into the ableist ideological underpinnings of these "curative" practices. According to medical professionals and the broader ableist culture, blindness is a disabling lack or loss that must, if possible, be avoided or cured.[7] Given this understanding, "the collective representation of blindness," disability studies scholars Rod Michalko and Tanya Titchkosky (2001, 215) explain, is that "of a 'need for help.'" Hence, similar to the ways that many other blindness metaphors function, labelling these people's vaginas "blind" is an ableist tactic to reaffirm the supposed necessity of "curative" dilation and/or vaginoplasty.[8]

Vaginoplasties and/or dilation, so the ableist metaphoric logic goes, will cure or give "sight" to "blind" vaginas. So what is the vagina apparently blind to? What sort of "cataracts" do these vaginas have? What do they need to see? Laura Inter's (pseud.) (2015, 96) experience can help to answer these questions: "One doctor explained that after the surgery I would have to use dilators and then I would be ready to 'have sex normally, with your husband, when you get married.' What the doctors didn't know ... was that since I was very young I had been attracted to women." These vaginas are "blind" to their supposed (passive) feminine function. "Sight," in this context, means the ability to engage in heterosexual, penetrative sex. The end goal of these de/reconstructing procedures is clearly to, in Kira Triea's (1999, 143) terms, "make the hermaphrodite fuckable" for prospective heterosexual men with penises. Or, in other words, vaginas are "usually created or deepened for the expressed goal of accommodating a penis, rather than for the satisfaction of the patients" (Arana and Human Rights Commission Staff 2005, 12). These vaginas apparently cannot "see" a "normal"-sized penis; they are too short to contain a penis. They are "blind" to the apparent wonders of heterosexual, penetrative sex. They are rendered disabled because they cannot fulfill feminine expectations and the cultural mandate of heterosexuality and dyadism. The fact that these procedures take place at all highlights the ableist, queerphobic, interphobic, and phallogocentric fear that a vagina will "go blind" (again) or "remain blind" to the phallic spectacle.

One may assume that "sight" would also involve the attempt to "fix" infertility. However, as noted above, vaginoplasties can cause infertility, effectively removing a possible life path by negating one's chance at biological reproduction. Drawing from David Mitchell and Sharon Snyder's (2000, 49) theory of narrative prostheses, I argue that disability and ableist rhetoric – in this instance blindness – is used as a "crutch" to justify curative violence and the legitimacy of compulsory dyadism and heterosexuality (see also Kelly and Orsini 2016).

The term "pouch" – which is typically used to describe a small bag or flexible receptacle that houses one's belongings and ephemera and is carried in one's pocket or attached to a belt – is also disconcerting. "Pouch" implies that vaginas are merely lithe repositories for a prospective penis – repositories or depositories that, given their tractability, can be moulded, de/attached, and re/formed for the user's purpose. However, the presumed user in this scenario is a prospective man with a penis. Access to this pouch, the contents of this pouch, or the future contents of this pouch are not attributed to the rightful owner. Discussing blind pouch vaginas on her YouTube channel Emilord, intersex activist Emily Quinn (2016) demands, "Please stop talking about my vagina like it's some weird purse" – a disabled pocket failing to hold the proper phallic contents.

As briefly noted above and outlined in more detail in the next chapter, the body-mind effects of dilation are disabling and traumatizing.[9] Claudia Astorino (2013) recounts her numerous dilation experiences:

I had a dilation procedure performed for almost every exam I had with intersex doctors from the time I was 8 until I was 16, so that they could check how long my vagina was as I grew. I absolutely hated these procedures. I mean, imagine a man as old as your father or your grandfather, who you don't know, inserting a medical dildo into you each time you saw him, knowing that you can't question the doctor's orders and just accept that you have to undergo these uncomfortable procedures for your health. Imagine a decade or so later, realizing that these procedures did nothing to track your health, and have everything to with grown men feeling good about the fact that you could fuck some dude someday like a "normal girl." That all those traumatizing procedures weren't actually medically relevant at all, and it was actually within my right to refuse those examinations.

In addition to, in Gina Wilson's (2012) words, the "pain of dilation and the indignity of it all," Astorino correctly points out that these procedures are medically unnecessary. Infants, children, and adolescents do not need to have a vagina that can accommodate a penis. Indeed, no one needs a vagina unless they express such a need and can fully consent to to the risks of surgery and/or dilation.

Referencing and building on the work of Maria Helena Palma Sircili and colleagues (2006) as well as the research of Elaine Maria Frade Costa and colleagues (1997), Berenice Bilharinho Mendonca and colleagues (2009, 184) claim, in stark contrast to intersex people's testimonies, that vaginal dilation is "an effective treatment choice ... resulting in good outcomes ... good cosmetic and functional results." However, the studies referenced have small sample sizes and are unclear, and the conclusions appear to contradict other elements of the studies. This is typically the trend: medical "research on intersex people is conducted by non-intersex clinicians, based on small samples and case studies of people who have been treated by the institution conducting the study. There is sample bias, and selection bias" (Carpenter 2013). In Costa and colleagues' (1997) study, only twelve people who had undergone dilation following a vaginoplasty were interviewed. The authors report that 87 percent of the participants had "satisfactory" sexual intercourse. However, "satisfactory" sex is not defined, and the study does not include *any* quotations from the interviews. Interestingly, Costa and colleagues (1997, 231) note that patients dealt with "anxiety" and "anguish" in relation to dilator use. Sircili and colleagues' (2006) study included only three people who had undergone dilation. Sircili and colleagues (2006, 209) claim that the participants had "good functional results." Yet the (phallogocentric) definition of good functional results appears to be that a "normal"-sized penis can fit inside the vagina. Good functional results (for prospective penises) are not the same as sexual satisfaction (for patients); the two should not be conflated. Moreover, participant details appear to contradict the claim that dilation had good results. Two of the three participants reported not engaging in sexual activity. Two of the three patients dealt with vaginal stenosis, symptoms of which included pain, dryness, burning, friable tissue (i.e., tissue that tears or bleeds easily upon contact), bleeding and discomfort during penetrative sex, UTIs, and urinary incontinence. And one of the three participants experienced pain during intercourse. These studies are misrepresentative, contradictory, and methodologically problematic. Even more, they do not demonstrate a medical need for such procedures. Rather, they clearly indicate the disabling nature of curative violence.

More recent studies contest the claim that dilation is successful. Having conducted a fourteen-year follow-up study on patients, Heng Zhang and colleagues (2013, 3) explain, albeit using problematic language, "For patients without vagina or with poorly developed vagina, vaginal dilation usually has unfavorable therapeutic efficacy." Likewise, Jatinder Kumar and colleagues (2012, 286) warn against dilating infants and children: "Vaginal dilatation should not be undertaken before puberty. Emphasis should be on functional outcome [i.e., "importance of clitoris for orgasm"] rather than [aiming] at strictly cosmetic appearance." A few biomedical texts also imply that consent is important. Indeed, Mendonca and colleagues (2009, 183) imply that consent is essential: "In patients who *wish* to initiate sexual activity, dilation of the blind vaginal pouch with acrylic moulds or [reliance on a] surgical neovagina promote[s] development of a vagina adequate for sexual intercourse" (emphasis added). Despite noting that it is vital and good medical practice to recognize the importance of patients' wishes, this iteration of consent reproduces heteronormativity and phallogocentrism. Successful, satisfying sexual activity or intercourse is conflated with heterosexual, penetrative sex. Any other kind of sex is not even recognized as sex. Employing this sort of discourse – when people are ready to have sex, they can choose dilation and/or surgery – while in conversation with intersex patients erases and delegitimizes queer, "blind," crip, and intersex life paths and sexual possibilities. This narrative unequivocally communicates to intersex people and their parents/proxies that they are innately abnormal and (hetero)-sexually unviable – which, in turn, can work to coerce people into "choosing" irreversible interventions that restabilize compulsory modes of being.

The more methodologically sound studies more accurately reflect many intersex people's experiences of trauma and body-mind disability and rightly emphasize the importance of the intersex person's (not a prospective penis's) pleasure, sensation, and orgasm. They also echo the report on intersex human rights by Marcus de María Arana and Human Rights Commission Staff (2005, 19): "There is no medical need for a preadolescent girl to have a vagina." That said, as noted above, there is no need for anyone to have a vagina unless one voices such a need and can appropriately consent to the risks of surgery and/or dilation.

Infertility

Some, but not all, people with intersex traits are born infertile or experience in/fertility issues. And, as noted above, surgical interventions can or inevitably do result in infertility. Despite the evident irony, medical professionals endorse invasive or disabling interventions to solve (potential) in/fertility problems. Concerns about in/fertility often crop up in conversations about hypospadias, Klinefelter syndrome, and partial androgen insensitivity syndrome (PAIS) diagnoses. Hypospadias ("hypo" meaning "under" or "beneath" and "spadias" meaning "slit" or "fissure") is characterized by the urethral meatus, or "pee hole," being situated on the underside of the penis. People with Klinefelter syndrome have XXY chromosomal formations; they may also have sparse body hair and muscle mass, "small" testes, and breast/chest tissue. Individuals with PAIS have the partial inability to respond to androgens, have variant genitals, and have testes that are, in Tamar-Mattis's (2012, 7) words, "often functional."

Many medical professionals and online fertility sources claim that people with hypospadias may have fertility issues given the location of their urethral meatus.[10] Relocating the urethral meatus will apparently solve this potential problem. For example, according to Sydney Chang who writes for the fertility company Progyny (2020),

> Hypospadias is a birth defect that affects the male penis ... Hypospadias can negatively impact male infertility in several ways: Since the urethra carries semen out of the body, the altered location of the opening can result in difficulties with ejaculation ... Males with hypospadias are also more likely to be born with an undescended testicle, which can also decrease sperm count ... Fertility problems should no longer remain after the hypospadias is surgically corrected.

These sorts of sources misrepresent in/fertility. Camilla Asklund and colleagues (2010) note that hypospadias in and of itself does not affect fertility because most people with hypospadias have fertile sperm. In other words, surgery will not make an infertile person with hypospadias fertile. Moreover, sources that endorse surgery also downplay the plethora of medical risks, the possible disabling outcomes, and the potential need to have subsequent surgeries. Occasionally, undescended testes (or cryptorchidism) accompany hypospadias, and this structural variation can affect fertility, but hypospadias (i.e., where the urethral meatus is located) does not. Drawing from Canadian infertility rates, pediatric urology experts Luis H. Braga and colleagues (2017, E252) state, "Any correlation of infertility with undescended testis (UDT) must be tempered by the fact that 15–20% of couples in the general Canadian population have difficulty conceiving, and there is often more than one factor involved."

According to Best Start: Ontario's Maternal, Newborn and Early Child Development Resource Centre and the Halton Region Health Department (2007, 78), Klinefelter syndrome is a "major congenital anomal[y]," defined as "an abnormal condition in a male characterized by two X chromosomes and one Y chromosome, leading to infertility, smallness of the testes, sparse facial and body hair." The words "major" and "anomaly," as well as the definition, are deceptive, if not false. Studies estimate that between 1 in 500 to 1,000 people have this variation (Bojesen, Juul, and Gravholt 2003; Fullerton, Hamilton, and Maheshwari 2010). Klinefelter syndrome is hardly anomalous. Hence, Gail Fullerton, Mark Hamilton, and Abha Maheshwari (2010, 588) refer to Klinefelter as "common" in the academic journal *Human Reproduction*. Moreover, "small" testes and sparse body hair cannot rightly be deemed major abnormalities or pressing medical concerns. Further, according to several studies, people with Klinefelter syndrome are not necessarily infertile.[11] People with Klinefelter mosaic cell lines may have reproductive sperm and can fertilize an egg without reproductive technologies. Additionally, with the development of microsurgical techniques and reproductive technologies, many people with Klinefelter syndrome can and do have biological children. Given these findings and developments, "the label of infertile should be reevaluated" (Fullerton, Hamilton, and Maheshwari 2010, 595).

The claim that medical intervention will "save" one's reproductive capacity is extraordinarily useful to medical professionals who want to maintain compulsory dyadism insofar as infertility is deemed to be innately disordered, pathological, and undesirable – and, therefore, to require a "cure." Infertility is not, however, inherently pathological; it is characterized in this way because of our cultural investment in compulsory reproduction, or in Lee Edelman's (2004, 11, 2) terms, the "absolute logic of reproduction" and "reproductive futurism." The cultural investment in, or

demand for, dyadic sex and, in turn, for heterosexual biological reproduction is not "natural" but an "unquestioned value" (Edelman 2004, 4).[12]
Infertility becomes pathological when fertility and (hetero)reproduction
are undisputed, taken-for-granted cultural values. In this context, intersex
people who may not be able to fulfill the heteronatural, pro-natal order of
things threaten "social order as such" (Edelman 2004, 11). Claiming that
intersex people who may not be able to reproduce must be "fixed" and rendered properly fertile becomes difficult to defend when one questions the
intersecting logics of compulsory reproduction, dyadism, able-bodiedness,
and heterosexuality. The main aim is not necessarily to ensure that intersex
people have access to a biological reproductive future but to safeguard pro-
natal ideologies and compulsory modes of being.

This agenda is clear given that intersex people are routinely sterilized.
Edelman (2004, 11) writes, "Whatever refuses this [reproductive] mandate
by which our political institutions compel the collective reproduction of
the Child must appear as a threat not only to the organization of a given
social order but also, and far more ominously, to social order as such." The
child, Edelman suggests, is not an actual child but an imaginary figure who
symbolizes the need to maintain social order; people are often compelled
to "think of the children" when folks threaten to disrupt the status quo. The
"whatever" to which Edelman (2004, 4) refers is the queer: "The queer comes
to figure the bar to every realization of futurity." Queerness disrupts the
social order and will irreversibly harm the Child. However, Edelman's account of the Child and compulsory reproduction is nuanced by "disordered"
or crip intersex people themselves and by the medical management of
intersex. In addition to the fact that intersex children themselves threaten
the Child because their body-minds threaten the social order, doctors do
not absolutely privilege compulsory reproduction given that they routinely
sterilize intersex people. One may be compelled to argue, in part, that doctors challenge the reproductive mandate because they sterilize intersex children. I posit, however, that rather than challenging compulsory reproduction,
they perform sterilizations to maintain compulsory dyadism. An intersex
person who has been "fixed" and rendered sterile is preferable to a fertile
intersex person with seemingly incongruous biological attributes, which
they might even have passed along if they were fertile. Medical practitioners
must privilege compulsory dyadism over compulsory reproduction; without the sex dyad, heterosexual cultural understandings of reproduction are
called into question.

Compulsory reproduction is typically associated with women. Rather than discussing "compulsory reproduction," scholars tend to explore "compulsory motherhood." Women's presumed "natural destiny" (Carroll 2012, 27) is to bear children. Women are culturally expected to perform the majority of child labour and caretaking (A.D. Watson 2020). Women apparently "feel" their biological clocks ticking and their "maternal instincts" kicking in. Hence, women "whose desires or social roles escape this [reproductive] function [e.g., spinsters] confound the ideological construction" that women's biological destiny is to reproduce and mother (Carroll 2012, 27). Given the cultural associations between women, reproduction, fertility, childrearing, and domesticity, fatherhood is rarely deemed compulsory (Bergman and Hobson 2002). However, in a perhaps unexpected turn, intersex fertility issues typically surround diagnoses given to and attributed to intersex people socio-medically assigned male. I suggest that this is the case because the procedures to render a socio-medically assigned girl intersex child "properly" feminine habitually result in infertility. That is, medical professionals' concern with fertility is not uniformly distributed and, therefore, must be questioned as disingenuous.

Tamar-Mattis (2012, 7) claims that "the fertility of intersex people is not being valued as highly as that of non-intersex people." Adding to this apt analysis, the fertility of intersex people socio-medically assigned female is not valued as highly as the fertility of intersex people assigned male. Medical professionals make this distinction very clear when discussing "treating" PAIS patients. Given that people with PAIS have variant genitals and testes (with, typically, fertile sperm), "there is still controversy and uncertainty about gender assignment in these cases, and it can go either way, depending largely on the doctor's judgment" (Tamar-Mattis 2012, 7). If the doctors decide to assign the child male, the testes will be left intact. If the doctors decide to assign the child female, the testes will be removed, rendering the child infertile. Tamar-Mattis (2012, 7), quoting Amy B. Wisniewski and Tom Mazur (2009, 5), explains the situation:

> One published article says: "At the present time fertility is challenging, but not impossible, for individuals with PAIS raised male. In contrast, fertility is not possible for individuals raised female" ... However, clearly the fertility does not depend on whether the child is raised as a boy or a girl. The authors quoted see fertility as impossible for a child with PAIS raised as female because they assume that raising her as female will include

removing her testes. This concept is so entrenched in the medical literature as to go unspoken.

In other words, fertility is not *im*possible because of the feminine rearing of a given child; rather, the child's fertility is contingent on – and becomes impossible because of – the surgeon's knife. Assigned girl children's testes must be exorcised because this biological attribute renders them queer, disabled, crip, incongruous, improperly feminine, and a heretic of compulsory dyadism. However, assigned boys can keep their testes and retain their fertility because they are not nearly as ideologically troubling as girls or women with testes. As Quinn (in Wall et al. 2015) states, "A lot of doctors are very uncomfortable with the idea I have testes and they are still trying to get them removed. But, I'm perfectly healthy and there's nothing wrong with them." Given that Quinn is a woman, she is deemed incongruous and in need of "fixing." Since medical practitioners are clearly working to uphold mandated ways of be(com)ing, "many doctors also do not see sterilizing surgeries as sterilization if the child would not have been fertile in the mode expected for the assigned gender" (Tamar-Mattis 2012, 7). Doctors most likely do not conceptualize sterilizations *as* sterilizations; rather, they understand these operations as reordering the disordered intersex body-mind.

As disability, trans, and critical race studies demonstrate, medical professionals are constantly trying to make calculations that will protect the Child. People with disabilities, trans individuals, as well as Black, Indigenous, and other people of colour (BIPOC) have routinely been sterilized. People with disabilities will presumably be unfit parents and may pass on their "undesirable" traits to their offspring. Trans folks supposedly ought not to reproduce because they will be inept parents, spreading their queer views to their children; and trans reproduction challenges deeply held beliefs about the nature of reproduction, motherhood, fatherhood, and parenthood. BIPOC, likewise, are presumably incompetent parents and may pass on their "objectionable" or "uncivilized" ways of life to their children. Although I have yet to come across anyone who explicitly claims that intersex people are or will be bad parents (and I hope that I never do), as noted above, intersex people, even if children themselves, threaten the Child because they challenge compulsory dyadism and, therefore, all other culturally mandated ways of being. To prevent this challenge, ableist discourses are mobilized. In turn, some intersex people's ability to biologically reproduce, typically that of socio-medically assigned girls, is sacrificed.

Gender "Affirmation"

The medical expressions "sex reassignment" and "sex change" have been used to describe medical procedures that some trans people undergo. These terms imply that medical intervention is "a means by which one moves from one sex/gender to the 'opposite' sex/gender" (Sullivan 2006, 553). In other words, they suggest that trans people are not really their genders unless doctors medically "reassign" or "change" their biological sex characteristics; the "truth" of one's gender is reduced to their genital formation. In turn, trans folks who cannot access or do not want certain medical interventions are, according to this discourse, not "really" their gender. Over the years, to avoid the problems noted above, these terms have been replaced with other expressions, such as "gender affirming/confirming health care" and "gender affirming/confirming surgery" (Baril and Trevenen 2014, 396).

Unlike trans people, who have to continually fight for medical interventions that they need/want and can consent to, intersex people are routinely subjected to procedures without consent. That is, trans people are forced to slow down possibly lifesaving and gender-affirming health care processes, whereas intersex people are deemed medical emergencies in need of a cure (G. Davis, Dewey, and Murphy 2016). Despite these differences, "sex/gender reassignment" has also been used, and is still used, to describe medical interventions performed on intersex infants, children, and adolescents. Employing this expression to describe these procedures is misrepresentative. Intersex people's sex or gender is not really being *re*assigned given that intersex is not recognized as a legitimate gender or sex category. Intersex infants and children are effectively deemed sexless or genderless until doctors medically assign a sex or gender. Nevertheless, the idea that medical interventions will affirm a child's gender is implicit. Echoing Inter's (2015) experience, noted above, Pagonis (2015b, 104) recalls that doctors were coming

> into the room to tell me what was going to happen next. "We noticed that your vagina is smaller than other girls'. While we're in the operating room fixing your urethra, we can also make a small incision in your vagina to make it longer. This way, you'll be able to have sex with your husband when you're older – Does that sound good?" I looked at my mom, who was in the prep room with me for this and wondered how to answer. I was only 11. I let out a shameful, "Yes." "Good then, we'll get that all taken care of for you as well during this procedure."

In other words, this operation would ostensibly enable Pagonis to perform their assumed heteronormative female gender. The procedure would effectively affirm or confirm their gender.

The idea that medical interventions performed on intersex people will, in no uncertain terms, affirm one's gender has been assumed. However, just as intersex is entering mainstream consciousness like never before and intersex people are testifying that medical procedures traumatized them and did not unproblematically affirm their genders or sexualities, gender-affirming language has recently been co-opted and explicitly used by experts in mainstream discussions. This co-option is a useful, albeit troubling, tactic for medical practitioners invested in maintaining compulsory dyadism and aligning intersex people's body-minds and identities with (hetero)normative ideals. In addition, the ways that "gender affirmation" is deployed effectively frame intersex people's protests to medical interventions as illogical, perhaps even as anti-trans or anti-queer.

Amid the tumultuous debates about sport sex testing and medically altering athletes (e.g., Caster Semenya and Dutee Chand) with intersex traits who apparently have an unfair advantage, gender-affirming terminology was mobilized. Representatives of the International Association of Athletics Federations (IAAF), Angelica Linden Hirschberg, Richard Auchus, and Stéphane Bermon, penned an open letter to the World Medical Association after it derided the IAAF's discriminatory policies that require women athletes with intersex traits to undergo medical intervention. Hirschberg, Auchus, and Bermon (2019) write that women athletes with naturally high levels of testosterone must "[reduce] serum testosterone to female levels by using a contraceptive pill (or other means)." They continue, "DSDs are associated with an increased risk of cancer ... A suitable form of treatment is recommended to lower the testosterone level, provided the patient accepts it herself. In worldwide clinical practice, male gonads are often removed, but pharmacological treatments to reduce testosterone levels are also used." They emphasize that "it is the athlete's right to decide (in consultation with their medical team)" and state that medical intervention "is the recognized standard of care ... These medications are gender-affirming."

Although I unpack the science behind, history of, and political implications of sport sex testing and medical management in Part 2, "The Racialized Intersex Spectre," for my purposes here, I analyze these professionals' mobilization of seemingly pro-feminist, pro-queer gender-affirming language in tandem with pro-consent care rhetoric. By co-opting gender-affirming discourse, the IAAF positions itself as gender-confirmatory or gender-supportive, all the while implementing discriminatory policies that force women athletes to undergo medical interventions that they do not want, that do not affirm their gender expression, and/or that may result in sterilization as well as a whole host of other life-long concerns. This policy does not affirm one's gender identity but undermines it by explicitly stating that these athletes are not "woman enough" to compete.

Moreover, intersex people's testimonies reveal that medical professionals are often not concerned with or do not consistently ask intersex people about which gender or sex they identify with or would like to embody. For instance, intersex activist, artist, and researcher Sean Saifa M. Wall was socio-medically assigned female and was subjected to "feminizing" intersex genital mutilation (IGM) even though this assignment did not reflect who he was, who he wanted to be, and how he related to his body. Wall (2015b, 118) writes,

> The pain that I felt following the surgery was perhaps the worst pain that I have experienced in my entire life. After surgery, my pediatrician prescribed estrogen and Provera as a hormonal replacement regimen. Fatty deposits changed the shape and contours of my face. Once robust and chiseled thighs now harbored cellulite. The beginnings of facial hair and prominent body hair became wispy and nonexistent. What was hard and defined became soft. *At no point did anyone ask me what I wanted to do with my body.* I actually missed the effects of my natural testosterone such as a deepening voice, increased hair and muscle mass.

Testimonies like Wall's reveal that medical interventions are not necessarily gender-affirming given that intersex people are not always or typically asked which gender or sex they are and would like to embody. The fact that the medical professionals associated with the IAAF employ gender-affirming language is disconcerting not only because this language does not represent many intersex people's experiences but also because endosex people unfamiliar with intersex issues may understandably assume that these medical professionals are uncontestable experts. Indeed, doctors and medical experts are presumed to be infallible, all-knowing, benevolent, godlike figures.

The IAAF's spokespeople also employ pro-consent rhetoric – "the athlete's right to decide" and "provided the patient accepts it" – to mask the fact that the policy creates an environment that does not leave room for one to fully consent or refuse. These athletes have no real choice. They cannot simply refuse medical intervention because, if they do, they cannot compete. And this situation is not simply about athletes being passionate about a sport and not being allowed to participate (on discriminatory grounds). If they refuse, this policy prevents them from engaging in a sport that secures their economic well-being and possibly that of their families. These athletes have no real choice.

That said, the IAAF implies that one would be unwise not to consent to "gender affirming" procedures, noting that intersex variations "are associated with an increased risk of cancer." However, as shown above, claims of intersex cancer risk are inflated and inconsistent. In fact, taking hormones for extended periods of time increases one's risk of developing certain kinds of cancers. Reproducing the false claim that intersex variations may cause cancer frames the athlete – or anyone who attempts to refuse medical procedures – as unreasonable for not consenting. According to the IAAF's faulty logic, the illogical party is the athlete who refuses, not the official who enforces discriminatory policy.

To reinforce the need for these athletes to agree to "affirm" their gender in order to avoid the supposed dangers of cancer, the IAAF tactically uses the word "medication." "Medication" implies a need, a way to get better and be cured. The IAAF, then, frames itself as caring for and curing athletes with potentially life-threatening conditions. However, athletes with naturally high levels of testosterone have no medical need for hormones; they require no cure. "Medication," like the cancer and gender-affirming narratives, functions to frame intervention as a kindness and a necessity.

The IAAF notes that athletes who "consent" will use "a contraceptive pill (or other means)." The "other means," which are strategically bracketed to de-emphasize the invasive nature of hormone intervention, may be skin patches, topical creams, vaginal suppositories, or injections. Additionally, failing to mention the possible side effects of these hormonal interventions – such as blood clots, stroke, cancer, heart attack, ir/reversible biological changes, and interference with other (necessary) medications – frames the intervention as "no big deal." Consequently, the unconsenting athlete is, once again, deemed unreasonable.

The gender-affirming and consent discourse also does not coincide with past or present intersex medical management. Framing intersex medical treatment as gender-affirming is misrepresentative because, historically, intersex children have been socio-medically assigned female in the Global

North. That is, vaginoplasties and clitoroplasties/clitorectomies have been considerably more widespread than phalloplasties. It is estimated that 90 percent of infants with variant genitals are assigned female (Chase 1998, 210). Intersex activist Cheryl Chase (2006, 302) (a.k.a. Bo Laurent) notes that "members of the Johns Hopkins intersex team have justified female assignment by saying, 'You can make a hole, but you can't build a pole'" (see also Bastien-Charlebois 2015; and Gurney 2007). Or, put in slightly different terms by John Gearhart (quoted in Holmes 2008a, 148), a pediatric urologist who worked with John Money, "it is easier to dig a hole than build a pole."[13] Typically, without much consideration for the intersex assigned girl child's genital sensitivity, these procedures – which maintain intersecting forms of discrimination, including interphobia, queerphobia, ableism, and phallogo-centrism (Bastien-Charlebois 2015) – take place because they are easier for surgeons to perform.

Outside of Western contexts, surgical trends can vary due to differing manifestations of interphobic, phallogocentric, and sexist ideologies. Consider, for example, China. Chinese intersex activist Small Luk (2015) writes, "Amongst the majority of families and parents, sons are more welcome, to continue the family line. Parents, family systems, communities, doctors and even the government tend to force intersex children, even intersex teens, to have genital 'normalising' surgery or medical intervention, to be men." Even though it may be "easier to dig a hole" and neglect assigned females' genital sensation, in China more intersex people are assigned male and surgically and/or hormonally altered. Compounding the issue in China, "the 'one child policy' has resulted in the abandonment and killing of baby girls, but also infants with intersex traits. Families in China have to pay the majority of medical expenses themselves, resulting in extreme poverty, or in rural areas, no treatment or surgery but a stronger likelihood of being killed or abandoned" (Luk 2015). Due to the instituted, but now phased-out, one-child policy, many culturally devalued children (i.e., intersex and girl infants) were killed or abandoned. Although there are significant differences between Western nations and China, phenomena of intersex surgical assignment are different manifestations of the same intersecting discriminatory ideologies.

Obtaining medical statistics concerning how often intersex infants and children are socio-medically assigned boys or girls is difficult. This information is typically kept secret. Patient confidentiality could figure in keeping this information privileged and private. Yet, for government budgetary and funding purposes, as well as for statistical purposes and public health, hospitals are often required to routinely release information without disclosing patient information. For example, the Canadian Institute for Health Information publicly releases provincial statistical reports for free online. These reports include, for instance, workforce information, access and wait times, how often particular procedures take place (e.g., cardiac implants, mastectomies, and abortions), and how often people are diagnosed with various pathologies (e.g., cancer and viruses). Information regarding DSD "treatment" remains absent from these types of documents.

In fact, a report of the Standing Committee on Health, authored by chair Bill Casey (2019), then a member of Parliament, offers up no statistics about how often these surgeries take place in Canada. The document, titled *The Health of LGBTQIA2 Communities in Canada,* is full of other valuable and troubling statistics concerning LGBTQIA2 people's health in Canada, but there is a glaring lack of statistics about intersex people and medical management. It stands to reason that there are no statistics available, that they are not deemed worthy of collecting, or that they are intentionally being withheld. At the "Public Consultation on Protection against Violence and Discrimination Based on Sexual Orientation and Gender Identity" (United Nations Human Rights 2017), Carpenter stated that nations typically do not disclose such information because doing so "discloses human rights violations." Keeping this information private – or refusing to gather such information – is both a means to protect hospitals and doctors from criticism and a means to deny abuses. However, given that approximately 1 in 2,000 babies are born with visible genital variations, public policy scholar Catherine Leigh Crawford (2019, 6) estimates that in Canada "around two hundred babies are evaluated annually" and may be subjected to surgery. Although this estimate is illuminating, there still are no definitive Canadian statistics about surgery rates, how often intersex infants are sociomedically assigned boys or girls, or whether surgical practices have changed in any considerable way.

However, there are some statistics from Europe. According to Ulrike Klöppel's (2016) study conducted in Germany, surgical practices are not improving. As described by Dan Christian Ghattas at the "Public Consultation" (United Nations Human Rights 2017), Klöppel's study

> is a retrospective, statistical data assessment from hospital statistics based on case flat-rates on feminizing and masculinizing genital surgeries carried out in that respective country's hospitals between 2005 and 2014. The study focuses on children under the age of 10 ... One of the key findings is

that the development of the relative frequency of so-called feminizing genital surgeries showed no significant decline.

In fact, the number of "feminizing" surgeries remained almost exactly same, and the number of "masculinizing" surgeries rose. Not only are Klöppel's observations troubling, but the data also do not support the idea that these procedures take place because they are gender-affirming. They are gender/sex-imposing or gender/sex-prescriptive. Moreover, given that surgical intervention typically takes place in one's infancy and childhood, one cannot properly consent to gender-affirming procedures.

Although the IAAF's open letter is just one case where gender-affirming discourse is deployed, I suspect that this rhetoric will be woven into the ableist language already adopted by medical professionals. Doing so is an effective means to obscure the queerphobic logics that have underpinned the history of intersex medical management; doing so also obfuscates the extent to which intersex people can resist having their body-minds invaded and cut up with impunity. Under the guise of affirmation, support, and care, compulsory modes of being are maintained; "the belief that physical sex, gender identity, and gender roles in an individual should all align to either masculine or feminine" is reaffirmed (Karkazis 2008, 248).

Conclusion

Most doctors probably believe that the procedures they endorse and perform are benevolent. They maintain that they are acting in the best interests of intersex infants, children, and adolescents. Given the intersecting logics of compulsory dyadism, able-bodiedness, and heterosexuality, medical professionals most likely regard curative medical approaches to intersex as the best course of action. Yet the health risks associated with intersex are at best contested and at worst exaggerated. As a result, the ableist narratives – and the emerging "gender-affirming" language – that they employ are not representative of intersex traits, intersex people's ability to consent, or the consequences of medical interventions. Rather, these discourses serve as a guise to maintain curative violence, they work to render intersex people illogical for challenging medical practitioners' course of "treatment," and they work to convince parents/proxies that irreversible procedures are necessary and will simply be forgotten by the child. Irreversible procedures are not forgotten. Intersex individuals become life-long patients, and the body-mind loss or acquired body-mind disabilities are inevitably enveloped into their be(com)ing.

Reflecting on the apparent need for curative medical practices in the documentary *Intersexion* (Lahood 2012), Bo Laurent (a.k.a. Cheryl Chase) states, "If I went around and said, 'Open heart surgery is a sham and nobody should do it anymore, we should just stop,' a whole bunch of people would come out and say, 'Well actually open heart surgery saved me, and I think we should not stop.' But that hasn't been happening around genital surgery [performed on intersex people]." If medical procedures were indeed medically beneficial or needed, finding an intersex person who has undergone such a procedure and is grateful that such an intervention occurred would be easy. It stands to reason that, since the Intersex Rights Movement is now a growing part of cultural consciousness, an intersex person who contests the claims of violence made by intersex activists and advocates would – even if anonymously – have come out of the woodwork. In fact, historian of science Alice Domurat Dreger (in Lahood 2012) confirms that people have searched for one such intersex person: "Journalists have gone for over a decade seeking one [intersex] person to go on camera, even behind a potted plant, and say, 'Yes, this [medical intervention] happened to me, and I'm glad my parents made this decision.' So where are all of these people?" Finding such a person appears to be an impossible task. Perhaps one does not exist at all.

Even with this utter lack of counter-testimony, the views of medical professionals who endorse intersex medical management without conclusive studies to justify interventions are typically privileged over the experiences of intersex people themselves. Not only do doctors hold esteemed socio-political positions that remain largely unquestioned by endosex, cisgender, heterosexual, white, thin, and able-bodied people, but folks with intersex variations also "spectacularly violate sacred ideologies of Western culture" (Garland-Thomson 2011, 26). According to compulsory modes of being, intersex people embody heresy. Hence, the exorcising curative violence performed is construed as an appropriate atonement or punishment for heretical embodiments that defy consecrated Western principles.

As a result, intersex studies scholars, activists, and advocates face a seemingly impossible task if they are to stop curative violence and undermine doctors' authority: they must convince lay endosex people that the sex dyad is a farce, convince them that medical practitioners – whom they trust and who may even have saved their lives – ought to be actively questioned and challenged, and convince them to be allies. I say "convince" them rather than "prove" anything because these scholars, activists, and advocates have already demonstrated the truth of their observations.

However, given the shifting discursive nature of intersex and its now intimate relationship with disability, intersex studies scholars, activists, and advocates need a new tactic. I propose cripping intersex. At this juncture, undermining compulsory dyadism is impossible without also undermining compulsory able-bodiedness. Rather than distance from disability, intersex studies and activism ought to embrace and celebrate the necessary theoretical and methodological tools offered by feminist disability and crip studies.

2

Medical Interventions and Acquired Body-Mind Disabilities

"Curative" Medical Interventions and Acquired Body-Mind Disabilities

Intersex activist, artist, and researcher Sean Saifa M. Wall (2015a) explains, "Surgeons are still mutilating children who don't look 'normal' ... Some feel they have the responsibility to mutilate children's bodies, in order to uphold antiquated notions of sex and gender, preserving a strict male/female binary." Echoing Wall, many intersex people who have endured medical interventions, intersex studies scholars, nongovernmental organizations (e.g., StopIGM.org and Organisation Intersex International), and intergovernmental organizations (e.g., the United Nations) claim that these interventions, or their consequences, constitute intersex genital mutilation (IGM), torture, inhumane practices, violence, sexual assault or rape, invasion, and human rights violations.[1] Some of the consequences are genital pain, (painful) scarring, loss of sexual sensation or ability to orgasm, anesthetic neurotoxicity, incontinence, inability to urinate without assistive devices or discomfort, infection, fear of intimacy, depression, anxiety, post-traumatic stress disorder, and suicidal ideation. Intersex individuals who live with these haunting effects of medical management are keenly aware that these procedures constitute curative violence. They rightly urge medical professionals to stop performing nonconsensual, irreversible, and humiliating procedures on people with intersex characteristics.

Some scholars have also employed the language of queering to describe and theorize the outcomes of medically managing intersex. Sociologist Katrina Roen (2005, 270), for example, argues that medical interventions that are intended to "straighten out" intersex people's anatomy – and, in turn, their gender and sexuality – "inevitably create newly queer beings" because they fail to set things straight. These discourses have been and continue to be fundamental in the battle against intersex curative violence. However, cripping intersex – approaching the medical management of intersex through a disability studies lens – requires us to contend with the fact that medical interventions are often disabling. Interphobic curative violence is a disability issue.

This chapter, therefore, bears witness to many intersex people's testimonies regarding the disabling nature of curative violence. Although the language of, for example, queering, mutilation, torture, rape, and sexual assault is apt and indispensable in the context of projects that combat compulsory dyadism and curative violence, I argue that folks invested in a crip intersex politics should also explicitly narrate the consequences of curative violence as disabling. They constitute gratuitously acquired body-mind disabilities. Narrating the consequences as disabilities or disabling underscores the horribly ironic fact that in the attempt to "enable" supposedly disordered intersex people – in the attempt to enforce compulsory modes of being – intersex people are actively disabled by medical interventions. Acknowledging the trauma as incurred disabilities unequivocally demonstrates the productive potential of an approach rooted in crip intersex studies that conceptualizes intersex as a disability issue, and it identifies a locus where intersex and disability issues align.

In the language of haunting, the various disabling outcomes that many intersex people "live with and through" (Holmes 2008b, 175) can be understood as "way[s] in which abusive systems of power make themselves known and their impacts felt in everyday life, especially when they are supposedly over and done with" (Gordon 2011, 2). J. David Hester (2006, 48) observes in Sharon E. Sytsma's edited collection, *Ethics and Intersex*, that the biological "liminality" of intersex traits "is not erased by this intervention, but is reinforced through a pathology of medical practices that renders the body of the intersexed unnatural and suspicious, even after intervention."[2] The intersex "phantasm" (Holmes 2002, 175) haunts the intersex child even if that child was surgically "fixed" or hormonally altered in the past. The discursive and literal work to declare – constitute – the intersex child a boy or girl "necessarily fails since the intersex body, both pre- *and* post-surgical inscription, is still, always already, a site of contested being, a locus of 'embodied becoming' (Roen [2009]). The intersex body is not ontological, but rather hauntological" (O'Rouke and Giffney 2009, x).

Prior to surgical and/or hormonal inscription, the intersex child is a site of contested being because *it* is "sexless" (Preves 1999, 52). The child is understood to be and is often made to feel like, as Martha Coventry (1999, 73) testifies, "a sexual failure." Echoing philosopher Judith Butler (1988), Coventry (1999, 52) writes that the child's "entrance into the social world may be halted until the child is sexed." Until such children are "properly" sexed and therefore gendered via socio-medical means, they are treated as a *disabled* medical emergency. They are a threat to compulsory dyadism, heterosexuality, and able-bodiedness and must be actively disabled, re-ordered, and rearranged. That is, an intersex child is not an innate medical emergency but a "social emergency in which medical experts are called to intervene" (Karkazis 2008, 96). As a result, even if medical intervention is completely medically unnecessary and is purely cosmetic, the intersex spectre must be exorcised via various procedures because "the intersex body haunts, spectralises, conjures up unimaginable futures" (O'Rouke and Giffney 2009, x). The assumption is that such children, if left unaltered, could never lead normal, heathy lives or be loved as they are. If left unaltered, they have no clear future or "no good future" (Kafer 2013, 3). Nevertheless, to borrow Joshua Gunn's (2004, 109) phrase, "exorcism is futile." Socio-medical assignment does not necessarily render one a sexual "success" or a nonemergency given the disabling nature of curative violence. Intersex traits always remain a hauntological threat.

The intersex phantasm cannot and never could be entirely cast out of one's body-mind. It lingers in the form of, for example, disabilities, memories, scars, body-mind pain and anguish, stigma, shame, and stolen futures. Moreover, given that the spectre always threatens to resurface and reveal itself again – for instance, as one goes through puberty – one must be constantly surveilled and must endure repeated medical visits and examinations, more operations, dilation routines, and/or hormone replacement therapy (HRT) routines. The spectre must be constantly deferred because it can never be completely cast out. Scars may fade, but they may never disappear; routines may cease, but the memory and disabling embodied consequences may or will not. Intersex need not be conceptualized as a frightening spectre requiring violent exorcisms. Rather, intersex characteristics ought to be understood as world-re/making, generative, beautiful, and worth celebrating.

This chapter addresses four commonplace medical protocols: HRT, surgeries, gratuitous genital examinations and displays, and explicitly deceiving, lying, misinforming, or withholding information from intersex patients and/or their parents/proxies. By attending to many intersex people's testimonies, I frame their embodied, ongoing experiences of curative violence as disabilities. Doing so offers generative connections between intersex and disabled embodied experiences and demonstrates the necessity of crip intersex studies. Although I maintain that underscoring the disabling nature of interphobic curative violence is imperative, my analyses do not prove that living with disabilities is inherently undesirable, negative, or bad. Interphobic medical management needs to stop because it is nonconsensual and violent and because it reinforces compulsory dyadism, able-bodiedness, and heterosexuality. I underscore the disabling nature of interphobic curative violence to demonstrate that intersex studies and activism must be politically linked; crip intersex studies is crucial.

Hormone Replacement Therapy

Many people with intersex variations are coerced into taking medically unnecessary "female" or "male" hormones – HRT – so that their embodiment "coincides" with or emphasizes their assigned sex/gender (see G. Davis 2015; Kessler 1998; Klöppel 2009; and L.S. Long 2015). HRT is common medical practice. I begin with HRT because its disabling or mutilating consequences are not often the focus of anti-interphobic projects; rather, the consequences of surgery typically garner the most attention.

HRT became a common treatment method in the 1950s. Steroid hormones were "discovered" and subsequently sexed and gendered (i.e., labelled male or female, masculine or feminine) in the 1920s.[3] Or, more accurately put, hormones were *invented*: "Preexisting ideas about masculinity and femininity caused scientists to look for, create tests for, classify, and perceive steroid hormones in a way that fit them into a dualistic system of sex" (Jordan-Young 2010, 16). Socio-political ideologies about gender led scientists and doctors to label testosterone as male and estrogen as female. This labelling re/stabilized the notion that girls/women and boys/men are fundamentally different (Eckert 2009). With this in mind, we can see that "sex is in some important sense, an effect of gender" (Jordan-Young 2010, 17). Dominant ideas about gender are discursively and literally prescribed into or onto sex traits. Sex is a social construction and phenomenon. This proposal does not deny the materiality of people's morphologies, differences between people's biological characteristics, or the complex relationships that people have with their biologies. Rather, quoting Butler (1993, 29), Anne Fausto-Sterling (2000, 22) explains that the idea of sex as a social construct reminds us that "every time we return to the body as something that exists prior to socialization, prior to discourse about male and female ... 'we discover that matter is fully sedimented with discourses on sex and sexuality that prefigure and constrain the uses to which that term can be put.'" One's anatomical and biological attributes are material entities that continually re/produce and are re/produced by discourses. And, if one's characteristics are presumed to violate compulsory modes of being and are subsequently pathologized – as is the case with intersex variations – one may be literally re/produced and de/reconstructed by a variety of "curative" interventions.

All that being said, the invention of "sex" hormones was, and continues to be, destabilizing. These hormones weakened the already fragile, but nevertheless supported, foothold of compulsory dyadism (Klöppel 2009). For example, this discovery revealed that sex hormone levels – or more accurately put, steroid hormone levels – varied widely within and between (assigned) sexes/genders. "Male" hormones do not necessarily counter or prevent "female" characteristics, and "female" hormones do not necessarily counter "male" characteristics.[4] Nevertheless, the belief in the sex dyad persisted, and the idea that hormones fundamentally shape one's male or female heterosexual gender identity was established, primarily by John Money and his colleagues, within the medical community and in mainstream culture.

"Normal" steroid hormone levels were assumed to be essential for "normal," heteronormative gender and sexual-identity formation. Since intersex people are perceived as developing abnormally – or to use Kathryn Bond Stockton's (2009, 1) term, "sideways" – HRT emerged alongside surgical treatments in the 1950s. At this time, the pediatric Endocrine Clinic of Johns Hopkins Hospital in Baltimore outlined a "novel treatment plan ... that scheduled 'corrections' of intersexual genitals and hormone therapy in early infancy in order to assure an unambiguous rearing as boy or girl and thereby a 'normal' psychosexual development" (Klöppel 2009, 173). Almost a century after the invention of hormones, many medical professionals still maintain that one's gendered performances and mannerisms are effects of the prenatal hormonal environment that they were exposed to (G. Davis 2015). This belief is called brain organization theory.

Brain organization theorists maintain that steroid hormones literally form the brain to have male or female and gay or straight brain structures.[5] Hence, tinkering with hormone levels prenatally or postnatally will apparently shape one's brain structures and, therefore, one's gender and sexuality. And the presumed best outcome of such interference is cisheteronormative behaviours and desires. Yet a comprehensive meta-analysis of brain organization studies demonstrates that there is no solid evidence to support this theory: "evidence that human brains are hormonally organized to be either masculine or feminine turns out to be surprisingly disjointed, and even contradictory" (Jordan-Young 2010, 3). Such a theory could never be properly proven anyway because it does not take into account social, cultural, discursive, environmental, or political variables. It fails to consider the ways that gender, sex, and sexuality are ongoing social constructs. It presupposes the legitimacy of the sex, gender, and sexuality binaries. It neglects the fact that people's socio-cultural experiences also literally shape people's brains and influence their sexed, gendered, and sexual behaviour. This theory also problematically assumes that the only "normal," and nonpathological way of being is heterosexual, cisgender, and gender-conforming. Even though there are evident methodological and theoretical failings and a lack of evidence, many medical professionals and scientists imply that this theory is a settled scientific fact. This is deeply worrisome, as "the stakes involved in prematurely promoting this theory to a 'fact' of human development are high, both for the advancement of science and for social debates that draw on science" (Jordan-Young 2010, 3). The stakes are high for LGBTQIA2 communities. The stakes are particularly high for intersex people. This misguided theory haunts academic and medical halls as well as intersex medical management, and it has made its way into mainstream consciousness, further sedimenting and propagating unsubstantial claims (see O'Keefe 2016; and Villarreal 2022).

In certain circumstances, HRT is medically necessary for intersex people. For example, people with congenital adrenal hyperplasia (CAH) who have intersex traits typically need to take a variety of hormone replacements (e.g., hydrocortisone, prednisone, and fludrocortisone) throughout their lives to ensure metabolic balance. In other circumstances, however, hormones are not medically necessary but are prescribed to reinforce one's assigned sex and gender. These circumstances illustrate the stakes and the violent, disabling consequences of nonconsensual or coercive HRT management. Consider intersex activist David Cameron's (1999, 2007) story. Medical professionals assured Cameron and his family that he was a "normal" boy even though he appeared different, more feminine, than other boys his age. Yet, when he was twenty, Cameron learned of his intersex variation, Klinefelter syndrome (or 47,XXY). Cameron was told that he was sterile and had "abnormally" low testosterone levels. Cameron was then construed as queerly disordered, and his doctor advised him to start HRT injections right away. This advice was given without psychological or emotional counselling *and* without discussing Cameron's gender identity. Cameron (1999, 91, 93) "always felt caught between the sexes," "more feminine." His doctor also advised him to take HRT without fully informing him of the various side effects that testosterone would have on his body-mind: "I was told that my 'sex drive would increase,' I would 'gain weight and my shoulders would broaden,' and that I would have to do this every two weeks for the rest of my life" (Cameron 1999, 91). His doctor did not tell him that he "was about to go through puberty again *with a vengeance* ... in my thirties" (Cameron 2007, 164). The doctor also did not communicate that the ultimate goal of HRT was to reorder his body-mind in order to better approximate "hegemonic masculinity" as well as compulsory dyadism (Connell and Messerschmidt 2005, 829). Wanting to increase his sex drive, Cameron followed the doctor's orders.

Cameron enjoyed his (temporarily) increased sex drive and his budding beard. To his consternation, however, his body was soon blanketed with hair and his head started to bald. His prostate also enlarged considerably. It grew so large that Cameron required medication that would enable him to urinate. These changes were, in Cameron's (2007, 164) words, "[altering] my sense of self." And, in turn, they caused long-term "emotional issues" (Cameron 1999, 93). As his prostate continued to grow, he was finally informed of some of the long-term effects of his HRT injections, including increased risk of developing prostate, breast/chest, or testicular cancer. He began to embody and comprehend the violence of "cure." Understandably, Cameron (1999, 93) started to view "the testosterone as a poison" and to question whether the doctor's (coercive) advice was correct or in his best interest.

Even with the current and prospective disabling effects, Cameron's doctor urged him to continue with the HRT injections and encouraged him to enhance the masculinizing process by undergoing testicular-implant and breast/chest-removal cosmetic surgeries. He decided against these seemingly more invasive interventions. However, because he heeded the medical advice to continue with testosterone injections, his prostate and urinary problems persisted, and Cameron (1999, 94) was "put on another drug to try and compensate for the side-effects of the testosterone." After nineteen years of injections, he decided to stop. Coming off HRT, Cameron (1999, 94) experienced "fatigue, mood swings, depression, [and] more difficulty urinating." In an effort to combat these disabling side effects, he later began using daily androgen patches. The patches, however, did not alleviate his depression or mood swings. The visibility of the patches also made Cameron (1999, 95) self-conscious, and the patches produced "constant skin rashes and itchiness." The epidermal problems prompted another medical treatment: hydrocortisone cream. This skin ritual was a haunting daily reminder to Cameron (1999, 95) that he "was different." He defied compulsory modes of being and, therefore, had to be punished; his intersex traits needed to be exorcised. His depression intensified, and two large fat deposits formed: "one on the back of my neck ... and the other in the form of a spare tire under my navel" (1999, 95).

The ongoing and compounding body-mind effects, the constant medical management and surveillance, and the "curative" rituals were aimed at keeping the intersex spectre at bay. Cameron's doctor worked to continually defer and cast out the intersex phantasm at the expense of Cameron's body-mind health, self-determination, and sense of gendered self/identity. Reasonably, Cameron (1999, 95) wanted "more control over [his] destiny"; but he was acutely aware that he could never return to what his body-mind was before these coercive, irreversible medical interventions. Despite medical professionals' efforts to make Cameron (1999, 96) into a "proper" man, he is still "a unique blend of ... female and male essences"; he is, and is legally recognized as, a "non-binary person" (Lindahl 2017). Finding the now closed Intersex Society of North America helped Cameron to trust his own embodied experiences and to challenge both curative violence and the idea that doctors are infallible gods. "My endocrinologist was not God," Cameron (2007, 164) writes,

> although I trusted that he knew what was best for me at the time ... I feel that I was rushed into an experience that I wasn't ready for and that my doctor deceived me. Doctors do not have all the correct information on sex, gender, and sexuality diversity. Not everything needs to be pathologized just because it is *different*. I've learned to trust my own life experience, not fitting into our "two sex/two genders: Western binary system" ... After that first intersex support group, I learned that, for me, my sense of gender as a "blend" is okay.

Cameron's story illustrates that medical professionals do not always have one's best interest in mind, even if they believe that they do. Rather than supporting one's well-being and providing all the relevant information for proper consent, a doctor's advice may primarily work to uphold valued cultural mandates and may result in re/emerging body-mind disabilities.

In many situations, HRT is medically unnecessary, but intersex patients and/or their parents/proxies are coerced into agreeing, often without all the information. Patients and/or parents/proxies of intersex children understandably trust doctors; they are godlike, benevolent cultural figures after all. In other circumstances, the medical need for hormones is created. As noted in the previous chapter, Karen A. Walsh (2015, 122) had to begin a life-long HRT regimen because of a medically unwarranted gonadectomy:

> I know now that it was not necessary to remove my gonads – my only source of endogenous hormones. [Because of the unnecessary gonadal removal,] I am at extraordinary risk for osteoporosis, as well as problems with libido. Additionally, I had problems feminizing during my "puberty," since the Premarin was not well absorbed. It is a myth in the treatment of intersex that exogenous hormones work as well as endogenous ones. This is a lifelong problem for me ... I wish I had been given the choice to keep my testes with regular monitoring instead of rushing to surgery. Hormone replacement therapy is a poor substitute for the real thing – especially at age 15 with a long life ahead.[6]

Because doctors needlessly rushed to exorcise Walsh's testes because they violated cultural expectations and standards, Walsh must always remain on HRT and anticipate/confront various disabilities.

Wall, diagnosed with androgen insensitivity syndrome (AIS), was similarly forced to undergo HRT. Even though Wall had always identified as male, medical professionals maintained that he was and ought to be sociomedically assigned female. He was subjected to "feminizing" surgery at the age of thirteen and was put on HRT to reinforce his assigned female gender and sex. As quoted in the previous chapter, Wall (2015b, 118) explains,

> The pain that I felt following the surgery was perhaps the worst pain that I have experienced in my entire life. After surgery, my pediatrician prescribed estrogen and Provera as a hormonal replacement regimen. Fatty deposits changed the shape and contours of my face. Once robust and chiseled thighs now harbored cellulite. The beginnings of facial hair and prominent body hair became wispy and nonexistent. What was hard and defined became soft. *At no point did anyone ask me what I wanted to do with my body.* I actually missed the effects of my natural testosterone such as a deepening voice, increased hair and muscle mass; when I asked if I could take both testosterone and estrogen after surgery, my mother remarked, "You would look too weird." The hormone therapy was coupled with intense social conditioning. I feel as if the social conditioning for young women raised

with AIS is suffocating. When doctors prescribed hormones for me to take, my mother constantly reminded me how "beautiful" the little yellow pills would make me.

At the age of twenty-five, Wall decided to no longer conform to his imposed and inscribed socio-medically assigned sex and gender. The effects of the intense social conditioning and curative violence – surgery and HRT – were evidently profoundly painful for Wall. His embodied becoming was non-consensually being literally de/reconstructed in ways that did not reflect his needs, wants, or gender identity.

These sorts of testimonies necessitate fundamental changes to inter-sex HRT prescription practices and philosophies about brain organization theory. HRT may or may not be required or desired. Intersex people's needs, identities, and desires must be centralized so they can live comfortably in their body-minds and the world. The end goal of medicine should not be to violently force people to embody an ideology, a sex, or a gender that is not their own. Doing so can cause them to experience profound body-mind disabilities, such as anxiety, depression, dysphoria, and dissociation, as well as unnecessary (prospective) disabling illnesses like osteoporosis and cancer.

Surgeries

Surgically altering people with intersex characteristics to "cure" them of their perceived malady began in the mid-twentieth century alongside HRT. Alice Domurat Dreger (1999a, 11) refers to the era in which surgery became common medical practice as the "Age of Surgery."[7] Surgery became the conventional medical response to individuals with intersex traits, partly because new technological and surgical tools were developed that could readily detect and (attempt to) exorcise the intersex spectre. Perhaps more importantly, surgery became routine because of the popularization of the views held by John Money and his colleagues about, as the title of one of Money's (1968) books puts it, "sex errors of the body." According to Money and his associates, surgery is paramount because a child must have "normal"-looking genitals to develop a "healthy," heteronormative gender identity and sexuality. Surgeries can include building up phallic tissue (i.e., phalloplasty), creating a vagina (i.e., vaginoplasty), amputating clitoral tissue (i.e., clitoroplasty/clitorectomy), relocating the penile urethral meatus, or "pee hole" (also known as hypospadias repair and masculinizing corrections), and removing gonads (i.e., gonadectomy). Although Money's epistemological reign is over because his theories about sex and gender proved to be incorrect, surgical practices are still very common today. The idea that children must have "normal"-looking genitals to, for instance, avoid teasing and develop "properly" persists despite the fact that intersex people have been, for decades, attesting to the gratuitously disabling and violating nature of nonconsensual surgery.

Some medical professionals claim that surgery should continue because there is not enough data suggesting that surgery is not the best course of action. For example, in a report published by Human Rights Watch and interACT: Advocates for Intersex Youth (2017), a gynecologist remarks, "I really think that we don't have great data on if we don't do surgery, is it better than if we do surgery." The report also quotes a urologist: "In terms of medical necessity ... I think drawing a hard line without hard data might just alienate many [practitioners]." However, the report contends that

> a lack of data on outcomes for intact children does not support defaulting to conducting irreversible and medically unnecessary surgeries that carry the potential for harm. Indeed, the available medical evidence points overwhelmingly in the opposite direction: that the well-documented harms of these operations should be a primary factor in doctors' recommendation to defer them until the patient can understand and consent to the procedure.

Not only does the available evidence overwhelmingly suggest that surgery actively and gratuitously disables, harms, and traumatizes intersex people, but claiming that we need more data before surgery can be stopped also does not create the conditions needed to accrue more data proving the violent nature of intersex genital mutilation. In addition, doctors' potential feelings of alienation should not be privileged. The purpose of medicine and changing medical practices is not to make doctors feel good. Medical professionals and practices are supposed to privilege patients' feelings and well-being. And, evidence suggests, surgery actively isolates, shames, alienates, and disables intersex people.[8]

But how common are these surgical practices? As noted in the previous chapter, obtaining information regarding how often IGM occurs is difficult; such information is typically not publicly released. That being said, citing Anne Fausto-Sterling (2000), Rainbow Health Ontario (2011, 1) notes, "It is estimated that 30–80% of intersex children undergo more than one surgery and some have as many as five surgeries." Some people with intersex traits have been subjected to well over a dozen surgeries. Recently, many medical professionals claim that the number of surgeries performed on unconsenting intersex infants and children are declining. Nevertheless, Morgan Carpenter noted at the "Public Consultation on Protection against Violence and Discrimination Based on Sexual Orientation and Gender Identity" (United Nations Human Rights 2017) that the "rhetoric of changes to medical practices remain[s] unsubstantiated."[9] Despite many doctors' seeming devotion to data, there are no data to back up their claims that the number of surgeries has declined.

In fact, Peter A. Lee and colleagues (2016, 167), authors of "Global Disorders of Sex Development Update since 2006: Perceptions, Approach and Care" – the 2016 report that follows up on the "Consensus Statement on Management of Intersex Disorders" (I.A. Hughes et al. 2006) – note that there is a "high prevalence of normalizing surgery," even though "adults' dissatisfaction with their early surgery is high." Yet the report does not condemn surgery. It merely suggests delaying procedures and combining them with psychological evaluations: "HRT and surgery *should* commence only after a full psychological evaluation at the appropriate age for each fully informed patient" (Lee et al. 2016, 172–73, emphasis added).[10] However, being informed does not equal informed consent. One can be well informed about the logistics of surgery, but having this knowledge does not mean that the patient has fully consented or has the ability to do so. Despite medical professionals' public proclamations and seemingly productive conversations about due process, data collection, and policy, no evidence can corroborate the claim that current medical practices are the best route to take or that medical practices have changed in any significant way.

The fact that surgical practice has not changed prompts me to question policies that claim to benefit, represent, and protect intersex people. For example, countries like Australia, Canada, and Germany, states like California, and provinces like Ontario and British Columbia have instituted a third "X" or "U" gender/sex identification option on certain legal documents. "X" stands for indeterminate, unspecified, or intersex. "U" stands for unspecified or unknown. Many have argued that these changes benefit and destigmatize intersex, trans, nonbinary, and genderqueer people. I understand why many people – including myself – get excited when these options become available. Legal recognition and representation are important. However, these third options are not nearly as important to intersex people as some suggest since most intersex people identify as women or men, which the traditional "F" (female) and "M" (male) options cover.

Hence, these third options do not benefit intersex individuals nearly as much as many people claim or assume. Indeed, intersex activist groups around the world have not endorsed and do not embrace the idea that justice for intersex people will be solidified with more gender/sex designations on identification documents. Importantly, since IGM takes place in all the locations noted above, these third options – which are typically presented as benefiting trans, nonbinary, genderqueer, *and* intersex people – are in part simply a symbolic gesture at intersex inclusion and acceptance.

That being said, having the "U" stand for unspecified seems like a good option since it implies that one (reasonably) does not choose to disclose their anatomical characteristics or gender identity. A "U" could also potentially benefit people at borders. When one's gender presentation does not seemingly align with their documents that state "F" or "M," they are more likely to be subjected to violence. One's gender presentation cannot really be incongruous with a "U" if it means unspecified. However, "U" fails to name other sex/gender identifications and can imply that one simply does not want to disclose their "true" male or female sex/gender. It also seems peculiar to me that "U" is also used to mean unknown and that the letter "X" is the most popular unknown variable in algebra. Although not all people want to be intelligible (Butler 2006), "indeterminate" and "unknown" are dehumanizing terms in this context since they indicate that one is illegible, indecipherable, and not properly human. Rather than adding more options, removing sex/gender as a category on identification documents all together is, I maintain, the best recourse. Vancouver-based lawyer Barbara Findlay (in Givetash 2017) and the chair of the Trans Alliance Society in Vancouver, Morgane Oger (in J. Armstrong 2015), also advocate for removing sex/gender from birth certificates and other identification documents. They argue that in Canada one's race or father's occupation is no longer recorded on birth certificates because these practices were discriminatory; sex/gender should also be excluded for the same reason. Rather than instituting more options, governments should abolish sex/gender from legal identification. Rather than simply praising countries for gestures of inclusion, diversity, or acceptance, we should condemn them for reaffirming the sex dyad in surgical theatres and beyond.

In addition to instituting third sex/gender options, other policies claim to benefit and protect intersex people. For instance, Ontario's Bill 33, *Toby's Act (Right to be Free from Discrimination and Harassment Because of Gender Identity or Gender Expression), 2012,* claims to represent and protect intersex people (as well as other marginalized individuals) from discrimination and violence. Legislation like Bill 33 benefits certain manifestations of discrimination. However, since IGM is legal in Ontario (and across Canada) under the *Criminal Code,* this bill is not all-encompassing. Subsection 268(3), "Excision," of the *Criminal Code* criminalizes wounding, maiming, excising, infibulating, or mutilating

> in whole or in part, the labia majora, labia minora or clitoris of a person, except where (a) a surgical procedure is performed, by a person dully qualified by provincial law to practice medicine, for the benefit of the physical health of the person or for the purpose of that person having normal reproductive functions or normal sexual appearance or function; or (b) the person is at least eighteen years of age and there is no resulting bodily harm.

The *Criminal Code* criminalizes female genital mutilation/cutting but does not criminalize intersex genital mutilation even though it involves wounding, maiming, excising, infibulating, or mutilating genital tissue and results in body-mind harm and disabilities. Borrowing from critical ethnic and queer studies scholar Jasbir K. Puar (2017), I argue that Canada has "the right to maim" intersex individuals via surgery and to deny the debilitating and disabling consequences for the purpose of maintaining compulsory dyadism.

"Curative" surgeries performed on intersex infants and children do not legally count as criminal discriminatory harassment, mutilation, or violence. Rather, having intersex characteristics that defy compulsory dyadism is seemingly a crime; and the punishment is curative violence. In a report of the Standing Committee on Health, chair Bill Casey (2019, 7), then a member of Parliament, suggests that the Government of Canada should reconsider Subsection 268(3) of the *Criminal Code,* which legalizes "genital normalizing surgeries on children." Rather than simply advocating for reconsideration of the *Criminal Code,* Casey should have advocated for immediate policy changes criminalizing these surgeries. Owing to the *Criminal Code,* Bill 33 is in part merely a gesture at intersex acceptance and inclusivity. It offers the guise of intersex protection. It does not protect intersex people from one of the most contested forms of compulsory dyadism: surgical biological exorcisms.

Speaking before the San Francisco Human Rights Commission in 2007, intersex activist, author, and artist Thea Hillman (in Clearway 2007) describes some of the disabling consequences of surgery:

I've heard of people being taken to the hospital with no idea why and waking up with bandages around their genitals. I've heard stories of friends being born with genitals that had sexual function and sensation and then being given surgery that took both away. I've heard of people who received so-called "repair" surgeries and the next surgery failed and the next surgery failed and they were on their sixteenth surgery in twenty-three years. I've heard stories about loss of continence from surgery, chronic infections, and illness due to surgery, and I have heard stories of surgically created vaginas that leak, that smell, and that come unattached from the body.

Given that surgical practices have not changed in any significant or perceptible way, intersex activists and scholars are still reporting these sorts of life-long disabling effects.

Providing more specific testimony, Tiger Devore (in G. Harrison 2011) recounts some disabling effects of undergoing several surgeries:

I would go back to school [from summer holiday], and I would have a tube running into my body with a sack on my leg underneath my pants that would collect my urine. So I didn't use boys' bathrooms. I didn't use girls' bathrooms. I had to go to the nurse's office ... to empty out this sack. So I didn't really have a sense of belonging to a sex on the basis of bathroom choice particularly. But also, instead of playing baseball or football and put[ting] my body at risk, I would play jacks with the girls or I would jump rope with the girls. So there was this confusion about how masculine I'm supposed to be, how feminine I'm supposed to be, what rules do I play by, which games do I choose, because the messages were very confusing. Of course, I could never tell anybody what was happening ... I always had to keep it a big secret ... I couldn't tell anybody that I was having surgery "down there," where I'm not supposed to talk about, where I'm not supposed to touch. Going back and forth to the doctors, which happened all the time, because there were infections and complications and breakdown of wounds ... I was enduring a lot of pain and very invasive procedures ... Unless there is a medical necessity to change the appearance of those genitals, I don't think they should be cut on at all. I think they should be prevented from being cut on. It's the kids' genitals. It's not the parents' genitals. It's not the doctors' genitals. It's the kids' genitals. And when they're young adults, they're going to want their genitals to work.

Devore's account illustrates that the genitals re/created by surgeons without consent do not "normalize," enable, or cure the apparently disordered intersex patient but cause confusion, shame, and a host of body-mind disabilities that haunt people for their entire lives. As Devore (in G. Harrison 2011) states, "I lost a tremendous amount of feeling tissue that I would like to have still. And that was taken from me." All of the things that were stolen from Devore – possible futures and literal biological attributes – haunt.

Many medical professionals claim that surgical techniques have improved since the advent of the Intersex Rights Movement in the 1990s. They claim that surgery may not or will not cause a patient to, for example, lose sensation or orgasm capacity. I do not doubt that surgical techniques have improved since surgery became common practice in the 1950s. However, surgery *always* carries risks. Even before the scalpel touches skin, long-term disabling consequences can begin to occur. General anesthesia and sedation can have long-term neurodevelopmental effects on infants' and children's developing brains (Baratz 2017). Even though medical professionals know that the use of anesthesia should be limited to "serious or life-threatening congenital conditions for which there are no alternative treatments and for which treatment cannot be delayed" (Andropoulos and Greene 2018, 906), intersex infants and children are routinely anesthetized. Rather than threatening a child's life, intersex traits threaten compulsory modes of being. As a result, their neurodevelopment is put in jeopardy or sacrificed for the "myth of dyadic sex" (Costello 2009).

Furthermore, cutting into or cutting off intersex children's delicate flesh always carries risks of infection, loss of sensation, scarring, and infertility. And surgeries unequivocally communicate to children that they are wrong and freakish and cannot be loved the way that they were born. Improved techniques also do not negate the fact that infants and children cannot consent to cosmetic surgery. Improved surgical techniques do not negate the fact that intersex folks wish that nonconsensual surgery never took place. And improved techniques do not compensate, recognize, or help to restore those who live with body-mind disabilities created by this violent, curative model.

Ultimately, as Cheryl Chase (1999, 151) (a.k.a. Bo Laurent) articulates, claiming that "'surgery is better now,' is a strategy for silencing intersexed adults: it relieves surgeons indefinitely of the responsibility of listening to any former patient." Adult intersex people's testimonies to acquired body-mind disabilities are seemingly discredited when medical scholars note that surgical techniques have changed. Chase (1999, 151) continues, "If genital surgery is indeed 'better now' and getting better all the time, that is actually a strong argument for allowing intersex children to be free of non-consensual early surgery." Given that surgical techniques tend to improve over time, waiting until one can properly consent to or reject surgical intervention makes logical sense.

To be clear, I do not oppose improving surgical techniques. Consenting intersex, trans, genderqueer, and nonbinary people who seek such interventions can benefit tremendously from surgical improvements. However, unconsenting infants and children do not benefit from unnecessary surgeries that typically result in a variety of body-mind disabilities. Rather than surgically altering intersex people's anatomies, it would be beneficial to emphasize consent and to reinforce that their body-minds are theirs to control, are magnificent and gorgeous, and are not shameful.

Genital Examinations and Displays

In addition to surgery and HRT, medical professionals have carried out other violent practices that result in body-mind disabilities, such as unnecessary genital examinations, also known as "medical display[s]" (Koyama 2003, 2) and "shaming examinations" (Lind and Brzuzy 2008, 272).[11] Many intersex infants, children, and adolescents have been subjected to numerous medically unnecessary genital examinations and displays without being told why such procedures took place and, in many circumstances, why they took place so frequently. These procedures perpetuate the idea that intersex traits are shameful, pathological curiosities. They teach intersex people to be embarrassed of their anatomical characteristics, effectively remove body-mind autonomy and integrity, and result in a plethora of body-mind disabilities.

These examinations contribute to "the social processes of enfreakment" (Garland-Thomson 1996b, 10), which include voyeuristically objectifying and, therefore, dehumanizing people perceived to be monstrous, deviant, queer, disabled, and/or pathological.[12] Racialized people, disabled folks, fat individuals, noncitizens or foreigners, women, people with intersex traits, and LGBTQIA2 folks have historically been, and currently are, the groups typically subjected to the processes of enfreakment.[13] Disability and gender studies scholar Margrit Shildrick (2002, 9) explains that people prone to enfreakment "show themselves in many different and culturally specific ways, but what is monstrous about them is most often the form of their embodiment. They are, in an important sense, what Donna Haraway [1992] calls 'inappropriate/d others' in that they challenge and resist normative human being, in the first instance by their aberrant corporeality." "Monstrous" people and/or ways of being in the world are "located outside the boundaries of the proper" (Shildrick 2002, 5). They defy culturally mandated ways of being and are subsequently subjected to intersecting forms of oppression and violence that are punishing, objectifying, and criminalizing.

A person is often enfreaked during cultural rituals of observation and objectification. The perhaps most obvious example of enfreakment is the presumably antiquated freak show. However, freak shows did not fall out of fashion but morphed alongside shifting cultural sensibilities and technologies into, for example, talk shows, reality shows, pornography, bodybuilding events, medical theatres, and documentaries (Chemers 2008; Clare 2009; Garland-Thomson 1996a). In addition to entertaining audiences, freak shows (contemporary or otherwise) primarily function to validate the spectator's sense of normalcy. Spectators assume that they are observing "a freak of nature" as opposed to "a freak of culture" and, therefore, are "[assured] that they are not freaks" (Garland-Thomson 1996b, 10). The freak's "monstrous" quality is presumed to be innately pathological, inferior, or degenerative rather than constructed by and evaluated against cultural ideologies of normality or the dominant "schemes of recognition" (Butler 2006, 2). Intersex people are acutely aware of this process. Intersex activist Kimberly Zieselman (2015, 124), for example, has been made to feel like "a real freak of nature, damaged and alone."

Suzanne J. Kessler (1998, 5) draws attention to some of the specific ways that intersex people are enfreaked in more contemporary venues in *Lessons from the Intersexed*:

> Television talk shows parade the real people who are living in intersexed bodies for the entertainment of an audience that is motivated like any old-fashioned sideshow crowd to gawk at the bizarre. Unlike a real sideshow, though, the remarkable genitals are not on view, and the audience is titillated only by the idea of intersex. Producers and consumers of pornography are intrigued by intersex genitals ... The viewer can think: Look at how many different sexual acts can take place at the same time! I can watch "homosexual acts" without my heterosexuality being called into question (or vice versa) because the gender of those people on the screen is (in some sense) both or neither.[14]

One can also consider how intersex people and other people with (perceived) disabilities have been objectified and enfreaked by medical photography.[15] Since these photographs are in medical texts and are displayed in medical settings, the "objective" medical guise and gaze partially mask or dispel viewers' anxieties about objectifying and staring at the intersex and/or disabled "freak." In fact, the medical photographs often explicitly block out the intersex and/or disabled gaze so that viewers can comfortably stare without having to meet and therefore register a human gaze; they can stare and effectively not see a human. The photograph incites viewers to interpret the intersex and/or disabled person as a freaky object to be observed. Gawking at, even being titillated by, objectifying representations of intersex people reaffirms viewers' sense of normality and their investment in the ideology of "normal."

Even though the audience may be relatively small, I conceptualize clinical settings in which repeated unnecessary genital examinations take place as sites of re/enfreakment that actively disable intersex subjects for the purpose of maintaining compulsory modes of being. Positioning people with intersex traits as freaks in clinical settings during shaming examinations and displays does not merely work to validate the viewer's sense of normalcy, re/legitimize consecrated Western ideologies, or "educate" accompanying medical professionals, students, or residents. Enfreaking intersex people in these circumstances is also a means to frighten parents/proxies and to convince them that their child is a freaky, disordered anomaly who therefore needs ongoing medical surveillance and intervention. In these circumstances, medical professionals teach parents/proxies to view their child as a freak; they create an emergency, a "state of exception," which then "lay[s] the groundwork for justifying medically unnecessary interventions" (G. Davis 2015, 23). The body-mind disabilities unduly caused by being enfreaked during these examinations are profound.

Many intersex people attest to the body-mind disabilities caused by or during unnecessary genital examinations. For instance, Konrad Blair (2015), Lynnell Stephani Long (2015), Wall (2015b), and Joan Whelan (2002), among many others, recall doctors, medical residents, and students performing or observing mortifying genital examinations on them without conveying why such exams were happening.[16] In Blair's (2015, 90) words, no one explained "why I had to be humiliated and ashamed, again and again." Long (quoted in Arana and Human Rights Commission Staff 2005, 43) recounts, "The most horrible experience I remember is laying in bed with IV's in both arms, having my doctor and at least fifteen student doctors stare at my genitals, and leaving without pulling down my hospital gown. I laid there exposed for over an hour until the nurse finally came in to change the IV bag." These medical displays inevitably cause intersex people to feel "different" (Wall 2015b, 117) and "freakish" (K.A. Walsh 2015, 120). These moments are undeniably "devastating and dehumanizing" and detrimental to one's body-mind well-being (Koomah 2017).

"Many intersex adults report that it was not necessarily the surgery that was most devastating for their self-esteem." Rather, as Emi Koyama (2003, 2) explicates,

> for many, it is the repeated exposure to what we call "medical displays," or the rampant practice where a child is stripped down to nude and placed on the bed while many doctors, nurses, medical students, and others come in and out of the room, touching and prodding and laughing to each other. Children who experience this get the distinct sense that there is something terribly wrong with who they are and are deeply traumatized.

These demeaning practices are one of the many reasons why intersex people report experiencing depression, dissociation, anxiety, shame, self-loathing, and post-traumatic stress disorder. It is, therefore, vital to frame these examinations as enfreaking *and* disabling.

The examinations, considered alongside parental/proxy consent and some medical professionals' poor bedside manners, further illustrate how destructive these experiences are. Laura Inter (pseud.) (2015, 95) recounts,

> From the time I turned one, I was subjected to genital examinations twice a year, during which the endocrinologist would touch my genitals and look to see how they were developing. These unnecessary and intrusive examinations had a profound effect on me. As a young child, I did not understand why I had to lower my pants in front of a stranger – the endocrinologist – and let him touch me. The fact that my mother was present, and approved of this was something that made me feel completely helpless. All this seemed very strange to me; I found it confusing, and terribly uncomfortable, and I just felt it wasn't right. I remember the doctor always spoke as if I wasn't right there, and I did not always understand everything the doctor said when I was young, because of all the medical terms he used. I grew up with a feeling of being "inadequate," of having a sense that something

was wrong with me, though I didn't know exactly what. These exams lasted until I was about 12 years old. Years later, as I began my adult, sexual life, I realized how much those displays had affected me emotionally.

When children witness their parents/proxies agree to and be present during these examinations, not only are they bewildered and scared, but they may also feel, as Michel Reiter (in Lahood 2012) felt, betrayed by their parents: "I had about 200 examinations in my life. I didn't want these examinations, but my mother took me to them. I didn't trust her. I saw her collaborating with my enemies."

Moreover, failing to meet intersex patients as people rather than objects to be viewed, manipulated, and fixed – such as speaking as though the patient is not even there – denies their subjectivity and humanity. Janet Green's (in G. Harrison 2011) subjectivity and humanity were effectively denied when "nobody [in the hospital] was looking into my eyes ... Nobody actually looked at me other than up the sheets." It is perhaps unsurprising that some medical professionals fail to meet the gaze of intersex people because the photographs of intersex people with blocked out eyes in medical texts have taught them to resist meeting the intersex person's gaze. These accounts illustrate that there is an important distinction between the physical characteristics of intersex people that are looked at and those that are not looked at. Intersex people are being examined and looked at (as disordered, freaky objects) while not being looked at (as humans worthy of self-determination).[17] Ultimately, a trusting relationship is not cultivated between patient and doctor as well as between child and parent/proxy in these circumstances. Rather than privileging these important relationships and protecting the patient's autonomy, compulsory modes of being and medical authority are privileged.

Some medical examinations cause other sorts of body-mind disabilities. Intersex activist Daniela Truffer (2015, 111) recounts an exam that caused life-long urinary problems:

During my childhood, I spent a lot of time in doctors' offices and hospitals, suffering countless examinations of my genitals and urethral opening. When I was two, our family doctor stuck his finger into my urethral opening; I was screaming very loud, my father says. My mother had to put me into warm water because every time I had to pee I screamed in pain. Later I was hurried to the hospital with a bad infection. Still today my urethra often hurts after going to the toilet. I knew early in my life that I was different. I learned fragments of the truth only after decades of ignorance and denial.

Manipulating children's delicate genital tissue repeatedly for no apparent medical reason can result in life-long disabling issues, as Truffer's testimony demonstrates.[18]

Medical spaces where intersex patients are subjected to objectifying, medically gratuitous genital examinations and displays are sites of contemporary freak shows. The medical context, however, offers a guise of objectivity and care so that the displays are not immediately perceived as enfreaking at all. In addition to enfreaking the intersex patient, they unequivocally teach patients, their parents/proxies, and any additional accompanying medical personnel to view intersex people as innately wrong, shameful, and disordered. This instruction coerces parents/proxies into agreeing to additional interventions, ensures that future medical professionals will continue this violent work, and actively disables intersex individuals in the name of compulsory dyadism, heterosexuality, and ironically, able-bodiedness.

Deceiving, Lying, Misinforming, or Withholding Information

Deceiving, lying to, misinforming, and withholding information from intersex patients and their parents/proxies about diagnoses, the effects of intersex traits, and procedures have also been integral to curative projects, along with surveilling, erasing, and disabling people with intersex characteristics. Since the "Age of Surgery" (Dreger 1999a, 11) began, lying to or deceiving patients has been standard practice.[19] Although lying to intersex patients and their parents/proxies is no longer widely endorsed, "in some cases, [lying] is still common practice today" (G. Davis 2017). Although lying or withholding information is typically not immediately conceptualized as (potentially) disabling, intersex people's testimonies reveal that one must approach doctors repeatedly lying to intersex patients and family members as a disability issue. The act of deceiving or lying to intersex patients causes health issues in and of itself; it is not simply an avenue that leads to disabling curative violence.

One of the proposed reasons for deceiving intersex patients is that they will not be able to handle the news. Learning about their characteristics will apparently be too upsetting. As expressed by David James Burrows Ashley (1962, 289), learning "the nature of his defect ... may cause great distress." Anita Natarajan (1996) similarly claims that learning of one's intersex diagnosis is too traumatizing, so withholding information is recommended. The paper where Natarajan makes this recommendation, arguably paradoxically, won an essay competition focused on medical ethics and was published in *The Canadian Medical Association Journal*. Dabbling in semantics, Natarajan (1996, 569–70) attempts to distinguish between lying and deceiving: doctors who withhold information are "not actually lying: they are deceiving." Whatever term one wishes to use, doing so is bad medical practice. Withholding information, especially from children, is also supposedly a patient-protection measure, a form of comfort. Doing so presumably will prevent patients from feeling freaky, abnormal, or defective. "Sometimes," pediatrician J.D. Lantos (quoted in Côté 2000, 199) states, "the best medicine might still be a comforting lie." However, as many of the testimonies accounted for thus far demonstrate, repeated hospital visits, genital displays, HRT, and/or IGM unequivocally communicate that something is wrong, freaky, and abnormal. Intersex people need not be verbally told that they are pathologized or "freaky"; the treatment that they endure communicates this assessment quite effectively.

As attorney and intersex activist Sherri A. Groveman (1996, 1829) explains, learning about an intersex diagnosis can be "traumatic," but discovering later in life that information was withheld causes more harm (G. Davis 2015, 2017; Karkazis 2008). Ama Kyerewaa Edwin (2008, 158) notes that, although lying to a patient is often done in good faith, doing so "may add considerably to a patient's distress and prolong the necessary adjustment process[,] thereby causing harm." Lesley J. Fallowfield, Victoria A. Jenkins, and Hazel A. Beveridge's (2002, 297) study about medical disclosure and dis/honesty confirms that being honest with patients may cause emotional pain, but "deceit hurts more." Deceit – as with the subsequent denial of a patient's self-determination – often causes a variety of body-mind issues since "a conspiracy of silence usually results in a heightened state of fear, anxiety and confusion," as well as depression, drug abuse, and stress, rather than producing a state of "calm and equanimity" (Fallowfield, Jenkins, and Beveridge 2002, 297). Reflecting on his own experiences, Catholic priest Spencer St. John (quoted in Arana and Human Rights Commission Staff 2005, 45) notes that deceit leaves "emotionally broken [intersex] adults in its wake," not comforted ones.

In addition to the body-mind disabilities noted above, deception can also contribute to the development or exacerbation of other disabilities and illnesses. Groveman (1996) was lied to by medical professionals about her diagnosis with androgen insensitivity syndrome. Like other intersex people who felt abnormal and sensed that they were being lied to, she headed to the library to conduct research about her experiences. On library book-shelves, she discovered truths about her body-mind. Outraged, Groveman (1996, 1829), among others, published a response to Natarajan's award-winning medical ethics essay and its endorsement of deceiving intersex patients:

> Learning the truth alone and scared in the stacks of a library is shockingly inhumane ... It is almost inevitable that the patient will learn the truth. The real question is how and when we want her to do so. When I discovered I had AIS the pieces finally fit together. But what fell apart was my relationship with my family and physicians ... I avoided all medical care for the next 18 years. I have severe osteoporosis as a result of a lack of medical attention. This is what lies produce.

Groveman's account effectively undermines Natarajan's claim that deceiving or withholding information from intersex patients is the best course of action. In doing so, she also draws attention to the disabling effects of lying to intersex people. Disabilities may not always appear immediately when one learns about years of deceit, but they may surface and be compounded due to a warranted distrust of medical professionals that causes one to avoid medical care when in distress.

Given the almost ubiquitous presence of the Internet and given intersex activists' online presence, people are learning truths about their intersex traits online. For example, at 4:00 in the morning in 2015, Irene Kuzemko learned that she was intersex by watching the online video "What It's Like to Be Intersex," which features intersex activists Sean Saifa M. Wall, Pidgeon Pagonis, Emily Quinn, and Alice Alvarez discussing their experiences of deceit and curative violence (S. Wall et al. 2015). Kuzemko saw herself and her experiences reflected in the video. Kuzemko learned that her doctors and father had been lying to her for years about her anatomical traits, why she had undergone surgery, and her subjection to HRT. Kuzemko (quoted in Strudwick 2018) recounts that the doctors "did all the tests ... And they never told me any results ... They would invite him [i.e., Kuzemko's father] into the office," but Kuzemko was never included in any conversations. She continues, "I never saw my medical records; nobody ever gave me a diagnosis." Given that she was never told anything, she had to fabricate a story when her schoolmates asked her why she had to go to hospital for surgery: "I couldn't explain properly because I didn't know myself ... so I lied and said I had a cyst on my ovary."

Despite the lies that were presumably supposed to comfort Kuzemko (quoted in Strudwick 2018), the surgery and the hospital visits that she endured communicated very clearly that she was fundamentally wrong: "On a deep level I thought, *I'm horrible and disgusting and shameful*. I felt like some kind of monster." As a result, Kuzemko reports struggling with depression, anxiety, self-hatred, and mental detachment from her body-mind and very existence: "My brain just couldn't comprehend what was going on ... And in order to continue living, my brain just stopped believing that any of this [i.e., her life] was real." These experiences were contextualized when she viewed the online video years later. Unlike what some medical professionals assume, learning that she was intersex did not trouble Kuzemko. She notes, "I never felt bad about it [i.e., being intersex]; I thought, *Wow! There is an explanation!* It felt so good to find the truth and find out I'm not alone." Although Kuzemko is proud to be intersex and is now a remarkable intersex activist who, in part, co-founded Intersex Russia in 2017, she explains that her "life could have been 100% different if one person would have told me the truth." If her doctor had told her the truth, like doctors are expected to do, so much disabling trauma could have been avoided.

Groveman's, Kuzemko's, and many other intersex people's stories about the disabling nature of lies and about the pieces finally coming together can also be read as instances of haunting, when something unclear – ghostly – begins to emerge. Once in view, new spectres form and surface: ruptured family ties, distrust and avoidance of doctors, or exacerbated illness. Experiences of trauma, intersex, and disability are neither distinct nor linear. According to Susannah Cornwall (2014, 56), the trauma caused by lying is "crippling." "Crippling," in this context, is not necessarily a problematic, ableist metaphor. The resulting trauma, embodied consequences, and compounded illnesses from lies are crippling disabilities, not metaphorical ones. Hence, Cornwall's comment on the "crippling" effects of lies and statements like "it felt insane to be walled in by secrets" (K.A. Walsh 2015, 120) need to be taken seriously; they require an approach rooted in crip intersex studies.

Many medical professionals believe that if intersex people learn of their intersex diagnosis, they may self-harm, experience suicidal ideation, and/or commit suicide. For example, when Rebecca (in Human Rights Watch and interACT: Advocates for Intersex Youth 2017) was a teenager, she was subjected to surgery in New York. As an adult residing in Arizona, she wanted to obtain her medical records, but the facility would not release them. Rebecca flew to New York and spoke with her doctor: "He said they were afraid I couldn't handle it – that I'd commit suicide." After her records were finally released to her, she returned to Arizona. However, she needed her doctor in Arizona to help her decipher the document. Like the doctor in New York, the doctor in Arizona "told me she wasn't sure if I should get the information – if I could handle it." The assumption that having intersex traits is such a bad thing that disclosure will cause self-destructive behaviour is not only unsubstantiated but also reproduces interphobic stigma and can make people feel "insane" (K.A. Walsh 2015, 120). As I and Meg Peters (Orr and Peters, n.d.) explain, "The fact that medical professionals withhold information reveals more about doctors' internalized discrimination and investment in compulsory dyadism than it does about patients' prospective emotional response."

Doctors also tell parents/proxies of intersex patients that their children will commit suicide if they learn of their intersex characteristics and are not surgically altered.[20] Angela Moreno's (in Coventry 1998) parents were told this lie and, unsurprisingly, followed doctors' orders. However, as Moreno (quoted in Coventry 1998) explains, she undermined her doctors' unsupported assumptions: "Although the doctors had claimed that knowing the truth would make me self-destructive, it was not knowing what had been done to me – and why – that made me want to die." Debbie Hartman's experience of being a mother to an intersex child, Kelli, also complicates the idea that honesty and no medical intervention will cause the child unbearable distress. Hartman (in Arana and Human Rights Commission Staff 2005, 48) was not provided with enough information to make an informed decision about surgery, and when she asked to speak with other parents of intersex children or intersex people themselves, she was told, "There is no one." Due to the fact that doctors withheld vital information, Hartman assumed that surgery was the right thing to do and agreed to the procedure on Kelli's behalf. Kelli "has endured unnecessary pain, confusion and severe emotional and physical scarring," Hartman explains. "My child has tried to commit suicide twice in her 10 little years because she says she hates her body," Hartman continues. "She constantly asks me why they ... cut up her genitals." Hartman reports Kelli stating, "They thought I was no good, Mom."

In addition to unnecessary medical procedures and surveillance, repeated lies and misinformation that emphasize difference, teach shame, coerce people into agreeing to irreversible procedures, and create body-mind disabilities are what cause suicidal ideation and self-destructive behaviours. Many intersex people report attempting suicide and/or struggling with suicidal thoughts and experiencing "shame, confusion, depression, anorexia, anxiety, insecurity, panic attacks, low self-esteem, explosive anger, [and] lack of trust and feeling of safety" (Ms. seMbessakwini, quoted in Arana and Human Rights Commission Staff 2005, 34). Although medical professionals have argued that such body-mind disabilities will arise if people learn of their intersex diagnoses or if their body-minds remain as they are, various disabilities in fact stem from lies, medical practices, and discourses that communicate that intersex people are, in Kelli's words, "no good." The practice of misinforming, coercing, and lying to patients or their parents/proxies is both disabling and a gross abuse of paternalistic power.

All that being said, according to Marcus de María Arana and Human Rights Commission Staff's (2005, 12) investigation into intersex human rights violations, intersex people "did not disproportionately ... attempt suicide." Nevertheless, they advocate for well-funded services in mental health, suicide prevention, and peer support for intersex people, particularly for intersex youth. More recent studies, however, suggest that intersex people are at an increased risk of self-harm and suicidal ideation. For instance, Tiffany Jones and colleagues (2016, 3, 122) report in their study concerning intersex people in Australia that "wellbeing risks were high – 42% of participants had thought about self-harm and 26% had engaged in it; 60% had thought about suicide and 19% had attempted it."[21] Contradicting doctors' claims, the study participants do not typically blame these thoughts and behaviours on their intersex traits in and of themselves but on interphobia, being subjected to curative violence, living with the disabling consequences of medical interventions, and mourning what was taken from them. Although it seems reasonable to claim that intersex people are more likely to self-harm, experience suicidal ideation, and/or commit suicide, we cannot reasonably assume – as many doctors do – that this behaviour is the direct result of knowing their diagnoses or medical history. It makes much more sense to assume that this behaviour is linked to the embodied impacts of compulsory dyadism, being lied to, and the disabling consequences of curative violence.

Again, although some may argue that a comforting lie is the best medicine, some of the lies told to intersex people and their families are not at all comforting. For example, some parents of intersex children have been told that their children will develop cancer and that, in order to prevent such a calamity, surgery is necessary.[22] Some parents, who have been blatantly lied to or who have been told only partial truths, are advised to perpetuate lies by telling their children that they had to undergo surgery because they had cancer. As discussed in Chapter 1, Pidgeon Pagonis and their family were told such lies. As a child, Pagonis (2015a) was told that they were born with cancer, whereas their parents were told that their child would develop cancer.

Lies about cancer are hardly comforting. As Pagonis aptly alerts readers, these lies are manipulative means to gain "consent" from parents/proxies for doctors to perform interventions that seek to re-enforce and restabilize compulsory dyadism. Doctors lie and exploit parents'/proxies' fear of illness, disability, and death so that culturally mandated ways of being can be upheld. And, ironically, because of the attempt to enforce the intersecting logics of dyadism, heterosexuality, and able-bodiedness by lying, intersex people live with body-mind disabilities, hormone dependencies, and futures that were stolen.

Conclusion

The language of mutilation, torture, rape, or sexual assault, among other examples, is accurate and indispensable to projects that combat compulsory dyadism as well as violent and deceitful medical practices. I do not suggest doing away with any of them. However, the testimonies offered up by intersex people demonstrate that the consequences also constitute body-mind disabilities. Disability, although very clear in many intersex people's testimonies, remains largely implicit. I suggest centralizing the gratuitously disabling nature of intersex curative violence. Supplementing the narratives that are often used when talking about disabilities is beneficial.

Claims of mutilation and torture, for example, are easier for authoritative doctors to discredit as sensationalized, hyperbolic, or inaccurate. Doctors are presumed to always care and cure, not mutilate or torture. Although incorrect, the general sentiment in the Global North is that genital mutilation and torture are entirely outlawed and happen "over there," not "over here." Given that all medical procedures come with (disabling) risks, a conversation may not be immediately shut down if the language of disability is deployed. In addition, naming intersex curative violence and explicitly framing the consequences as disabling may, in certain circumstances, better highlight the horribly ironic fact that in the attempt to enable or reorder supposedly disabled or disordered intersex people – in the attempt to enforce compulsory dyadism – intersex people are actively disabled by medical interventions. In an effort to exorcise the intersex phantasm, medical professionals violently create newly disabled beings and ghosts via HRT, surgery, lies, and so on. The very institution that claims to heal, cure, and safeguard contributes to gratuitously disabling intersex subjects. Moreover, the language of acquired/created body-mind disabilities may resonate with many intersex people's embodied experiences of curative violence.

In turn, one may be more willing to forge alliances and share knowledges with disability groups. Acknowledging the trauma as incurred disabilities unequivocally demonstrates the productive potential of an approach rooted in crip intersex studies that conceptualizes intersex as a disability issue, and it identifies a locus where intersex and disability issues align. Indeed, the intersex people's testimonies explored in this chapter reflect and add a nuanced layer to many disability studies scholars' and activists' proposals that embodied disabled experiences are not static. Disabling trauma or violence can be an ephemeral phantasm, its consequences nonlinear; it can remain undetectable for years or can compound in unexpected ways.

3

Is There Medical Recognition of the Disabilities Created?

Doctors "Do Not Realize" the Harm Caused

Given that intersex medical management often disables intersex people's body-minds, do medical professionals really not realize this fact? Sean Saifa M. Wall (2015a) posits that "many surgeons and specialists do not realize the life-long emotional and physical impact of performing irreversible surgery on intersex people such as myself." If they do not realize the harm caused, perhaps all one can do is classify intersex medical management as a medical mistake. Indeed, a few doctors who have realized and openly recognized the disabling nature of intersex curative violence claim that they made mistakes (see Carmack 2014; G. Davis 2015; and Truffer 2015).

I suggest that the disabling consequences of intersex medical management are spectral and embodied evidence of discriminatory medical malpractice – "unresolved social violence" (Gordon 2011, 2) and curative violence – not indications of medical mistakes. Without a doubt, errors and mistakes are endemic to the practice of medicine. As explained by the late sociologist Marianne A. Paget (2004, 17), medicine and medical care are "process[es] of discovery and response, of risked action and error"; as a result, medical mistakes are "an existential reality."[1] Consequently, many people acquire and are haunted by body-mind disabilities because of such mistakes, and some family and friends are haunted by the loss of a loved one because a mistake was made. However, framing the decades-long, violent, disabling, and non-evidence-based medical treatment of intersex people as a mistake is grossly inaccurate. In addition, construing this treatment as a mistake, rather than as medical malpractice, is a discursive means that any remorseful doctor can use to skirt responsibility, legal or otherwise. Individual doctors, like the medical field as a whole, are protected by the mistake narrative. The curative violence that intersex people are subjected to constitutes systemic discriminatory medical malpractice, which is tolerated, taught, encouraged, and carried out to maintain compulsory dyadism, able-bodiedness, and heterosexuality.

Many doctors typically do not explicitly acknowledge – indeed, they often deny – the harm caused and body-mind disabilities created by this interphobic medical malpractice. Yet I question whether medical practitioners actually do not realize this fact. That is, there is a difference between realizing and openly acknowledging that intersex curative violence actively and gratuitously disables people. Of course, openly acknowledging this fact would render one and the medical field vulnerable to, for example, radical systemic change and legal retribution. The clinical term "hypospadias cripple" suggests that medical professionals comprehend the disabling consequences a lot more than they let on. Hypospadias is an intersex variation. The ureteral meatus, or "pee hole," of intersex people with hypospadias is not at the exact tip of the penis. Even though hypospadias, in and of itself, rarely causes medical or health issues, surgical "hypospadias repairs" or "masculinizing corrections" are performed on unconsenting infants and children so that one will be able to stand to pee and able to ejaculate out of the tip of the penis (Bauer and Truffer 2015; Craig et al. 2014; Orr 2019). These people's penises are pathologized because they undermine compulsory modes of being and hegemonic masculine behavioural expectations (Orr 2019). Interestingly, however, not all people with hypospadias are deemed crippled. Medical professionals reserve the expression "hypospadias cripple" for those who have undergone failed "repairs" or "corrections" and who experience short- and/or long-term disabilities. Hence, even though medical professionals often refuse to explicitly and publicly acknowledge the disabilities created, this descriptor is an unequivocal admission. Medical professionals know that surgery will likely "cripple" the unconsenting intersex patient, yet they perform the surgery anyway. It is integral that we name the current medical management of intersex people as medical *malpractice* and reject the idea that doctors are simply unaware or that they make mistakes.

Medical Recognition (or Lack Thereof) of the Disabilities Created: Hypospadias Cripple

Medical professionals, by and large (with some notable exceptions), deny or refuse to explicitly acknowledge the traumatizing effects of and body-mind disabilities created by "curative" interventions.[2] However, the clinical term "hypospadias cripple" signals otherwise. Even though "cripple" is typically deemed an outmoded socio-medical descriptor and is not usually found in medical scholarship or uttered in clinical settings, Katrina Roen (2009, 21) notes that clinical texts "refer to intersex people in terms such as 'hypospadias cripple." Nevertheless, contrary to what Roen implies, not all intersex people with hypospadias are labelled "crippled." Intersex people with hypospadias who have undergone failed surgical "hypospadias repairs" or "masculinizing corrections" resulting in various disabilities are deemed "crippled."[3] This term is a form of recognition of the disabling nature of intersex medical management and intersex genital mutilation (IGM).

"Hypospadias" is the medical/izing term used to describe a cosmetic, intersex genital variation. "Hypo" means "under" or "beneath," and "spadias" means "slit" or "fissure." Hypospadias, therefore, is characterized by the urethral meatus being situated on the underside of the penis. Depending on where the urethral meatus is located, the type of hypospadias may be medically referred to as distal or glanular (i.e., near the head of the penis but not at the tip of the glan), midshaft (i.e., middle or lower on the underside of the penile shaft), penoscrotal (i.e., where the penis and scrotum join), or perineal (i.e., behind the scrotal sac). There are no worrisome medical or health concerns associated with hypospadias itself. When left alone, people with hypospadias are entirely capable of orgasming and urinating without issue.

Nevertheless, people with hypospadias are routinely "crippled" by curative violence, which involves "dissection of the penis to 'relocate' the urinary meatus" to the tip of the penis (Bauer and Truffer 2015, 30). In fact, according to intersex activists and researchers Markus Bauer and Daniela Truffer (2015, 30), hypospadias "is arguably the most prevalent diagnosis for cosmetic genital surgeries." In part, this diagnosis and this "reparative" procedure are so common because hypospadias is very common (Fichtner et al. 1995; C.J. Long et al. 2017). It is often estimated that, globally, between 1 in 125 and 1 in 300 people born with a penis have hypospadias (Griffiths 2018). However, this oft-cited estimate is contestable. Jan Fichtner and colleagues (1995, 833), in the Department of Urology at the University of Mainz Medical Center, noticing the high prevalence – 70 percent – of glanular and midshaft hypospadias in their pediatric hypospadias patients, decided to "study the meatal location in normal men [i.e., men never medically diagnosed with hypospadias] to investigate if meatal advancement [i.e., surgery] in all patients with anterior [i.e., glanular and midshaft] hypospadias can be justified when the wide variation of meatal locations in normal men are considered." If "normal" people's meatal locations vary considerably, according to Fichtner and colleagues (1995, 833), the necessity of surgery should be reconsidered. "Of the 500 'normal' men" whom Fichtner and colleagues (1995, 833) observed, "the meatal location varied widely with only 55% [or 275 people] of all meatus at the tip of the glans." Hence, 45 percent of apparently "normal" people with penises are actually not "normal" by dominant medical standards. In fact, some of the undiagnosed people had "significant hypospadias," but they did not have "complaints about cosmetic or functional aspects" of their penises (Fichtner et al. 1995, 833). Hypospadias does not appear to cause people marked distress, and according to medical standards, hypospadias is arguably the "norm." Despite this revealing research from over two decades ago, medical standards and conceptions of "normal" have not changed in any significant way.

Even though hypospadias is common, people with hypospadias diagnoses all across the globe are habitually subjected to gratuitous operations that routinely fail. In fact, many medical professionals "advise early surgeries, usually *between 12 and 24 months of age*" (Bauer and Truffer 2015, 30). People with hypospadias typically experience several surgeries throughout their lives, "with increasing numbers of repeat surgeries the older the children get" (Bauer and Truffer 2015, 12). Bauer and Truffer (2015, 30) report that people with hypospadias are, on average, subjected to 5.8 surgeries; however, "a dozen or more repeat surgeries are not uncommon" because surgery often fails. For example, Tiger Devore (in G. Harrison 2011), diagnosed with severe hypospadias, has undergone well over a dozen surgical procedures. "They [i.e., doctors] performed 10 operations by age 10, pretty regularly once a year," Devore (1999, 79) explains. Likewise, interviewee James (in Chapman 2016) recounts, "I started seeing a doctor from about six months old. I had about 16 or 17 operations over the next 13 years, in batches. It was corrective surgery to try and repair what had happened before." More often than not, the failure to "repair" or "masculinize" requires repeat, redo procedures.

Although follow-up studies concerning rates of hypospadias surgical complication have declined in the past several years, the available studies indicate that complication rates are 50 percent and higher (Bauer and Truffer

2015; C.J. Long et al. 2017). According to a study by Christopher J. Long and colleagues (2017, 852), surgical complications are more frequent in midshaft, penoscrotal, and perineal repairs compared to distal repairs, but the "overall complication rate was 56%." Among people who have been subjected to surgeries intended to repair their ostensibly disabled penises, 56 percent have dealt and/or continue to deal with various disabilities.[4] The complications, disabilities, or impairments include urethral strictures and urinary fistulas (also known as rectourethral fistulas), urethral hairballs and stones, and ventral curvature.[5] To clarify some of these medical terms, urethral strictures are scars that develop in the urethra. They narrow the urethra and can cause swelling in the penis, blood and discharge, pain in the pelvic area, and problems with urination, including pain upon urination or the complete inability to urinate. Urinary fistulas are holes that form between the urethra and the rectum. These holes can cause urine to pass through the rectum, infections, swelling, pain, and discomfort. Urethral hairballs occur when hair-bearing skin is used when reconstructing the urethra. They can cause pain and discomfort when urinating, chronic pain and swelling, and chronic urinary infections, and they can contribute to urethral stone formation. Urethral stones, hard masses that form in the urinary tract, can cause pain, bleeding, and infection, and they can block urine flow. Ventral curvature is caused by scar tissue and makes the penis point or curve downward. It can result in erectile dysfunction, pain, and infection. All of these problems may necessitate additional operations, which carry their own risks.

In various medical texts, people with hypospadias who have undergone failed surgeries and experience these sorts of disabilities are referred to as "hypospadias cripples."[6] Samuel A. Amukele, Jeffrey A. Stock, and Moneer K. Hanna (2005, 1540) explain that "hypospadias cripples" is a term reserved for people with hypospadias who have undergone "at least 2 failed attempts at hypospadias repair."[7] Not all intersex people with hypospadias are labelled "crippled." Although all people with hypospadias are conceptualized as disordered, disabled, or diseased, medical practitioners do not deem them "crippled" prior to curative violence. People disabled – "crippled" – by curative violence are referred as cripples.[8] Ultimately, the fact that medical professionals have a term – "hypospadias cripple" – for patients who live with these disabling consequences indicates that medical professionals clearly comprehend the disabling nature of interphobic curative violence.[9]

Although some medical scholars suggest that doctors "should probably" avoid the "somewhat pejorative" term "cripple" (Craig et al. 2014, 196), many medical professionals continue to use the term. In most circumstances, "cripple" is construed as an offensive and outmoded descriptor; it is not merely "somewhat pejorative." Expunging the term from medical discourse is wise, not simply "probably" a good idea. Nevertheless, removing the term from medical discourse does not negate the fact that the term's development and deployment are a blatant recognition of the disabilities that curative violence causes. Moreover, since intersex is understood as a disability by medical professionals, the term emphasizes that although surgical interventions may further disable intersex people, doctors choose to perform surgeries anyway. Highlighting medical professionals' recognition is a useful tactic in combatting nonconsensual, medically unnecessary procedures in all their forms, especially given that many medical professionals typically publicly deny the harm caused. Underlining this recognition emphasizes not only that doctors' curative medical approach, one that is supposed to heal people, violently disables intersex people's body-minds but also that, nevertheless, doctors continue to be invested in this approach and continue to perform these procedures. Medical professionals effectively, violently, and *knowingly* create newly disabled beings to maintain intersecting discriminatory logics.

Given that doctors understand the crippling nature of these sorts of treatments, why do they continue to conduct them? One of the primary ideologies that motivates hypospadias repairs or masculinizing corrections is the cultural demand that (assigned) boys and men must stand up to urinate (Bauer and Truffer 2015). Standing to urinate is a sign of "proper" hegemonic heteromasculinity. Alice Domurat Dreger (2017) summarizes,

> Most hypospadias "repairs" performed by surgeons occur because of an untested, Freudian belief that you can't grow up to be a "real man" if you urinate and ejaculate from somewhere other than the very tip of your penis. Urology texts of the past made it pretty plain: if you don't "fix" hypospadias, a boy might be so messed up in his gender identity that he'll grow up gay. Few urologists today seem to believe that sexual orientation is caused by how one pees, but many still think boys' psychological health absolutely depends on being able to pee standing up. There's no evidence for this.

Also noting the outdated "Freudian obsession regarding the presence/absence of the phallus," sociologist Stephen Craig Kerry (2014, 216) writes, "While there is considerable attention given to the (hetero)sexual function of the phallus, what is also implied is that a 'boy' or 'man' who is unable to urinate from the tip of their penis, and in the standing position, is considered 'abnormal.'" Sitting to pee, interpreted as failed masculinity, is deemed pathologically feminine or queer. The cultural demand for assigned boys and men to pee standing up has resulted in countless nonconsensual surgeries. These surgeries are risky, and many of them result in short- and/or long-term body-mind disabilities. That is, socio-medically assigned boys' well-being is sacrificed for hegemonic masculine standards rooted in compulsory dyadism, heterosexuality, and able-bodiedness.

Another ideology that informs hypospadias "repair" is the heteromasculinist cultural demand that assigned males must be fertile and ejaculate at the exact tip of the penis. Since infertility is often pathologized in our pronatal, pro-reproductive culture (Edelman 2004; Gentile 2016; Riggs and Peel 2016), concerns with in/fertility crop up in conversations about hypospadias. If a boy or man is infertile, not only will he "fail" the pro-natal demand to heterosexually reproduce, but his very belonging to the category "male" will also be called into question. Male infertility poses "a particular threat to conventional views of masculinity" (Gannon, Glover, and Abel 2004, 1169) – that is, a threat to "heterosexual desire and potency, [and] fatherhood" (Shumka, Strega, and Hallgrimsdottir 2017, 4). Given that male infertility is "conflated with impotence," when a (presumed) boy or man is infertile, his masculinity is "in crisis" (Gannon, Glover, and Abel 2004, 1169). One is construed as failing to be a "real" man; one's sense of belonging in the sexual and reproductive economy is threatened.[10] Because of the looming threat of failed masculinity and, in turn, of pathologically queer masculinity, people with hypospadias must be "fixed"; their masculinity must be surgically salvaged.

Nevertheless, Camilla Asklund and colleagues (2010) note that hypospadias itself does not necessarily affect fertility. Yet some online, mainstream fertility sources claim that fertility is affected and that surgically relocating the urethral meatus will solve this problem. For example, according to Sydney Chang (2020),

Hypospadias is a birth defect ... [in which] the opening of the urethra ... which is normally found on the tip of the penis, is located instead on its underside ... Since the urethra carries semen out of the body, the altered location of the opening can result in difficulties with ejaculation ... Fertility problems should no longer remain after the hypospadias is surgically corrected.

These sorts of sources misrepresent in/fertility. Most people with hypospadias have fertile sperm. Hence, the masculinity issue is not simply about fertility itself but also about precisely where the sperm is ejaculated from. Sperm is deemed properly "potent" and masculine only insofar as it is ejaculated from the exact tip of the penis. The location of evacuation matters to the hegemonic construction of heteromasculinity. On rare occasions, cryptorchidism (i.e., undescended testicles) accompanies hypospadias, and this structural variation can affect fertility, but hypospadias itself does not. Sources that promote hypospadias repairs also downplay the plethora of medical risks and problems associated with surgery. All that being said, infertility is not inherently pathological or something that must be avoided or "fixed." When left alone, people with hypospadias are entirely capable of orgasming, ejaculating, and urinating. Unfortunately, people with hypospadias are all too often subjected to curative violence that results in various short- and/or long-term body-mind disabilities that, paradoxically, may actually prevent them from fulfilling this pro-natal, hegemonic masculine demand.

Ultimately, how common hypospadias variations are, the lack of genuine medical issues associated with hypospadias, the discriminatory logics that fuel surgery, *and* the high prevalence of "crippling" surgical complications are all indications that we should not simply, as Fichtner and colleagues (1995, 834) conclude, "narrow our indication for meatal advancement [surgery]." Rather, medical professionals should first do no harm, as they have pledged to do (Pagonis 2017b); patients should be old enough to fully understand the risks associated with this kind of cosmetic surgery and have the chance to consent to or reject such intervention. Moreover, hypospadias (like all other intersex variations) demands that we completely reject compulsory dyadism, compulsory able-bodiedness, compulsory heterosexuality, heteromasculinitist logics, and the concept of normality. There is no "normal." We must divest ourselves of the "quest for normalcy" (Surina Khan, quoted in Karkazis 2008, 1) – from the ideology, "tyranny" (Fiedler 1996; Silvers 1994), and "empire of the 'normal'" (Couser 2000, 305). If we remain invested in essentializing morphologies and remain on this quest for normalcy, people deemed abnormal will be continually read as "medical crises that demand normalization," even if said normalizing projects are disabling and medically unnecessary (Garland-Thomson 2005, 1567).

Hida Viloria's account of being interviewed by a correspondent of the news program *20/20* alongside a medical professional who endorses irreversible and nonconsensual interventions also draws our attention to another way that medical professionals, perhaps inadvertently, admit or recognize that these disabling procedures are for social, not medical, reasons. Viloria (2017, 193–94) explains that, during the interview, the doctor was "condescending":

> In response to watching a clip of me saying how happy I am that I didn't have a clitoral reduction surgery, he says he still thinks he could have helped me. Even better, when the interviewer asks him why he believes these surgeries are necessary despite what he's heard from people who have experienced it and from me, he answers, "Society can't accept people of different colors, and now we're supposed to accept somebody with genitalia that don't match what their gender is. I do not believe society is ready for it" ... I'm ... fascinated by how the doctor's racism analogy reveals that social prejudice – not medical necessity – is what is truly at the heart of these procedures. It's actually one of the most honest statements I've ever heard a doctor make about what we are subjected to. His analogy makes it easy to see why the practice is misguided.

Viloria's analysis of this doctor's analogy is apt. It highlights the fact that although some medical professionals understand that disabling interventions are for social, ideological reasons and although they are aware that intersex people testify to the harms of such interventions, doctors continue to conduct these surgeries.

Furthermore, since medical professionals regard intersex people as disabled *and* knowingly "cripple" or (further) disable intersex people, intersex and disability scholarship and activism have good reason to align in order to combat curative violence in all its forms. An approach rooted in crip intersex studies is necessary. Indeed, the term "hypospadias cripple" is a means to open up a conversation about intersex-as/is-disability and the disabling consequences of curative violence. In fact, "crip" or "cripple" could be re/claimed by some intersex people, if they so chose.

Medical Mistakes, Medical Malpractice

According to urologic surgeon Adrienne Carmack (2014, 67–68), many medical interventions performed on people with intersex variations have been mistakes: "The approach by medical doctors to assign a gender, and then administer irreversible treatments to support that gender, is fundamentally flawed! No matter the original logic behind this treatment model, it is now apparent that in many cases it was a *mistake*. Yet, surgeries are still being done based on what is thought to be the gender a child will relate to" (emphasis added). Carmack suggests that many procedures performed on intersex infants have been mistakes. Even before a treatment "mistake" occurs, doctors first "mistakenly" assume that it is unproblematically possible to determine one's gender identity and what anatomical structures one will want to have. Similarly, the gonadectomy that Daniela Truffer (2015, 111) was subjected to was deemed a mistake:

> When I was two months old, and still in the hospital, doctors opened my abdomen and found healthy testes, which they threw in the garbage bin. According to my medical records, my parents had not provided consent. Further tests showed I am chromosomally male. Later the "castration" was declared a "mistake": one doctor said I was a boy with hypospadias. As they had already removed the testes, however, they would have "to continue this way and the small patient must be made a girl."

Truffer's doctor seems to think that the castration was a mistake because her "male" testes aligned with her "male" chromosomes. Although I am encouraged that the doctor reconsidered the efficacy of the surgery, I am discouraged that it was deemed a mistake only because Truffer could or should have been "made" into a boy in the first place. The mistake, as this doctor saw it, had nothing to do with violating and irreversibly altering Truffer's body-mind without consent.

Nevertheless, is "mistake" an appropriate or accurate characterization of past and present intersex treatment? When considered alongside the numerous testimonies explored in this book thus far, the Intersex Rights Movement, and a differentiation between mistake and maltreatment, this query demonstrates that the disabling consequences cannot be construed as mistakes, no matter how good-intentioned the initial interventions were. Given the fact that procedures are performed on unconsenting intersex children and are overwhelmingly medically unnecessary as well as the fact that interventions occur for reasons that are social, not medical, they constitute institutionalized medical malpractice, medical abuse, and in some circumstances, sexual assault. In other words, given the evidence that these procedures are harmful, the situation is not about, to use Paget's (2004, 12) terms, the fact that "something we initiated went wrong" but instead is about the fact that although "something" is known to be violent and motivated by discriminatory ideologies, medical professionals continue to initiate it.

Paget (2004, 17) explains that mistakes in medicine are inevitable because medicine is a cultural "process" always under revision. Hence, the fact that many medical mistakes are discovered retrospectively is unfortunate, sometimes even macabre. A quick look into past popular medical theories, diagnoses, procedures, and cures for various (perceived) illnesses, diseases, disorders, and disabilities demonstrates that medicine is precisely about learning from mistakes. Developing and espousing evidence-based medicine have been integral to avoiding many, but not all, mistakes. Mistakes are endemic to the practice of medicine. Yet, as Paget (2004, 8) notes, mistakes, abuse, and discriminatory, institutionalized medical malpractice "are not identical issues." Making a mistake is not the same as medical malpractice. A mistake is an adverse result of human error, a miscalculation of sorts. A doctor unknowingly doubling the dose of a patient's medication would, for example, constitute a mistake. Such a mistake could seriously harm a patient, cause death, and result in legal action, but it is not an example of medical malpractice. Institutionalized medical malpractice or abuse includes established, systemic discrimination, negligence, and denial of evidence that typically result in harmful, disabling, or poor medical care.

The disabling procedures enacted on countless intersex people are not mistakes. They are institutionalized malpractice or abuses for the following reasons: (1) for decades, intersex people and their advocates have clearly and unequivocally demonstrated that nonconsensual, medically unnecessary procedures are discriminatory, harmful, disabling, and mutilating; (2) there is no evidence to suggest that nonconsensual, cosmetic treatments benefit intersex people; (3) for decades, activists associated with the Intersex Rights Movement, intergovernmental organizations, nongovernmental organizations, and intersex studies scholars have urged medical professionals to cease such interventions because the evidence demonstrates that they are gratuitously disabling, mutilating, and tortuous; (4) medical professionals recognize and confront the "crippling" consequences of these procedures; and (5) despite all of these points, these practices continue. Systemically and systematically mutilating intersex children and knowingly creating body-mind disabilities are not mistakes. These interventions are medical malpractices, not evidence-based medicine.

In addition, various "curative" procedures constitute "ritualistic sexual abuse of children" (Koyama 2003, 2) and, therefore, medical malpractice. Emi Koyama (2003, 2) explicates,

Adult intersex people's stories often resemble [the stories] of those who survived childhood sexual abuse: trust violation, lack of honest communication, punishment for asking questions or telling the truth, etc. In some cases,

> intersex people's experiences are exactly like those of child sexual abuse sur-
> vivors: when they surgically "create" a vagina on a child, the parent – usually
> the mother – is required to "dilate" the vagina with hard instruments every
> day for months in order to ensure that the vagina won't close off again.

Medical practices like dilating a child with a medical dildo-like device are
not simply like sexual abuse but are "institutionalized sexual abuse" (Betsy
Driver, in Arana and Human Rights Commission Staff 2005, 31) and "medical rape" (Monro, Crocetti, and Yeadon-Lee 2019, 789). Taking seriously
the idea that medical professionals have systematically sexually assaulted
intersex people, Karsten Schützmann and colleagues (2009) conducted a
study. Highlighting the fact that both intersex people and women who have
endured sexual abuse report being touched and examined against their will,
Schützmann and colleagues compared and contrasted the mental health of
intersex people and women who have experienced sexual abuse. The authors report that both groups of people exhibit similar self-destructive behaviours and mental health disabilities (e.g., depression and anxiety).

Various "treatments" are sexual abuses and, therefore, medical malpractice. In recognizing this fact, one must keep in mind that intersex people are
construed as disabled by medical professionals and that people with disabilities – children and adults – are at increased risk of being subjected to sexual assault and chronic sexual abuse.[11] Some studies estimate that children
with disabilities are two to three times more likely to be sexually assaulted
or abused than are able-bodied children (Gorey and Leslie 1997; Kvam
2008). Children with disabilities are particularly vulnerable to abuse because, for example, they may be inter/dependent on others, they may be
institutionalized, and they are often in literally and metaphorically vulnerable positions in medical/izing settings (Putnam 2003). Hence, many of-
fences are committed by health and service providers and occur in contexts
of medical care. Such abuses are infrequently reported and seldom result in
conviction. In fact, sexual assault and abuse are rarely even recognized as
such unless they are "quite obvious" (Kvam 2008, 1073). Often, they are not
"quite obvious" given that children with disabilities are not seen as credible
sources because they may not have access to certain discourses to express
their experiences, because they may have troubles effectively communicat-
ing to adults, and/or because, as with intersex children, the medical protocol or prescription may be the act of sexual assault. Dilating a child is not
seen as sexual abuse or medical malpractice because it is narrated as medical care – a medical necessity (Orr 2018; Orr and Watson 2021).

Even though these practices are medical malpractices, most medical professionals cannot or will not recognize intersex curative violence as such. Not only do these doctors want to protect themselves, their careers, and the institutions that they are a part of, but their positionalities can also prevent them from fully recognizing the harm caused. As Paget (2004, 11) states, "interpretation is a communicative relation," by which she means that deciding whether or not a medical practice is harmful, abusive, or malpractice is an interpretative exchange (and sometimes a legal determination). Patients can claim that practices are harmful, disabling, or instances of malpractice – and evidence may even support this claim – but medical professionals may disagree and believe that their practices are helpful, reparative, and curative. The medical malpractices that intersex people endure are often not recognized as such because, according to many medical professionals, intersex is a disability, an "emergency," that necessitates curative action. Framing intersex in this way allows doctors to "abandon medical ethics" (G. Davis 2015, 23), thereby institutionalizing compulsory modes of being as well as medical malpractices that are violently disabling. This discourse masks the harm caused as care and cure. Consequently, medical professionals have been largely protected from mainstream criticism and legal action.

Doctors' tremendous amounts of authority, power, and cultural capital also protect them from considerable criticism. "The problem is," Viloria (2017, 150) explains, "whenever intersex adults step forward to say they were harmed by these surgeries, doctors often respond that intersex people would have been worse off if they had been left as they were, and sadly, because the social stigma against us is so strong, most people believe the physicians." In addition to the stigma against people with intersex traits, medical professionals are typically regarded as all-knowing, godlike truth tellers. This expert reputation works to effectively silence intersex people who contradict "expert" claims. Consider Wall's (in Wall et al. 2015) experience meeting with the doctor who mutilated him: "The doctor had no regrets. He was very condescending. He [said,] 'You intersex activists don't know what you're talking about.'" This exchange was not just a failed communication or an instance when the trauma caused to Wall's body-mind was denied or not recognized. This sort of exchange is about power; it is about who has the power to tell truths (see van Heesch 2009). Doctors can easily exploit their position of power and claim authority over the truth about intersex people's body-minds, their experiences, and the theoretical futures stolen from them. Denial of the fact that intersex people – as well as other marginalized people, such as disabled folks, fat individuals, women, LGBTQIA2 folks, and people of colour – have authority over their body-minds, experiences, identities, and futures has been and continues to be an enormous hindrance to rectifying institutionalized discriminatory and oppressive medical malpractices.

The procedures performed on unconsenting intersex people are rarely recognized as mistakes and are not recognized as medical malpractice within the medical field because intersex is construed as a disability, disease, or disorder. Disability, disease, and disorder, according to ableist medical logics, demand curative interventions. The medical logics surrounding intersex-as/is-disability typically fail to consider the ways that discriminatory ideologies inform medical/izing responses. If medicine is "a practice of responding to the experience of illness" (Paget 2004, 21) and if intersex is deemed an illness of sorts for defying culturally mandated ways of being, medical professionals are expected to and "must" intervene. Since medical professionals are taught to view intersex in this manner, invasive interventions are rarely construed as mistakes or malpractices but are instead deemed proper, curative, beneficial medical protocol.

One the one hand, there are a handful of doctors who insist that mistakes have been made and who, by extension, imply that medicine is an ongoing, cultural process that is always under revision. On the other hand, in spite of all the sound evidence and countless intersex people's testimonies to trauma and incurred disabilities, there are doctors who insist that invasive intervention is the best course of action. By extension, these doctors imply that the evidence and intersex people's testimonies are unreliable or hyperbolic; these medical professionals either fight against the revisionist process of medicine or remain largely apathetic to this process when it comes to intersex variations, as well as other culturally devalued and pathologized traits and ways of being. Many doctors are not especially invested in, or they remain ambivalent toward, questioning compulsory ways of being and their commitment to them. Or perhaps these doctors are content to live with the cognitive dissonance of believing that they are acting in the best interest of their intersex patients and claiming to be invested in evidence-based medicine even as they ignore all the evidence suggesting that current (and past) intersex medical management is discriminatory, violent, and disabling medical malpractice.

Conclusion

The culture of silence, abuse, shame, and unquestioned medical authority surrounding intersex is changing because of the Intersex Rights Movement, growing mainstream media attention, and intersex studies scholarship. Although those of us doing this work continue to contest medical malpractice, attend to the haunting effects of curative violence, and seek restorative justice for intersex people, major challenges remain. As long as medical professionals retain the status of all-knowing, infallible experts who impart the truth, intersex people's human rights and self-determination will be denied and medical malpractice will continue. Altering the unquestioned expert status of medical professionals, recognizing that intersex people are the predominant authorities on intersex and their own experiences, and changing both the medical response to and the construction of intersex-as/is-disability are the shifts required in light of the analyses and testimonies presented thus far.

Intersex studies scholars and activists must reject the narrative that medical professionals make mistakes and must insist that the procedures imposed on intersex people's body-minds undoubtedly constitute gratuitously disabling medical malpractice. There is no doubt that intersex medical management constitutes medical malpractice for the following reasons: sound research and intersex people's testimonies illustrate that nonconsensual, medically unnecessary procedures are discriminatory, harmful, disabling, and mutilating; medical professionals have been urged for decades to cease such interventions because they are gratuitously disabling, mutilating, and tortuous; medical professionals are fully aware of and face the "crippling" consequences of these procedures; and, yet, these practices continue. Systemically and systematically mutilating children and knowingly creating body-mind disabilities are not mistakes. These interventions are medical malpractices, not evidence-based medicine.

That said, I understand why doctors may choose to claim that they made a mistake. A mistake is presumably forgivable, an unfortunate accident of sorts. Claims of medical malpractice can open one up to legal issues and possible medical disbarment. However, at this time, disbarment is unlikely given that intervention is deemed the best course of action. Moreover, when doctors claim that they made a mistake, they are humanized. Many intersex people's accounts effectively dehumanize and demonize doctors; as noted in Chapter 1, many intersex people's testimonies "paint a disturbing image of half-crazed doctors running down hospital corridors wielding knives" (Karkazis 2008, 2). I recognize the ableist implications of representing doctors as "half-crazed," and I am aware that doctors have benevolent intentions.[12] Yet framing doctors in this way makes sense to many traumatized, disabled, "crippled," and scarred intersex people. I do not suggest that intersex people should necessarily change their stories or alter how they perceive the doctors who mutilated, disabled, or "crippled" them. However, I do suggest that when repentant medical professionals claim that they made a mistake, they can effectively undercut intersex people's rightful anger. When respected and revered doctors claim that they made a mistake, we often presume that they deserve forgiveness because they must not have known better; they did not mean to cause harm. In turn, intersex people's resentment may be construed as merciless or spiteful, even though their resentment is entirely valid given that doctors do know better. Hence, employing the discourse of medical malpractice can help to undercut the bourgeoning narrative of mistakes. The mistake narrative can undermine intersex people's claims, and it obscures the fact that intersex curative violence *is* medical malpractice.

Interestingly, however, the mistake narrative can provide one with enough leverage to challenge the idea that doctors are infallible, objective "gods" (Cameron 2007, 164), unerring experts who always know best and who, therefore, do not or cannot make mistakes. When doctors claim that they made a mistake concerning intersex patients, they effectively admit that medical practitioners are not objective or absolute arbiters of the truth. When it comes to intersex medical management, doctors cannot pick and choose when they want to be seen as human mistake makers and when they want to be seen as infallible truth tellers. Even the claim of only a few medical professionals that they made a mistake demonstrates that medicine, medical care, and medical practitioners are not, never have been, and never could be objective.[13] Intersex people, activists, and advocates as well as intersex and disability studies scholars continually battle against the image of doctors as all-knowing, faultless, objective experts in order to underline the need to question medical protocol concerning supposed abnormal and deviant embodiments. Drawing attention to the mistake narrative can aid in this battle and can lead to fruitful conversations about the difference between mistakes and medical malpractice. Lastly, given that we can assume the long-term consequences of medical malpractice – disability, trauma, and stolen futures – naming intersex medical management as such reflects the violence, the haunting, and the nonlinear effects and affects of intersex medical malpractice. The phantasms that haunt intersex people are embodied remnants, reminders, or remainders of discriminatory medical malpractice.

PART 2

THE RACIALIZED INTERSEX SPECTRE

4

Temporarily Endosex

A disability adage reminds us that able-bodied people are only ever *"temporarily* able-bodied" or *"enabled"* (Clare 2009, 82). Able-bodied people can become disabled or acquire a disability at any point in their lives. Able-bodied people enjoy a state of "mythic health" (Chen 2011, 273) or a false sense of independence because they are currently enabled by ableist systems, such as infrastructure. In other words, "the spectre of disability" (Belser and Betcher 2013, 344) "haunt[s] us all" (Garland-Thomson 1997, 9). Reworking this adage and continuing with the language of haunting, I suggest that endosex people are only ever temporarily endosex, "normate" (Garland-Thomson 1997, 8; Wilkerson 2012, 183), and not "gender-disabled" (K.P. Morgan 2005, 301). Endosex people merely temporarily fulfill the strict demands of compulsory dyadism. The "spectre of intersex" (Sparrow 2013, 29) haunts ostensible endosex people. That is, the possibility of having anatomical traits categorized as intersex – the possibility of experiencing the medicalizing "process of intersexualization" (Eckert 2009, 64) – haunts all people.

People can learn that they have intersex characteristics at any point in their life and, subsequently, be at the mercy of compulsory dyadism, the process of intersexualization, and curative violence. As an elusive, queering, cripping ghost, intersex confirms that our body-minds are not fully "transparent and knowable" to us (van Dijck 2005, 6); they are not objectively or definitively inter/sexed, dis/ordered, dis/abled, or racialized. "What you are and what you are not," what you think you are or will become, and what you think you are not and will not become "[fold] into each other" (McRuer 2006, 71). The spectre is not and cannot be contained. Everyone is always and already contested. Endosex people who appear to embody compulsory dyadism are merely temporarily seemingly embodying said mandate. Compulsory dyadism is not simply an event or distinct policy; it is an ongoing process.

If intersex haunts all people, however, it apparently does not haunt all people equally. For centuries, the intersex spectre has historically been racialized and feminized. Western, colonial forces have consistently imagined sexual "ambiguity" in racialized nations and people, specifically racialized women (Magubane 2014). The ongoing institutional and mainstream media focus on and fascination with alleged intersex athletes suggests that the broader cultural imaginary assumes and represents intersex as overwhelmingly haunting elite athletes. More specifically, the phantom is currently represented as haunting women track athletes of colour in colonized nations of the Global South, most notably Caster Semenya (b. 1991) of South Africa but also, for example, Santhi Soundarajan (b. 1981) of India, Francine Niyonsaba (b. 1993) of Burundi, Margaret Wambui (b. 1995) of Kenya, and Dutee Chand (b. 1996) of India.[1] And, as the symbolic and/or literal violence enacted on these women suggests, they haunt and deceive the apparently honest, fair athletic world. Race, gender, and nation are central to the construction of sexual "ambiguity," intersex, and disorders of sex development (DSDs).

Despite the fact that intersex has been discursively created and attached to certain people, races, and geographical locations, there are ongoing debates about who is intersex and who is endosex. How many people are intersex? How common are intersex variations? Where does the border between intersex and endosex begin and end? Who can claim intersex as an embodied reality or identity and, therefore, occupy intersex spaces and speak to intersex experiences? These questions concern intersex activists, especially because there are accounts of ostensible endosex people claiming to be intersex and, at times, misrepresenting curative violence as a kindness. I am sympathetic to concerned intersex activists. However, as Hida Viloria (2017) observes, more people desiring to identify as intersex counters interphobic beliefs that no one would want to be intersex because intersex is innately undesirable. Reading supposed endosex people's claims to be intersex alongside the transability phenomenon (see Baril 2015a, 2015b;

J.L. Davis 2012; and Stevens 2011), I question whether excluding supposed endosex people from claiming to be intersex is de facto good, sustainable, anti-interphobic, and grounded in anti-essentialist theorizing.

The Dangers of Universalizing Intersex

The idea that intersex haunts endosex individuals is arguably a rather unnecessarily emphatic and dangerous proposal. Seemingly universalizing intersex – claiming that intersex haunts all endosex people – is politically risky. I claim that the *possibility* of having anatomy currently classified as intersex and be(com)ing intersexualized haunts all people, but I do not argue that everyone should claim intersex as an identity, assume to have intersex variations, or claim to have uniquely intersex experiences. I celebrate intersex identity and identification. Yet, as I discuss at length below, claiming an identity (or embodiment) requires accountability and a critical examination of the social, material, historical, and political power relations that mould the identity (see Linton 1998; Mollow and McRuer 2012; and Viloria 2017).

My proposal that the possibility of having anatomical traits categorized as intersex haunts all people comes from a place that challenges the notion of essential, distinct body-mind classifications and recognizes that theorizing about the precariousness of embodiments, classification systems, and identity remains politically and theoretically useful. Doing so can be illuminating and liberatory. This sort of theorizing enables us to un/do, perform, and think of new modes of relating, organizing, identifying, and becoming different gendered, sexed, dis/abled, queer, and racialized subjects. Doing so helps us to imagine and construct new, less oppressive worlds by bringing into focus the political and marginalizing nature of the current classification systems. In some respects, I echo Robert McRuer's (2006, 57) statement that it is theoretically and politically "important to raise issues about what it means, for the purposes of solidarity, to come out as something you are – at least in some ways – not."

In addition, claiming that intersex haunts endosex people is potentially worrisome because said claim could be misconstrued. I do not mean to imply that endosex people should care about intersex issues because they may have intersex traits, simply do not know of such traits, and may be subjected to dehumanizing violence in the future. And I do not suggest that people should be invested in intersex human rights issues because they may learn that they have intersex traits in the future or may experience the processes of intersexualization. People should be invested in all people's human rights because all people are innately valuable and deserve human rights, dignity, and body-mind autonomy.

Exploring the idea that people are temporarily endosex and only ostensibly embody compulsory dyadism is perhaps troubling and potentially risky. However, doing so is worth the risk. Doing so helps me to move away from dichotomous reasoning – the intersex-endosex and disabled-enabled binaries. The language of hauntology is particularly helpful here. The language emphasizes how intersex – like gender, disability, race, and sexuality – moves discursively and seemingly literally through time and space. Who we think is or is not intersex is, and always has been, complicated and contested across, for example, racial, national, and gender borders. Employing the discourse of haunting is not intended to diminish or ignore people's lived experiences of interphobia by only functioning within the theoretical realm. Although I employ the language to highlight that all body-minds are contested, I also, arguably more importantly, use hauntology to highlight how interphobic violence and compulsory dyadism circulate and collude with other forms of oppression.

Temporarily Endosex

The fact that people can discover that they have intersex traits at any stage in their life suggests that the phantasm haunts all endosex people. The now closed Intersex Society of North America (n.d.) explains, "Though we speak of intersex as an inborn condition, intersex anatomy doesn't always show up at birth. Sometimes a person isn't found to have intersex anatomy until she or he reaches the age of puberty, or finds himself an infertile adult, or dies of old age and is autopsied. Some people live and die with intersex anatomy without anyone (including themselves) ever knowing." For those who have not been medically diagnosed or subjected to curative violence, for those who do not know that they were diagnosed and were lied to by medical professionals and family members, for those who (will) learn something new about their anatomical attributes later in life – for all people – intersex is a ghost that is, to borrow from languages, literature, and cultures professor Colin Davis (2005, 373), "neither present nor absent, neither dead nor alive."

As noted in Chapter 2, there are countless testimonies of medical professionals withholding diagnoses and lying to people about their intersex traits, what procedures were done to their body-minds, and why interventions were done. However, I will offer another example to contextualize my claims here. Karen A. Walsh (2015, 120) writes,

Truthful disclosure didn't come to me about my biology and what was done to me as an infant until I was 33, when I forced the issue by removing my medical records from my endocrinologist's office. I learned that there was never full disclosure to my parents either, and therefore there was no informed consent for the "corrective" surgeries performed on me as an infant. My parents were only told that their little girl would get cancer and would not have a normal development as a girl unless her "deformed ovaries" were removed, and that they should never discuss these problems with me. Thus, after having presented with an inguinal hernia and having exploratory surgery at the age of 16 months, my intra-abdominal testes were removed in a second surgery two months later. I was pronounced a "male pseudohermaphrodite," a diagnosis that was shared neither with my parents or me.

Like Walsh, many other people learn that they have/had intersex characteristics later in life, a discovery that may contextualize medical trauma and body-mind disabilities.

However, some assumed endosex individuals who discover that they have intersex traits have different experiences. Consider the thirty-seven-year-old "ordinary bloke" Rob (pseud.). After undergoing cancer screening, Rob found out that he, as described in the *National Post*, had a "full set of female reproductive organs" (Sawer 2015). "'Ordinary bloke' prepares for hysterectomy after doctors discover womb during bladder cancer test," Patrick Sawer (2015) reports. Understandably, this discovery was shocking to the apparently "ordinary businessman" (Sawer 2015) – the self-described "regular red-blooded guy" (quoted in McDermott 2015). Rob (quoted in Sawer 2015) explains,

The diagnosis came as a bombshell. I've never seen myself as anything but an ordinary bloke who has a normal sex life. I was shocked when the consultant said I had a fully functioning set of women's reproductive organs, and I was even having periods. It appears I could even potentially get pregnant. But I've been told by the doctors I'll be having a hysterectomy in the next few weeks. Bizarrely, that could lead to menopause.

Indeed, Rob was not as "normal" as he thought. For decades, Rob was ostensibly endosex, but he housed an undetected intersex ghost. And that ghost was to be cast out via a hysterectomy. After the operation, Rob likely experienced menopause symptoms, such as hot flashes, fatigue, and mood changes, ghostly reminders of his tenuous endo/sexed and gendered existence. Whether or not the hysterectomy was medically necessary is not explained in the articles that cover Rob's story. The procedure is presented as an assumed given to "align" his body-mind. That said, Rob (quoted in Smith-Squire 2015) clarifies that he wants to undergo the operation because the biological attributes and capacities in question do not align with his gender identity: "It appears I could get pregnant. But as much as I would like a baby, getting pregnant would feel too weird. Instead I hope that getting the female reproductive [organ] removed will improve the quality of my own sperm and I have a baby as a man."

Rob's experience and anatomy were recounted in and circulated by many online magazines and newspapers, including *Cosmopolitan* (R. Rose 2015) and the *Sun* (McDermott 2015). As I discuss below, intersex variations are not uncommon. Nevertheless, Rob's experience was represented as rare, odd, unnatural, freaky, *and* comical. For example, the article about Rob's experience featured in *Cosmopolitan* is accompanied by an image from the cisgenderist and queerphobic 1994 romantic comedy *Junior* (Reitman 1994) depicting Larry Arbogast (Danny DeVito) rubbing the pregnant stomach of Alex Hesse (Arnold Schwarzenegger). In the film, Hesse, a scientist, becomes the world's first pregnant man in order to test a drug that he designed for pregnant people. Coupling Rob's story with this film effectively enfreaks him. He becomes a freakish, comedic "Wonder womb man," as Nick McDermott (2015) describes in traditional sideshow style for the *Sun*. Such a representation is alarming for a number of reasons, one of them being that it is traumatic for many supposed endosex people to (finally) learn about their intersex embodiments later in life and about possible past medical curative violence. Although in some ways it is not impossible to imagine that people who learn of their intersex traits might find the situation amusing, such a comedic representation glosses over and effectively erases the trauma and shame that are experienced by so many people with intersex variations due to intersecting discriminatory logics and compulsory modes of being. In addition, the comedic tone functions to quell assumed endosex readers' discomfort with confronting the fact that perhaps the intersex spectre haunts and dwells within them as well – the ideas that perhaps they are not as "normal" or "ordinary" as they believe. Nevertheless, Rob's experience reminds us that intersex is an elusive queering, cripping ghost that tells us that our body-minds are not transparently or definitively sexed, dis/ordered, or gendered.

Unlike Rob, who learned of his intersex variation from his doctor during cancer screening, some presumed endosex people have learned of their intersex traits from at-home genetic testing kits. Dawn Covino is one such person. When she was thirty-eight years old, Covino found out that she has "male" XY chromosomes after using a 23andMe kit. Covino initially was interested in 23andMe so that she could learn more about her adopted twin daughter and son. Covino explains (quoted in R. Weiss 2019), "I sent it in for the kids and said, 'I'm just going to do it on myself to see if it's accurate, see if it can tell me that I'm half Polish.'" Like all other 23andMe users, Covino offered her sample and filled out the required form, which asked her to disclose her (presumed) sex: female. When the results came back, she was informed via email that her listed sex and test results were incongruous. After providing another sample, a 23andMe geneticist called to inform Covino that she has androgen insensitivity syndrome (AIS), an intersex variation. People with AIS have XY chromosomes and testes; however, their bodies are insensitive to – do not respond to or register – "masculinizing" hormones like testosterone. As a result, people with AIS may appear like a typical endosex girl or woman.

Covino (quoted in R. Weiss 2019) remarks of the situation, "You think you know yourself right?" Indeed, people typically think that they know what biological characteristics they have, and given that people's identities are so bound up with and often dictated by their sexed and gendered biological characteristics, they think that they know who they are. Many people take for granted the presumed fixed nature of their sexed and gendered selves. Even though Covino (quoted in R. Weiss 2019) was understandably stunned by the results, she states that they "gave me a sense of relief." Learning of her XY chromosomes and AIS diagnosis contextualized an operation that she had endured when she was fifteen. At the time, she "didn't know the specific nature of the procedure" (R. Weiss 2019). She now knows that the surgery removed her undescended testes. The intersex spectre was presumably cast out of Covino's body-mind via the gonadectomy. Given that very few people's chromosome formations are tested by their general practitioner, Covino's doctors presumably thought that the phantasm would never resurface or be rediscovered – that she would never learn about her diagnosis, her intersex anatomy, and why the operation took place. Yet, as tests like 23andMe become increasingly accessible and popular as personal explorations and gift options for friends and family, people are learning more about their biologies. Covino's experience with 23andMe reveals that one is perhaps only temporarily endosex. The intersex spectre lingers, takes different forms, and may reveal itself in unexpected ways.

There is no geographical border or sexed, gendered, or racial category that contains the spectre. Any person born could theoretically have/develop intersex characteristics or be subjected to the process of intersexualization. As a result, people who apparently embody compulsory dyadism are only ever temporarily doing so. In other words, compulsory dyadism and, therefore, compulsory able-bodiedness and heterosexuality are innately unstable and consistently challenged. Pathologization, enfreakment, and curative violence seek to restabilize the tenuous nature of culturally mandated ways of be(com)ing.

(Racist) Historical Conceptions of Intersex and Temporarily Endosex

The anxiety concerning the temporary nature of endosex embodiment and the tenuousness of compulsory dyadism are not new phenomena triggered by contemporary advancements in genetic and medical technologies. Worries regarding the intersex spectre, the limits of the male-female dyad, and the ability to develop new or "ambiguous" biological characteristics have a long historical tradition. Not only have these fears challenged the sex and gender dyads and been fuelled by sexism, but they have also challenged racial categories and been fuelled by racism. That is, the intersex spectre is feminized and racialized; it has been – and still is in some regards – often explicitly discursively attached to women's body-minds, particularly racialized women's body-minds.

Western European colonizers have been, to use Lena Eckert's (2009, 62) term again, "intersexualizing" the Other for centuries. They have consistently placed the intersex spectre "over there" in racialized nations and women. For example, there is a long Western, colonial, imperial, and scientific history of labelling African women's genitals – particularly South African women's genitals – ambiguous, primitive, degenerate, and malconformed.[2] Quoting Theodor Waitz's (1863) *Introduction to Anthropology*, sociologist Zine Magubane (2014, 769–70) explains,

> One thing that South African, US, and European medical texts from the seventeenth century through the twentieth seem to agree on was the fact that malformed or ambiguous genitalia ... were particularly common among women of African descent – a 'fixed peculiarity of race' (Waitz 1863, 107). The science of comparative anatomy in Europe owed a significant debt

to naturalists' descriptions and travelers' tales about black South African women.

Alfred A.L.M. Velpeau, Magubane notes, is one such medical scholar. Velpeau (1845) explicitly acknowledges in his book *An Elementary Treatise on Midwifery; or, the Principles of Tokology and Embryology* that he drew from said naturalists' descriptions and travellers' tales and concludes that racialized women are more likely to have sexually ambiguous characteristics. Quoting Velpeau (1845, 58), Magubane (2014, 770) writes that Velpeau "claimed that the labia of women in Persia, Turkey, and Africa were 'naturally much longer than in our European regions.'"

Like Waitz and Velpeau, Hubert von Luschka and colleagues (1868), William Henry Flower and James Murie (1867), Johannes Müller (1834), Theodric Romeyn Beck and John B. Beck (1863), Georges Cuvier (1817), and Adolf Wilhelm Otto (1816) all concur that racialized women – particularly African women, and even more specifically, South African women – are more likely than European women to have "*unusual formations of the generative organs*" (Beck and Beck 1860, 176). The supposed ambiguities or malconformations (also known as "Hottentot aprons") included "excessive" clitoral length and/or labia minora visibility. These scholars further theorized that these malconformations were literal markers of these women's innate degeneration, primitivism, and perverse, insatiable sexuality. As a result, an African woman "becomes her genitalia" (Gilman 1985, 90). And these genitalia were used as justification for myriad forms of literal, discursive, and epistemological dehumanizing, racist violence.[3]

The authors of these texts did not necessarily deny that European women can also have such traits. However, as Beck and Beck (1860, 175–76) claim, "it is not common in Europe, but is quite frequent in warm climates ... This malconformation rarely occurs in temperate climates." In addition to the assertion that these characteristics are literal markers of racialized women's degeneracy and lower status on the evolutionary scale, these writers maintain that temperature has a significant impact on how one's genitals develop and present themselves. Warmer temperatures apparently lead a woman to develop more barbaric, protruded, visible, or prominent genitalia. In turn, cooler temperatures lead a woman to develop more advanced, desirable, subtle, or flat genitals.

To contemporary readers, the suggestion that weather has any bearing on how genitals develop is likely bizarre. Nevertheless, centuries before the writers above made their claims, temperature was deemed crucial to one's biological sex development. These authors were informed by, for example, Aristotle's and Galen's claims that women and men develop different genital formations due to temperature and humidity. Political science and philosophy scholar Georgia Warnke (2011, 30) recounts, "Men's bodies were hot and dry, women's bodies were cold and moist, and because they were, women's bodies lacked sufficient heat to force the organs to their proper place on the outside. In the end, for Galen (here following Aristotle), women were simply imperfect, outside-in men ... If [the body] lacked adequate warmth, it would become only half-baked." If one did not have the necessary warmth to push their genitals out to their "correct" position, they would remain inside, underdeveloped. Given the supposed crucial nature of temperature, people were at risk of changing sexes or becoming sexually "ambiguous." If a woman, for instance, was in a warmer climate or took part in physical, "manly" activities that caused the body to heat up, her biological sex may slip from its "sexual anchorage" (Laqueur 1992, 124). The belief in the importance of temperature persisted for centuries and was used to discursively create and maintain the idea of pathological or "ambiguous" sex as well as to justify sexism, racism, colonialism, and imperialism. The conclusion was not that supposed sexually ambiguous African women were closer to embodying the "perfect" male body but rather that they were uncivil, evolutionary degenerates who were not properly women.

The connection between race and sexual "ambiguity" persisted even after medical professionals rejected the importance of climate and temperature theories. Texts published into the twentieth century, Magubane (2014) notes, perpetuated the false idea that African people and other Black people are more likely to have sexually "ambiguous" traits. Echoing Waitz, obstetrician, gynecologist, and general surgeon Godfrey Charlewood (1956, 12) wrote in 1956 that intersex "abnormalities" are more frequent in "Negroes and related races." In the late 1980s, geneticists Michèle Ramsay and colleagues (1988, 9) similarly claimed that "ambiguous genitalia [seem] to be much more common in blacks than in whites." This belief impacted how intersex was "treated" in medical settlings, namely who was "treated." When surgery became common practice in the Global North in the mid-twentieth century, the idea that Black people are more likely to be sexually "ambiguous" was still being circulated. Discussing the rise of intersex medical management in America, Magubane (2014, 771) writes that surgery on white patients was imperative to establish the normality of whiteness. An ambiguously gendered white body needed to be corrected to retain its whiteness, whereas an ambiguously gendered black body was seen as confirming the essential biological difference between whites and blacks. Equally important was the need to use surgical correction to further secure the gendered distribution of racially exclusive social privileges such as the right to inherit and own property, the right to vote, the right to marry, and the right to education. These social privileges were extended only to whites and, therefore, it was a political imperative that their bodies be identified as either male or female and, once identified, be surgically and socially forced to conform.

The white intersex body-mind must be rendered invisible. Hence, "curative" surgery was presumed crucial for white intersex children. White children needed to become or appear endosex in order to preserve their whiteness and, therefore, their rights as white people.

Although most medical professionals now advocate for "normalizing" procedures for all people with intersex variations and no longer maintain that racialized people are more likely to have intersex traits, racist conceptions of sexual "ambiguity" are still perpetuated, namely in the sports world. As I explore at length in the next chapter, women athletes of colour in colonized nations of the Global South are currently targeted for sport sex testing because of their supposed manly and incongruous bodies and abilities, most notably, as stated above, Semenya of South Africa but also, for example, Soundarajan of India, Niyonsaba of Burundi, Wambui of Kenya, and Chand of India. And, as the symbolic and/or literal violence enacted on these women suggests, they haunt and seek to deceive the apparently honest, fair athletic world. The claim that these athletes are dangerous gender cheats is a contemporary iteration of the old trope that "hermaphrodites" are "deliberately deceptive or shady character[s]" (Reis 2005, 412). For centuries, there were anxieties concerning dishonest "hermaphrodites" – "brute animals" (Reis 2005, 418). "Embedded in many of the medical accounts," historian of medical ethics and gender Elizabeth Reis (2005, 428–29) writes, "were worries going beyond the threat of dishonesty and illicit sexual relations to the far more troubling threat of inexplicable sexual transformation." That is, some believed that "hermaphrodites" could "[shift] back and forth between genders at will" for nefarious purposes (Reis 2005, 429). Of course, rather than deceiving or cheating anyone, historical figures with intersex traits, like contemporary (suspect) intersex athletes, were simply trying to live without oppression, intervention, and discrimination.

Sean Saifa M. Wall (2016) states, "I am not just intersex. I am Black and I am queer." Here, he is not simply listing off his identities but also drawing attention to the fact that his identities and the forms of discrimination that he is subjected to cannot be understood in isolation. Wall (2015b, 117) states elsewhere, "I stand at the intersection bearing witness to how [racist] violence has incarcerated my friends and loved ones as well as being subjected to [interphobic] medically unnecessary surgical intervention." The logics of interphobia, racism, queerphobia, and ableism interconnect and fuel all sorts of violence: racist science, enslavement, colonialism, incarceration, pathologization, medical malpractice, and curative violence. Hence, it is vital to underscore the racist historical construction of sexual "ambiguity" and how that construction has maintained compulsory dyadism for centuries.

Race, gender, and nation are central to the construction of sexual "ambiguity," intersex, and DSD. As a result, we must fully acknowledge that racism, ableism, queerphobia, and interphobia are not distinct forms of oppression. We must take nationality, gender, and race into account when considering the complexities of socially constructed intersex and endosex classifications. Even though historical and contemporary iterations of intersex have been racialized, Pidgeon Pagonis (2016) observes that intersex activist and support spaces have been predominantly white, that white intersex people tend to neglect the ways that racialized intersex people's identities and experiences overlap, and that white intersex people can and do perpetuate racism. The Intersex Rights Movement is not immune from reproducing discriminatory logics: racism, ableism, sexism, or otherwise. Intersex activists Lynnell Stephani Long, Wall, and Pagonis (2016) remark,

> As intersex people of color, we acknowledge that we cannot have intersex liberation if we are not in alliance with other oppressed peoples fighting for liberation across multiple movements. As such, we are committed to expanding the conversations about bodily integrity and autonomy so that our movement as intersex people of color can align with reproductive justice activists, the transgender community, those who are incarcerated, disabled, undocumented, and anyone else fighting for sovereignty of their bodies, communities, and sacred lands.

My arguments echo Long's, Wall's, and Pagonis's commitment to pay particular attention to how all forms of oppression uphold interphobia. Compulsory dyadism and interphobia cannot be effectively dismantled if compulsory able-bodiedness and heterosexuality, racism, colonialism, imperialism, cisgenderism, and sexism are not central to anti-interphobic projects.

Claiming Intersex: Who Is Intersex or Endosex?

Intersex and endosex are socially constructed categories that have shifted through time and place. Given the instability of these categories, there have been and still are ongoing debates about who is (not) sexually "ambiguous," who is (not) intersex, who is (not) endosex, who might be "masquerading" as intersex, and who, therefore, can occupy intersex spaces. Some intersex activists are concerned with endosex people claiming to be intersex and, in turn, appropriating intersex experiences, pain, or expertise. Yet we must ask who – what groups, organizations, or institutions – ought to have the authority to determine who is endosex or intersex. Who can claim endosex or intersex as a biological reality or an identity? Not all intersex people, intersex studies scholars, or medical professionals agree. Nevertheless, as Viloria (2017, 204) suggests, the blurriness between endosex and intersex is "okay." Rather than resisting the ambiguity between the endosex-intersex binary, thinking about the productive ways to navigate this complexity is imperative. Comparable to trying to maintain the homosexual-heterosexual or enabled-disabled binaries, attempting to uphold the intersex-endosex dichotomy is theoretically and pragmatically untenable. The intersex-endosex binary also does not reflect all people's identities, histories, or relationships with their body-minds. The intersex-endosex binary can function to invalidate these people's identities, histories, and body-mind relationships. The binary is limiting.

In this section, therefore, I seek to traverse the complex endosex-intersex binary. To do so, I first address the disputed question of how common intersex traits are. The inability to conclusively define or agree on male, female, endosex, and intersex categories problematizes the project of gaining statistical knowledge about intersex and determining who is (not) intersex or endosex. Second, I address debates concerning whether or not people with polycystic ovary syndrome (PCOS) or with Mayer-Rokitansky-Küster-Hauser (MRKH) syndrome are intersex or can rightly claim intersex as an identity or biological reality. Third, I examine the ways that some people have been excluded from intersex spaces because they, for example, do not have medical records or have not undergone curative violence. Fourth, I unpack some intersex activists' concerns that endosex trans people are claiming to be intersex, are identifying as intersex, or are "posing" as intersex online. Some intersex activists maintain that these people ought to be excluded and that they pose a danger to the Intersex Rights Movement. Lastly, I sympathize with these intersex people's worries. I wonder, however, whether this exclusionary position is sustainable, de facto good, and entirely rooted in anti-discriminatory politics. Drawing from Viloria's (2017) arguments concerning supposed endosex people claiming to be intersex and from disability studies scholars' analyses of transability, I propose that the claims of ostensible endosex people to be intersex should not be considered inherently dangerous, undesirable, or menacing.

What counts as intersex and endosex anatomy is, and has historically been, hotly disputed. This point is illustrated by the now defunct Intersex Society of North America's (n.d.) response to the question of how common intersex traits are:

> To answer this question in an uncontroversial way, you'd have to first get everyone to agree on what counts as intersex – and also to agree on what should count as strictly male or strictly female. That's hard to do. How small does a penis have to be before it counts as intersex? Do you count "sex chromosome" anomalies as intersex if there's no apparent external sexual ambiguity?

No one can agree on these questions. As a result, there are several different estimates. Intersex variations are typically assumed to be uncommon because one misrepresentative statistic is frequently referenced. Viloria (2015) explains, "Some groups use an old prevalence statistic that says we make up 1 in 2,000, or .05% ... of the population, but that statistic only refers to one specific intersex trait, ambiguous genitalia, which is but one of many variations which, combined (as they are in medical diagnostics and coding), constitute the 1.7% estimate" provided by Anne Fausto-Sterling (2000). Melanie Blackless and colleagues (2000) claim that 2 percent of live births have intersex anatomy. According to these statistics, intersex traits are as common as twins and people with red hair (at 1 to 2 percent of the population) and much more common than other well-known variations or disabilities such as Down syndrome (at 1 in 800 to 1,000 births) and albinism (at 1 in 20,000 births). Kristin Zeiler and Anette Wickström (2009) as well as Brendan Gough and colleagues (2008) estimate that up to 4 percent of people have intersex traits. However, Jan Fichtner and colleagues' (1995) study concerning hypospadias, as referenced in Chapter 3, contests this estimate. Among the 500 apparently "normal," endosex, cis men with penises whom they studied, 45 percent were not actually found to have "normal" penises according to dominant medical standards. Given these sorts of studies, intersex and trans activist and scholar Cary Gabriel Costello (2012a) concludes that a "conservative estimate is that more than 1 in 150 people are born with intersex bodies."

The inability to conclusively define or agree on male, female, endosex, and intersex categories problematizes the project of gaining statistical knowledge about intersex and determining who is (not) intersex or endosex. Even if there were "a large, representative, random subpopulation of people to agree to be genitally examined, hormone-screened, genotyped, CAT-scanned, and to have their gonads biopsied," Costello (2012a) notes, researchers would likely "rely on medical diagnostic categories that purposefully deny that many people with sexually-intermediate bodies are 'really intersex.'" Purposefully denying how frequently sexually intermediate characteristics manifest is useful to those invested in maintaining compulsory dyadism. If intersex traits are so uncommon – for example, 0.5 percent – the medical community can argue that they are rare aberrations, flaws, disabilities, or malformations that require cure.

Having a sound statistic is pragmatically and theoretically beneficial. Pragmatically, a reliable estimate proves that a relatively large portion of the population is not recognized – indeed, intersex people have been actively silenced – and do not have full rights as human beings or citizens. In contrast to some intersex people's experience of being told by medical professionals that there is "no one" else like them (Debbie Hartman, in Arana and Human Rights Commission Staff 2005, 48), a sound statistic demonstrates that this is not the case. They are not "real freak[s] of nature, damaged and alone" (Zieselman 2015, 124). Theoretically speaking, a statistic concerning how frequently intersex traits manifest demonstrates that the male-female sex dyad is a farce and that compulsory dyadism is not "natural" or inevitable.

Nevertheless, attempting to determine how frequently intersex traits manifest comes with dangers. As noted above, doing so requires strict boundaries between female, intersex, and male. That is, doing so relies on biological essentialism and gendering body parts. In addition, trying to determine how common intersex variations are can problematically fall into dichotomous thinking: endosex-intersex. Given the pragmatic benefits, I do not propose that researchers abandon attempting to estimate how frequently intersex traits manifest. That said, intersex activists and intersex studies researchers should be wary about and pay attention to the tenuous endosex-intersex dyad.

The fragile nature of the endosex-intersex binary is clear when one attends to specific disputes regarding biological variations and identity claims. For example, there are debates within intersex communities concerning people with polycystic ovary syndrome (PCOS). People with PCOS have higher than typical "female" testosterone levels and may exhibit sex/gender-variant or "masculine" secondary sex characteristics, namely "male-typical body and facial hair; masculine facial features and musculature; [and] male-pattern baldness" (Vidya 2010). Should people with PCOS be considered intersex? Can they claim intersex as an identity? Some claim that PCOS is not an intersex variation because medical professionals do not categorize or diagnose it as a DSD (Brunner et al. 2015; Trans Brain FX n.d.). However, this logic problematically and ironically supports the medical industry as the gatekeeper and producer of "real" intersex knowledges. Yet some intersex folks and people with PCOS think that it should be classified as an intersex variation. As a result, they argue that the category of intersex should be expanded, not limited or exclusionary. Vidya (2010), a person with PCOS, writes that even though PCOS "is usually not grouped under an intersex classification, I see no obvious reason that it should not be ... I can see an intersex identity being advantageous in the sense of helping me/others become more open and public about the 'male' characteristics ... that many of us possess but generally minimize/hide." Likewise, Gillian Giles (2020) argues that intersex as a category should be expanded to include PCOS because people with PCOS, like people with intersex traits, are pathologized for blurring and undermining the sex and gender binaries. In addition, Giles notes that many people with PCOS experience social stigma and curative violence because of their physical characteristics. That is, some people with PCOS may experience interphobia whether or not they are medically deemed intersex or claim intersex as an identity or embodiment. Giles (2020) concludes, "Under an expanded intersex spectrum that acknowledges the social constructs of gender and includes people with PCOS and other biological variations, our preoccupation and reliance on who fits where dwindles drastically ... Even without an expanded understanding of intersex, these shared experiences alone are a call and case for greater intersex solidarity within PCOS Advocacy." Giles offers convincing reasons why people with PCOS could claim intersex, can be construed as intersex, and can experience interphobia, as well as revealing that the intersex-endosex binary is tenuous.

In addition, there are questions about people with Mayer-Rokitansky-Küster-Hauser syndrome. Should they be considered intersex? Would they want to be considered intersex? Viloria (2017, 204) writes of these questions,

> There has always been confusion and debate over which variations should be considered intersex. For example, there's a variation called Mayer-Rokitansky-Küster-Hauser syndrome, or MRKH, in which people are born with bodies that look typically female but have a small or absent uterus and a short or absent vagina. I had wondered whether these people should be considered intersex, or would they want to be, and I learned that most of them didn't because they identified as women. Conversely, I learned that there are people who *don't* have visibly androgynous sex anatomy and *do* consider themselves intersex ... So yes, it's confusing trying to figure out who and what is intersex, but to me, that's okay.

Like Giles, Viloria implies that the intersex-endosex binary and the intersex-endosex identification are difficult to navigate. People's biologies and identification desires are diverse and complex. Yet I am inspired by Viloria's comfort with the messiness of it all, by their dedication to respecting how people want to identify, and by their openness to expanding the definition of intersex and, in turn, endosex.

Some intersex activists are particularly concerned with people who have not been subjected to curative violence and/or do not have medical records or diagnoses. "I've come to discover that sometimes when people ... have tried to come out as intersex and join the intersex community, they've been turned away with accusations that they're not really intersex," Viloria (2017, 328) recounts; "I've received reports from intersex people who have tried to join other intersex organizations but were dismissed because, having escaped IGM [intersex genital mutilation], they don't have a medical diagnosis to 'verify' that they are intersex." Unsurprisingly, then, given that many intersex people have been and are subjected to curative violence and experience various body-mind disabilities, some people with intersex traits who have not experienced this disabling violence may question whether they rightly belong in intersex groups or if they are "intersex enough." Viloria is one such person. While on their first intersex retreat, Viloria thought (2017, 92–93), "I'm worried I'll be seen as too normal to be here. My genitals aren't scarred like the others"; maybe Viloria's clitoris was "not big enough to make me intersex."

Understandably, intersex people are protective of their systemically marginalized group. In addition, there are cases of people with, by all accounts, endosex traits who are claiming to have intersex traits/diagnoses.[4] As a result, some intersex people have developed a sort of vetting checklist to determine whether or not one is "really" intersex and can rightly enter intersex spaces. Some intersex people imply that medical verification, mutilation, and/or disabilities are prerequisites to claim intersex status and rightfully enter intersex spaces. Even though the intersex folks in these spaces combat pathologization, medical authority, and curative violence, some paradoxically rely on medical diagnoses and trauma to assess whether (possible) members truly belong. Medical diagnoses, body-mind disabilities, mutilation, trauma, scar tissue, intersex belonging, and intersex identification are understood as being intertwined. In addition, the demand that people "prove" their intersex status with medical diagnoses, origin stories, and trauma replicates the same problematic logic that other marginalized and oppressed groups face. For example, to receive the recognition, care, support, or accommodations that they need, disabled people – particularly people with invisible disabilities – are consistently called to "prove" their disabilities with origin stories, personal histories, medical or psychological documentation, trauma, and/or diagnoses.[5] Comparably, to receive recognition and the things that they need, LGBTQIA2 people are consistently called to "prove" their sexuality or gender with stories, histories, documentation, trauma, and/or diagnoses.[6] As a result, like Viloria wondering whether they are intersex enough, many disabled people ask, "Am I disabled enough? What story must I tell to be recognized?" Many LGBTQIA2 people wonder whether they are lesbian, gay, bi, trans, or queer enough. They ask, "What story must I tell to be accepted? What if my story differs from the dominant narrative?"

Drawing from the concepts of "transnormativity" (Johnson 2016, 1) and "paradigmatic" disabled people (Mollow and McRuer 2012, 12), we can understand that Viloria's accounts reveal that there is an internormative script or paradigmatic intersex person who is expected and accepted by some intersex people. Writing of transnormativity, sociologist Austin H. Johnson (2016, 1) states, "Transnormativity describes the specific framework to which transgender people's presentations and experiences of gender are held accountable ... Transnormativity structures transgender experience, identification, and narratives into a hierarchy of legitimacy that is dependent upon medical standards." For example, the "born in the wrong body" narrative is medically accepted and, in many respects, expected. Therefore, trans people must structure their personal narratives and identities around this narrative to "prove" or "authenticate" their genders if they are to receive the social recognition and gender-affirming care that they need, even when this narrative does not reflect their experiences or narratives. As disability studies scholars Anna Mollow and Robert McRuer (2012, 12) observe, some disability studies scholars and activists have proliferated the image of a "paradigmatic" disabled person: "His or her body manifests visible difference; physical suffering is not a primary aspect of his or her experience; and he or she is not seeking cure or recovery." In light of these apt reflections, there appears to be a paradigmatic intersex person or internormative script that is being created and supported by some intersex people, as illustrated by Viloria's accounts. This paradigmatic intersex person must be able to reproduce a script. This is a person who has been diagnosed by medical professionals and subjected to curative violence, who advocates against intersex genital mutilation (IGM), and who has the physical proof of trauma: medical records, scars, and/or disabilities. These experiences and physical/medical credentials presumably "prove" one's intersex status and claim to intersex identity. The paradigmatic person and script, to borrow from Johnson (2016), structure intersex "experience, identification, and narratives into a hierarchy of legitimacy that is," quite ironically, partly "dependent upon medical standards." They create a hierarchy of belonging and suffering. And, just like the paradigmatic disabled person and transnormative scripts, the paradigmatic intersex person and internormative script erase and can delegitimize intersex people with other experiences: those who escaped curative violence, those who lived in communities or rural locations where curative violence was unavailable or not even considered, those who were never diagnosed by medical professionals, those who cannot gain access to medical records, and those who learned of their intersex variations later in life. The paradigmatic person and script shut down – rather than open up – spaces for more voices to be heard and for more conversations about alternative intersex experiences that may not be fundamentally rooted in trauma. They also implicitly and paradoxically presume a constant stream of gratuitously disabled and traumatized intersex people. Although intersex activists rightly demand outlawing curative violence, undermining medical authority, and dismantling compulsory dyadism, the paradigmatic intersex person and internormative script run counter to these aims.

Arguably, the most heated debate concerning who is "really" intersex or endosex concerns trans people. "Certain community members have a fear that there are trans people pretending to be intersex and that it will be bad for the movement," Viloria confirms (2017, 328). "I've been hearing about this fear since I came out as intersex twenty years ago, and I still hear it to-day." The assertion that some trans people claim to be intersex in some respects is not unfounded. For example, as explained by Stella, a trans participant in Costello's (2016, 104) study,

> Being transsexual is really a type of intersexuality. I was born with a female brain in a male body. So I'm intersex, too. My condition is just as real, and needs treatment just as much. It's unfair, that all these barriers are put in the way of my getting the hormones and surgery I need ... They need to understand we have a kind of intersexuality. Then they'll treat us differently.

Repurposing the "born in the wrong body" narrative, Stella implies that if medical professionals view trans people as having an intersex disorder or disability, then medical professionals will more readily offer "treatment" or gender-confirming care. That is, Stella reproduces and relies on interphobic, ableist medical evaluations of intersex-as/is-disability that requires a "cure." The "treatment" imposed on unconsenting intersex people, however, does not constitute gender-confirmation procedures, as addressed in Chapter 1. The "treatment" constitutes curative violence, medical malpractice, mutilation, and so on. Given that Stella relies on medical professionals to grant her access to gender-confirming care, it is, at least in part, understandable why she thinks that claiming to be intersex is a means to get what she needs.

In Kenneth J. Zucker's experiences working as a clinical psychologist with trans adolescents, a minority of his patients have claimed that they have intersex traits. "One male-to-female patient," Zucker (2012, 97) reports, "told me that an endocrinologist had visualized ovaries during an ultrasound. A female-to-male patient told me that he had undescended testes. Another male-to-female patient claimed to have menstrual bleeding through the penis. Of course, when asked for medical documentation, it never materialized." Although an endosex trans person's intersex claims will not be confirmed or supported by medical professionals, there is a biological-essentialist allure or logic to this claim. Rather than struggling to navigate the cisgenderist social and medical world that denies trans people's genders at every turn, they can point to a supposed biological intersex trait that will justify their transition – a supposed literal feminine or masculine "born that way" biological marker. The allure is, at least in part, the presumed legitimacy of biological essentialism. If one is invested in dominant socio-medical conceptions that biological traits are a physical symptom of one's "true" male or female gender, then claiming to have a physically "real" feminine or masculine trait may seem compelling. In addition, the desire to claim to be intersex may intensify when speaking with someone – like Zucker – who is or is presumed to be integral to granting one's access to gender-confirming procedures.

In contrast to, for example, transexclusionary radical feminists' beliefs that trans men transition in order to gain access to male privilege and that trans women seek to invade women's spaces and appropriate women's experiences, the medical and psychiatric industrial complexes perpetuate the idea that trans people are pathological or disordered; they have gender dysphoria (formerly diagnosed as gender incongruence or gender identity disorder).[7] They are deemed disordered because of intersecting cisgenderist, ableist logics. "Stay[ing] in the 'natural' given body" and conforming to one's assigned gender are presumed de facto desirable, healthy, and normal (Baril and Trevenen 2014, 393). As a result, the medical and psychiatric world that many trans people navigate demands that "trans* people justify their transition in terms that are intelligible to medical, political and cultural norms" (Baril and Trevenen 2014, 393). Doctors expect and accept the ableist and cisgenderist narrative that trans people are disordered in some way. Trans people are often called to reproduce this narrative in order to gain access to the care that they need. However, even when trans individuals do reproduce this narrative, they are required to "slow down any requested medical interventions" (G. Davis, Dewey, and Murphy 2016, 493). In contrast, since intersex traits are deemed emergencies that require immediate curative intervention, intersex people are quickly subjected to medical interventions. That is, although both intersex and trans people are deemed disordered and pathological, intersex individuals are routinely subjected to "curative" procedures post-haste, whereas trans people must fight for years for these kinds of interventions.

Given that medical professionals readily perform procedures on "disordered" intersex children – procedures that may look a lot like gender-affirming procedures to some trans people – claiming intersex may look like a promising route. People might reason that deploying interphobic ableist narratives, rather than cisgenderist ableist logics, may grant them access to the medical care that they need much more quickly. Underlying endosex trans people's claims to be intersex is the, arguably misplaced, assumption they will be accepted and confirmed as their gender by professionals who are the gatekeepers to gender-confirming care and, perhaps as a result, by their community and family members.

Endosex trans people or trans people who are read as endosex by others but claim to be intersex are "received very poorly by intersex people" because they sometimes reproduce and exploit interphobic ableist conceptions of intersex and imply that curative violence is an essential kindness (Costello 2016, 104). As explained by Oscar (quoted in Costello 2016, 104), an intersex and trans person,

> I hate that whole argument, that TG [transgender] is an intersex brain state that 'needs' to be cured with genital surgery. Because the argument is saying that the surgery doctors force on intersex kids is necessary and good. Because it treats intersex people as lucky, not as victims. These people making this argument have no idea what our lives are like, but they're happy to use us, to say they speak for us ... The feminizing surgery that was forced on me as a kid mutilated me, but you're treating it as good. Don't you dare claim to speak for me.

Intersex communities and intersex studies scholars all agree: curative violence is horrific, torturous, violent mutilation. The discriminatory belief that IGM is a good thing should not be used to justify trans people's access to the medical and gender-confirming care that they may need. Access to these things can be justified without reproducing the medical industry's claim that curative violence is a necessary curative kindness.

The ability to potentially hide one's "true" identity online complicates this situation. Since the advent of the Internet, people have been troubled by the possible dangers of not really knowing who someone is online. And, of course, people lie about who they are on the Internet for all sorts of reasons: attention, trolling, catfishing, amusement, and money. Consequently, there is a fear that some endosex people, specifically trans endosex people, are masquerading as intersex online. In addition to noting that "anecdotally, intersex 'posers' ... represent a substantial fraction of participants in electronic discussion groups for the intersexed," semantic and intersex studies scholar, Peggy Cadet, and professor of psychiatry and psychology, Marc D. Feldman (2012, 93), offer three case studies of Internet intersex "posers." Each case involves a trans woman who claims to have or actually has transitioned. These people apparently have "factitious intersex conditions," which qualifies them as having Munchausen by Internet (MBI), a form of Munchausen syndrome (Cadet and Feldman 2012, 91). Drawing from Feldman's (2000) work on MBI, Cadet and Feldman (2012, 91) explain that MBI "refers to such deception taking place online, typically in special-interest or health-based support groups ... As in real-life cases of factitious disorder, individuals engaging in MBI behaviours falsify illness, disability, or crisis, typically to gain attention and emotional nurturance" and "self-aggrandizement." That is, Cadet and Feldman imply, these people are not only lying but are also pathological for doing so. As the authors explain, (1) these "posers" offer "implausible medical claims," (2) there is "contradictory third-party information," (3) there is "contradictory published information" (e.g., copying "nearly verbatim" an intersex person's story and diagnosis and claiming it as their own), (4) their appearance is inconsistent with claimed diagnoses, (5) they have a "false social history," (6) they make "inconsistent claims," and/or (7) they refuse to show medical documentation that would confirm their intersex claims because doing so would be "an invasion of privacy" (Cadet and Feldman 2012, 92–94). The cases and evidence of inconsistency are compelling.

The main aim of Cadet and Feldman's (2012) paper is not merely to detect lies. The authors are concerned that this "substantial" fraction of online "poser" participants takes away valuable space from "real" intersex people who need this space for community support. In addition, the authors explain, their inconsistent and false claims about intersex variations spread misinformation about intersex to both intersex and endosex people seeking accurate information. Cadet and Feldman's article received high praise from the nongovernmental organization StopIGM.org (2017): "Thank you Peggy Cadet and Marc Feldman! Instrumentalising intersex is NOT a victimless crime!"

Again, I do not deny that there are people on the Internet who pretend to be intersex – or pretend to have any other identity, diagnosis, or experience. However, it is worthwhile to unpack and be critical of the logics deployed here. It is worthwhile to ask and explore further. Given that it is reasonable to assume that an endosex cis person is capable of "posing" as an intersex person online, why is the debate always focused on presumably trans people? Is framing these ostensible endosex trans people as pathological liars representative of the situation? What would it mean to take a supposed endosex person's claim to intersex identification seriously? Can an ostensible endosex person legitimately identify as intersex? Can something positive come from this identification, or is this dangerous and frightening? I attempt to answer these questions in turn.

Endosex cis people can "pose" as intersex online. So why are these online people presumably trans? Cadet and Feldman (2012) presume that the people explored in their case studies are trans because each person claims to have or has transitioned from male to female. Moreover, they speculate that these people are lying about being intersex because they are in denial about being trans; they are struggling with internalized cisgenderism. That is, claiming to have an intersex variation may seem easier than asserting a trans identity. Perhaps this is, in part, the case. For them, like for Stella or for Zucker's patients, discussed above, maybe the allure of claiming to be intersex online offers a space to claim a material, biological feminine or masculine "born that way" marker that presumably validates their gender and transition. However, unlike Stella and unlike Zucker's trans patients who claim intersex status offline, endosex trans people who claim intersex status online may feel safer since they likely will not be challenged by medical professional gatekeepers, will likely receive support from others, and may skirt identity politics and "realness" debates.

Is framing these ostensible endosex trans people as pathological liars representative of the situation? Do they have MBI? Is the root of the problem some pathological impulse to lie? It seems to me that the root of the problem is a complex discriminatory medical system that pathologizes "disordered" intersex and trans people in different but extremely harmful ways. The medical system consistently challenges trans people's genders, expects them to reproduce pathologizing transnormative scripts that may not align with their experiences, and denies them the medical care that they need by obliging them to "slow down any requested medical interventions" (G. Davis, Dewey, and Murphy 2016, 493). Consequently, it forces trans people to find any possible alternative way to gain access to the recognition, support, and care that they need. If all responsibility is placed on "pathological" deceiving trans people, one neglects to pay attention to the systemic problem: the impossible position and the medical system that trans people often find themselves in. The underlying problem is not necessarily some pathological desire to lie or one's internalized cisgenderism but rather a cisgenderist, interphobic, heteronormative, racist, and ableist medical system that relies on biological essentialism and denies people – intersex, trans, queer, racialized, fat, and disabled people as well as women – body-mind autonomy, a system that then incites tensions and animosity between oppressed groups.

In addition to the fact that endosex cis people claiming or lying about intersex and/or trans online or offline is not out of the realm of possibility, the focus on alleged endosex trans people should prompt us to keep in mind that trans people – trans women in particular – have consistently been represented as dangerous deceivers, frauds, and cheats (Baril 2015a). They supposedly threaten "innocent" endosex cis folks with their gender lies. Trans people, trans women specifically, have been represented as "traps," "deceivers who lure straight [i.e., cis] men into sexual encounters" (Wodda and Panfil 2014, 932). Trans women have been characterized as predatory "male" frauds who seek access to women's bathrooms for nefarious purposes (Sanders and Stryker 2016). Trans women have been interpreted as male cheaters in the sports world, seeking an "unfair" advantage over "real" cis women (Sykes and Smith 2016). These accusations against trans people are unfounded and seek to reinforce the cisgenderist idea that trans people are not really their genders. Nevertheless, they persist, supporting the belief that trans people are, in some important sense, dangerous pathological liars who "threaten" cis people.

Similar logics are evident in some intersex people's fears that endosex trans people are pathologically lying about being intersex for self-aggrandizement purposes and to exploit intersex people for emotional support, nurturance, or intimacy. It is imperative to resist reproducing the narrative that trans people, particularly trans women, are threatening pathological liars who maliciously harm people for self-centred reasons. Resisting this narrative does not mean denying that some endosex trans people may lie on the Internet or have lied on the Internet about having intersex traits. Rather, doing so requires placing fears, accusations, and cases in conversation with the broader cultural anxiety that trans people are dangerous deceivers, frauds, and cheats. It requires thinking critically about the usefulness of labelling these alleged endosex trans people pathological and paying more attention to the reasons why they may claim to be intersex, lie about being intersex, or genuinely believe that they have intersex variations.

Doing so offers more nuanced explanations and can foster solidarity. The fact that the medical system effectively prevents intersex and trans people from exercising body-mind autonomy and self-determination comes into focus. Thinking more critically about the trope of the trans deceiver also prompts one to reconsider the fact that intersex people are similarly construed as dangerous cheats and said to be "deliberately deceptive or shady" (Reis 2005, 412). The groundless narrative about the malicious deceiver is deployed to oppress and foster discrimination against both intersex and trans people. This fact offers intersex and trans activists and scholars a site for solidarity building.

What would it mean to take ostensible endosex people's claims to be intersex seriously? Should people be fearful of supposed endosex people claiming to be intersex? Whether one identifies as intersex or not, it is dangerous to suggest that curative violence enacted on intersex people is a kindness. According to Viloria (2017, 328), claiming to be intersex but "not working against, or even talking about, the irreversible harms of IGM," while possibly "diverting the focus to other issues ... isn't great." Although I do not expect all people to become activists in the traditional sense, if the idea of intersex curative violence as vital and good is perpetuated, fearing for intersex people's well-being makes sense. I fear for them. However, if people are expected to at least understand and oppose the gratuitously disabling nature of curative violence, the fact that the socio-medical construction of sexual "ambiguity" and IGM has roots in racism – not just ableism and queerphobia – must be centralized. Moreover, lying about experiences or diagnoses and spreading misinformation about intersex are deeply troubling practices. The fact that intersex people have been consistently lied to about their own experiences, body-minds, and diagnoses may only compound the perceived severity of the deceit. Spreading misinformation also undermines the decades of work that intersex activists and scholars have done to distribute accurate and destigmatizing information to other intersex people and to the public more generally.

When people claim intersex status and seek out interventions to approximate a specific intersex variation, questions and fears concerning ostensible endosex people claiming to be intersex only intensify, and the boundaries between endosex and intersex and, as a result, between disabled and enabled only continue to blur. Consequently, it is pressing that we ask about the implications of taking claims to be intersex seriously. According to intersex activist Anunnaki Ray Marquez (2019b), intersex "should not be adopted by people who 'feel' like they are intersex, but have endosex (non-intersex) bodies." I wonder whether this exclusionary position is sustainable and de facto good. Drawing from Viloria's (2017) arguments concerning supposed endosex people claiming to be intersex as well as from disability studies scholars' analyses of transability, I remain unconvinced that ostensible endosex people claiming intersex status ought to be considered inherently dangerous, undesirable, or menacing.

Given that intersex is a presumed diagnosable condition and that many intersex people's experiences are bound up with navigating ableism and (living with) disabilities, thinking about the "dangers" of alleged endosex people identifying as intersex can be read alongside transabled people's claims. As defined by feminist, trans, and disability studies scholar Alexandre Baril (2015a, 689), transabled people are "considered able-bodied by others and want to become disabled or acquire an impairment by transforming their bodies."[8] Transabled people identify as disabled, present as disabled (e.g., use a wheelchair), and/or seek out ways to acquire a disability or impairment. A transabled person may, for example, desire or need to become deaf, paraplegic, or incontinent or seek to contract HIV. Analyzing presumed endosex people claiming to be intersex alongside transability offers up the opportunity to examine and contrast the arguments often deployed to delegitimize alleged endosex and/or able-bodied people's identity claims. In addition, endosex embodiment is bound up with able-bodied norms. Whereas endosex is deemed able-bodied, intersex is deemed disabled, disordered, or diseased. Therefore, presumed endosex people who identify as or want to acquire an intersex variation can be read with the transability phenomenon; indeed, they could be considered transabled.[9]

Echoing many intersex people's concerns with pathological intersex "posers," disability activists are suspicious of transabled people, regarding them as mentally unstable "wannabes" (J.L. Davis 2012, 319) who "pretend to be disabled" (Baril 2015a, 689). "We cannot tolerate psychologically unbalanced people pretending to share our obstacles," Rob J. Quinn (quoted in Baril 2015a, 692) remarks of transabled people. Reproducing these sorts of sentiments about transabled people feeds into medical professionals' assessments of transability as an innate pathological disorder. Medical professionals diagnose transabled people as having body integrity identity disorder (BIID). Like cisgenderist logics, transability is presumed to be a disorder insofar as the desire to transition one's abilities, identity, or physical characteristics is believed to be "less normal than a lack of desire to do so" (Baril 2015a, 698). The desire to change or not change one's body-mind traits or dis/abilities is not more or less natural or normal. Deeming one desire more normal is a cultural and ideological declaration, not an objective assessment. Further, Baril (2015a) notes that rejecting transabled people because they are "psychologically unbalanced" undermines the work done by many disability and mad activists who advocate for "mad" or mentally disabled people and fight against sanism.[10] Nevertheless, disability activists consistently exclude transabled people.

If we take earnestly the idea that presumed endosex people who claim to be intersex are transabled, then intersex activists' assertion that these people are pathological liars not only fuels the cisgenderist idea that trans people are maliciously deceitful but also fuels the medical industry's assessment that the desire to change one's traits or dis/abilities is unnatural. If, as I have argued thus far, intersex activism and scholarship ought to align with disability activism and scholarship, avoiding indirectly undermining disability and mad activists' anti-sanist work ought to be important. The transabled *and* transgender phenomena can also help intersex activists to draw attention to a paradox with medical professionals' approach to "disordered" people: they presume that one's lack of desire to change one's physical characteristics and abilities is normal, yet they impose such changes on intersex people. And they do so precisely because intersex variations are construed as disabled, disordered, or diseased.

As noted above, some intersex activists are concerned that people who "lie" about being intersex online take valuable space and resources away from "real" intersex people who need them. Similarly, many disabled activists maintain that transabled people "steal resources from disabled people" (Baril 2015a, 689). Resources for both intersex and disabled people are scarce. They are, however, not inevitably scarce. Rather than attempting to "establish hierarchies and priorities" – hierarchies of belonging and suffering – anti-interphobic, anti-ableist, and anti-sanist activists "must fight against political and economic austerity" (Baril 2015a, 693). Intersex activists have demonstrated that anti-interphobic resources and professional psychological support are not inevitably scarce. These resources and support are often actively hidden by medical professionals and denied to intersex people in need. Many medical professionals have consistently denied anti-interphobic resources and support to intersex people and their parents/proxies because these resources effectively undermine their authority and the "need" for curative violence.[11] Given the lack of anti-interphobic support offered by medical practitioners, an exorbitant amount of resources, support, and emotional labour is offered by intersex people themselves. The labour performed by these intersex people is invaluable and helps intersex communities to grow and strengthen. However, these folks likely cannot do this labour constantly without burning out. Resources and labour may seem scarce, but anti-interphobic support is not inevitably scarce. Medical professionals' approach to intersex ensures that these resources are inaccessible to many. Rather than attempting to establish priority and belonging hierarchies that will not contribute to systemic change, working to ensure that medical professionals who deny and withhold vital resources are held accountable is imperative.

Claiming an identity is an ethically complicated decision that requires accountability and a critical examination of the social, material, historical, and political power relations that mould the identity in question. From what has been recounted thus far, making this decision is not always taken as seriously as it ought to be by some people who claim intersex status. Nevertheless, Viloria (2017, 328–29) is wary that policing people's identities reproduces biological essentialism:

> I also don't think anyone has the right to tell another person that they have to be born with certain sex characteristics in order to identify as the gender associated with those sex characteristics. In fact, intersex people are living proof that gender doesn't always match biological sex. People with CAIS [complete androgen insensitivity syndrome], for example, are always assigned the female sex at birth, because they "look like" women [on the outside], despite their male biology [i.e., undescended testes] – so even the term *sex* does not always refer to actual biological sex, but gender! Therefore, at the risk of provoking the wrath of biological determinists, I feel compelled to point out that if both trans and intersex people demonstrate that neither sex nor gender is determined by one's biological sex at birth, why does being intersex have to be determined this way? ... I don't need people to prove that they're intersex.

Viloria's reasons for refusing to police how people identify are politically and theoretically compelling. If one is invested in anti-essentialism and recognizes how anti-essentialism figures in intersex, trans, queer, and disability scholarship and activism, policing who is (not) or who should (not) identify as, for example, intersex, endosex, trans, woman, man, genderqueer, nonbinary, dis/abled, or disordered becomes quite tricky, arguably indefensible. Moreover, the ways that some intersex, endosex, trans, genderqueer, nonbinary, disabled, or disordered people choose and consent to alter their body-minds for affirming or healing purposes should prompt us to reconsider where the supposed intersex-endosex and disabled-enabled boundaries are drawn. As noted above, these borders only get blurrier when a supposed endosex person identifies as intersex and undergoes confirmation procedures to approximate a certain intersex variation.

Moreover, even though disability studies scholars and anti-ableist activists have deftly challenged and blurred the disabled-enabled binary, the binary becomes rigid when transabled people seek to be included. Likewise, even though intersex studies scholars and intersex activists have challenged and blurred the endosex-intersex binary, the binary becomes rigid when an ostensible endosex person desires to identify as intersex and to be included. Attempting to reaffirm these rigid binaries by excluding people, policing how they identify, or policing how they may desire to modify their dis/abilities and anatomical traits undermines the ground-breaking theoretical work done by these scholars and activists; doing so feeds back into the essentializing of gender, sex, dis/ability, and body-mind traits.

According to some intersex activists and scholars, intersex "posers" fetishize and appropriate intersex people's experiences of oppression (Cadet and Feldman 2012; Marquez 2019a, 2019b). Transabled people are also often construed as "fetishizing, or appropriating marginalized realities" (Baril 2015a, 689). Rather than using the language of fetishization or appropriation, Viloria (2017, 328) suggests that a greater number of people wanting to identify as intersex is a positive thing and can do some important anti-interphobic work: "In the *long run,* given that intersex babies are operated on precisely because people think it's an undesirable way to be, it seems far from hurtful if adults who weren't born intersex nevertheless *want* to be identified as intersex. It demonstrates that it's actually something desirable (which personally I believe)." Viloria's position echoes that of both Bethany Stevens (2011), who writes that "transabled people depart from ableist compulsions 'to never want to be disabled,'" and Baril (2015a, 700), who states that transabled folks "disrupt metanarratives of disability as an undesired condition." Transabled individuals undercut the idea that no one would voluntarily want to occupy this marginalized position. Presumed endosex people who want to or do claim intersex depart from the interphobic assumption that being intersex is a terrible existence and, therefore, that no one would voluntarily desire or decide to be intersex. Or, if we regard these ostensible endosex folks who claim to be intersex as transabled because intersex is deemed a disability, they undermine both ableist and interphobic narratives.

The logical limits of excluding transabled people from disability spaces and, by extension, transabled "endosex" people from intersex spaces are further demonstrated by Baril's (2015a, 699) apt analysis of the exclusion of trans women from women's spaces:

> Just as trans women are not considered women (refusal of self-definition) and are accused of being men with male privilege who fetishize femininity, appropriate women's minoritized experience, and infiltrate women-only

spaces as sexual predators, transabled people are refused self-definition and perceived as able-bodied individuals with able-bodied privilege who fetishize disability, appropriate disabled people's minoritized experience, and infiltrate disabled people's groups to sate their perverse desires ... If trans people are often refused membership in the categories men/women, it is because an ontology of what men and women are regulates their exclusion. According to these ontological criteria, some men/women are real, authentic, and legitimate, while others are not.

This sex/gender ontology is deeply rooted in cisgenderist biological essentialism and functions to exclude trans people, deny their genders, and deem them dangerous fetishists. A similar ontology – the "ontology of disability" (Baril 2015a, 700) – controls understandings of disability. This ontology demands that disabled people have specific physical realities, traits, requirements, and experiences. Instead of feeding into this essentializing and limited ontology, Baril (2015a, 700) maintains that transabled people ought to be included: one should resist the "limited definition of what 'real' disabilities are and encourage a broader 'disabled' category that includes the experience of disabled people who fall outside the dominant ontology." Broadening this "ontology of disability" prompts one to reconsider transabled people's active exclusion, alleged endosex people's claims to intersex, and the overlap between disability, intersex, and trans identities, realities, and embodiments.

Like Baril, I sympathize with disability activists' disquiet with transabled people. Equally, I am sympathetic to intersex activists' worries regarding supposed endosex people claiming to be intersex. These activists share genuine reservations. Yet I am inspired by anti-essentialist arguments (Viloria 2017) and by Baril's (2015a, 695–96) observation that exclusion is "not an effective means to fight oppression. Violence towards transabled people does nothing to advance the battle against ableism." Hatred aimed at people perceived to be not intersex, not intersex enough, not disabled enough, or not traumatized enough is not a reliable tool to wield in the battle against intersecting forms of oppression and compulsory modes of being.

Conclusion

The apparently distinct category "intersex" breaks down when one scrutinizes what characteristics count as intersex, endosex, female, and male. Many scholars, medical professionals, and activists continue to draw (inconsistent) ideological, literal, and statistical lines between intersex and endosex and, in turn, between disabled and enabled. Yet, trying to contain these leaky, ever-shifting categories in an indisputable or unproblematic way is impossible. These lines cannot be drawn because people's anatomies are infinitely different. Morgan Holmes (2002, 175) notes, "When we appreciate that the difference between intersex and not intersexed can be only millimetres it seems clear that no one is truly intersex, but we are all, in our infinite differences from each other, intersexed." Likewise, when we appreciate that one can go decades, even an entire lifetime, without knowing that one has intersex traits and that one is not, as presumed, endosex, it seems clear that no one is truly endosex but rather that we all are, in our infinite differences, (not) intersex and endosex.

Human biologies are endlessly diverse. Hence, a boundary between endosex and intersex cannot be definitively and straightforwardly drawn because biological sex is a social construction informed by interphobia, ableism, racism, queerphobia, and sexism. Intersex is, after all, "nothing more than a perpetually shifting phantasm in the collective psyche of medicine and culture ... Intersexuality is a historical and cultural construction rather than a simple biological phenomenon" (Holmes 2002, 175). Therefore, who is (not) classified as intersex can and does vary depending on who is looking and what ideologies inform the gaze (Kessler 1998). As demonstrated by European colonizers' and scholars' racist and sexist evaluations of sexually "ambiguous" women of colour, both when and where evaluations are made have lasting and far-reaching impacts.

Intersex and endosex categories are continually kaleidoscopic discursive phantasms attached to certain people's body-minds, typically in order to maintain intersecting forms of oppression and compulsory modes of being. However, given that biological sex is a social construction, it can be – and is being – contested and restructured for anti-discriminatory purposes. Consequently, rather than attempting to maintain a rigid binary between endosex-as-enabled and intersex-as-disabled, I propose attending to the fact that definitive/objective endosex or intersex biology is an illusion. Intersex and/as/is/with disability is an elusive queering, cripping ghost that haunts all people. And if this spectre wants to be welcomed and claimed by presumed outsiders, there is radical political potential in exploring the pragmatic and theoretical benefits of said claims while maintaining anti-discriminatory ideologies. As people learn more about human biological diversity, as scholars and activists undermine biological essentialism, and as people engage more with medical technologies, it is revealed that there never was and never will be clear male-intersex-female, male-female, inter-sex-endosex, and disabled-enabled boundaries. Expanding – not limiting – how people's body-minds and identities are conceptualized is imperative.

5

Cripping Sport Sex Testing

In 2009, South African middle-distance track athlete Caster Semenya (b. 1991) was subjected to sport sex testing after her victory at the Berlin Olympics. Despite the fact that her test results were not officially made public, numerous news forums claimed to know her biology and published intimate details of her biology in articles with headlines like "Caster Semenya 'Is a Hermaphrodite,' Tests Show" (Hart 2009), "Caster Semenya Has Male Sex Organs and No Womb or Ovaries" (Hurst 2009), and "Semenya, Forced to Take Gender Test, Is a Woman ... and a Man" (Yaniv 2009). Like Semenya, other middle-distance women athletes – such as Santhi Soundarajan (b. 1981) of India, Annet Negesa (b. 1992) of Uganda, Francine Niyonsaba (b. 1993) of Burundi, Margaret Wambui (b. 1995) of Kenya, and Dutee Chand (b. 1996) of India – have been caught in the crossfire of sport sex-testing controversies, have been subjected to sex testing, and/or have publicly spoken out about how sport officials have pressured them to undergo "corrective" medical interventions, including disabling irreversible surgeries that constitute intersex genital mutilation (IGM).[1] Given that the intersex spectre haunts all people and is not bound to racial or geographical borders, why are women of colour in colonized nations of the Global South who run track at elite levels targeted for sport testing? Why are these specific athletes so central in mainstream representations of the pathologization of intersex variations? How can one effectively unpack the intersections of sport, track, intersex, gender, race, pathologization, dis/ability, location, colonization, and citizenship?

To answer these queries, I trace past and present sport sex-testing practices. I discuss the reasoning that sport governing bodies have used to justify sport sex testing as well as to render athletes (suspect) intersex. Over the decades, women athletes in particular nations have been targeted by sex testing and publicly slandered. Not all women and nations have been or currently are equally beset, maligned, and rendered (suspect) intersex. This history illustrates that anxieties about sex and gender shift and expand depending on the global political climate. Since the early 2000s, women athletes of colour in colonized nations of the Global South who run middle-distance track have been targeted and presumed to be intersex or gender-deceivers who cheat or have an unfair advantage. I determine that sex testing functions as a complex political multi-tool that aids in projects of war, colonialism, imperialism, sexism, racism, interphobia, and ableism. In other words, the employment of sex testing and the current targeting of these particular women athletes of colour reveal that sport sex testing not only upholds compulsory dyadism but is also a colonial tool and practice.

The shifting target – who and what nations are targeted – prompts me to question the presumed investment in the idea that sport sex testing ensures fairness. Despite the uneven deployment of sex testing, does sport sex testing make sport fair? Does it – or does it have the potential – to level the playing field? I determine that sport sex testing is fundamentally anti-science and does not and cannot ensure fairness. The evidence used to justify sex testing is not based in theoretically or methodologically sound medico-scientific evidence. In the name of "fairness" and "objective" science, compulsory dyadism, sexism, interphobia, racism, colonialism, and imperialism literally converge on and infiltrate these women athletes' body-minds and nations. That is to say, these discriminatory models are perpetuated and institutionalized by sport legislation.

This chapter concludes by asking, "What can a disability studies lens bring to sport sex-testing controversies? What would it look like to crip this site of compulsory dyadism?" Analyzing sport sex testing through a disability lens may seem like an unusual inclination. World-class athletes and Olympians are not typically construed as or imagined to be disabled, and (suspect) intersex athletes are presumed to have an unfair advantage. Nevertheless, cripping sport sex testing uncovers a troubling discrepancy: intersex is represented as an inherent, degenerate lack and is pathologized as a disorder, disability, or disease by medical professionals outside of sport contexts, whereas intersex traits are represented as both disordered, disabled, or diseased and (unfair) advantages inside of sports contexts. Cripping this site of compulsory dyadism provides the necessary tools for identifying the discriminatory and anti-scientific il/logics that sport governing bodies employ to uphold sex testing. Since these beliefs are the scaffolding that upholds this practice, sport must be cripped, queered, and decolonized. Sport sex testing must be abolished.

History of and Justification for Sport Sex Testing

The intersex spectre haunts all people. Nevertheless, the spectre is not represented as such. Looking at sport policies, particularly sex testing, highlights this representational discrepancy. In sport, the spectre seems to move and occupy different nations, people's body-minds, and geographical borders depending on the broader political climate. Sport sex-testing policies are strategically employed to maintain numerous discriminatory ideologies as well as to advance Western nations' political and economic goals.

During the 1920s, the first decade of the interwar period, women were entering the traditionally male domain of sport like never before.[2] Due to the belief that "real" or "hegemonic femininity" and athleticism were paradoxical (Krane 2001, 115) given that a "real" woman could not possibly excel in sport, many women athletes' sex and gender were called into question. When a woman athlete was deemed "too" masculine, muscular, or athletically inclined, the International Association of Athletics Federations (IAAF) and the International Olympic Committee (IOC) required a physical examination to "confirm" her sex and, therefore, her gender and ability to compete fairly. Decades later, in 1966, all women athletes, not just "suspect" athletes, were subjected to humiliating physical examinations that consisted of "nude parades." In the name of protecting women from male impersonators – who, it is implied, are innately physically superior to women and therefore will inevitably win – women athletes were required to "parade nude in front of a panel of doctors" (Cooper 2010, 246).[3]

Professor of sport management Lindsay Parks Pieper (2014) notes that there is only one case of a German man, Hermann Ratjen, masquerading as a woman, which occurred at the 1936 Berlin Olympics. Nazi Germany hoped that the Olympics would be a political showcase of their superiority. With the aim of winning the most medals, the Nazi regime instructed Ratjen, a Hitler Youth member, to live and compete as a woman. Adopting the name Dora, he lived and trained as a woman for three years. I cannot help but draw attention to the cognitive dissonance inherent in a queerphobic, sexist Nazi regime ordering Ratjen to cross-dress for years in order to prove the essential superior nature of the German people. At the Olympics, Ratjen did not win Germany a medal. This one case was not adequate to justify the institutionalization of demeaning nude parades. Nevertheless, these parades were instituted policy.

This "protectionist discourse" served to justify the invasion of women's privacy and body-minds with impunity (Dworkin and Cooky 2012, 22). The institutionalization of sex testing was not established to reflect innate physical capacities and differences between men and women but rather to preserve "images of male superiority" (McDonagh and Pappano 2008, 17).[4] As illustrated by countless scholars for decades, the belief that women are innately inferior at sport and must be protected from competing against men, trans women (who are presumed to be men by sport organizations), and "masculinized" intersex women has led to decades of literal, discursive, and symbolic violence against women athletes, including the underfunding of women's sport, markedly less women's sport coverage, sexist and objectifying sport commentary, queerphobic and interphobic sport commentary, inequitable gendered pay, and of course, sex testing.[5]

In 1967, a year after nude parades were instituted, they were abolished. Individual gynecological exams took their place (Simpson et al. 2000). Again, only women were subjected to such tests because the unsubstantiated belief that men are inherently better at sport persisted. After women athletes spoke out about how humiliating and intrusive these examinations were, the tests were changed again in 1968. Women athletes were then required to undergo a chromatin test in order to ensure that they had XX "female" chromosomes (Simpson et al. 2000). The aim was to test for "male pseudohermaphroditism," characterized by "feminized" external genitalia and the presence of a Y chromosome. Many scholars and scientists critiqued the test. Indeed, instead of the expected XX or XY chromosomes, some individuals have variations such as XXY, XO, and XXXY, some women have XY chromosomes, and some men have XX chromosomes. Ultimately, mounting evidence suggested that sex cannot be reduced to chromosomes and that sex is not definitely or objectively definable or dyadic. The IAAF stopped sex testing women athletes with chromatin tests in 1991. In 2000, the IOC followed suit.

Although in mainstream culture the myth persists that sex chromosomes are dyadic (i.e., XX and XY) and that they reveal one's "true" sex, this myth has been debunked for decades. Testosterone levels then became, and remain, the focus of the IAAF and the IOC and of conversations about sport. Exercise physiologist and sport science writer Ross Tucker (2017) explains that after Semenya was sex tested in 2009, "the IAAF response was to create a hyperandrogen policy." The policy required woman athletes to have testosterone levels below 10 nmol/L for at least twelve months prior to competition. It is important to note that people's testosterone levels fluctuate throughout the day and throughout their lives due to, for example, puberty, aging, pregnancy, depression, weight, illness, and mal/nutrition. Moreover, some women with XX chromosomes have naturally elevated testosterone levels, and some women with XY chromosomes have a natural insensitivity to testosterone. Nevertheless, at this time, the IAAF maintained that "normal" men have levels at or above 10.5 nmol/L and that "normal" women have levels that range from 0.1 to 2.8 nmol/L. Even if these are statistically average levels and account for how people's testosterone levels vary throughout their lives, it does not follow that men and women who fall outside of them (for whatever reason) "fail" their gender or are inherently abnormal, unfairly advantaged, or pathological. Yet the IAAF's proposed guidelines dictated that women had to maintain levels below 10 nmol/L because women with polycystic ovary syndrome have an average testosterone level of 4.5 nmol/L. To represent extreme outliers, the IAAF considered raising the level to 7.5 nmol/L. Further research revealed that if this level was the instituted standard, 16 out of 1,000 women athletes would be required to undergo hormone replacement therapy (HRT) for twelve months prior to competition. This number seemed much too high, so the IAAF settled on 10 nmol/L, a level supposedly "just below the bottom end of the normal male range" (Tucker 2017). The fact that the cut-off of 10 nmol/L was quite arbitrary is clear. Yet the IAAF remained invested in the idea that to be a "real" woman, one must have certain biological formations, even if people's biologies do not and cannot reflect the cultural ideology of "real" woman or compulsory dyadism.

When testosterone became the focus, sport governing bodies sought to expose women athletes with high levels of testosterone due to intersex traits that lead to hyperandrogenism, a biological variation that is characterized by naturally high levels of androgens. However, not all women athletes' testosterone levels were or are tested. Rather, Emily J. Cooper (2010, 247) explains in *The Journal of Gender, Race, and Justice*, the IOC and IAAF retained "the right to examine female athletes that raise suspicion." As explained in the IAAF's (2011, 3) regulations, "the IAAF Medical Manager may initiate a confidential investigation of any female athlete if *he* has reasonable grounds for believing that a case of hyperandrogenism may exist" (emphasis added). The "reasonable grounds" were overwhelming applied to women who appeared "too" muscular, manly, athletically inclined, and racialized. Additionally, the medical manager assessing these women's body-minds and claims to womanhood is presumed to be a man.

"The violation of privacy," anthropologist and bioethicist Katrina Karkazis (2016b) remarks, "has taken place in ways horrifying and yet predictable." Rebecca Jordan-Young and Karkazis (2012) explain that this violation was predictable given that privacy is "implicitly reserved for socially-privileged groups (male, white, heterosexual), and that living outside these interlocking privileges means inhabiting a body that is always, to some extent, 'public' and available for scrutiny, probing, and coercion" – available to be subjected to irreversible procedures. As a result, unfortunately to no surprise, specific women athletes' privacy was consistently violated. Indeed, several women athletes with intersex traits have been coerced into undergoing medically unnecessary partial clitorectomies and/or gonadectomies to become "proper" women and, therefore, "properly" competition-ready (Jordan-Young, Sönksen, and Karkazis 2014). That is, even though testosterone was the supposed culprit, many women athletes were coerced into undergoing other forms of curative violence. Annet Negesa is one of these athletes. Negesa was a hopeful 800-metre candidate for the 2012 Olympics. If she wanted to compete and avoid being banned from sport, she had to undergo medical interventions. Negesa (quoted in T. Morgan 2019) reports that her doctors coerced her into agreeing to a procedure that they did not fully explain: "They told me it was kind of an injection, they were pulling out my testosterone ... But that's not what they did. When I woke up in the morning, I had wounds." The doctors subjected Negesa to a gonadectomy. Negesa never competed again and now must take HRT for the rest of her life and live with the potentially disabling long-term consequences. Another athlete, who remains anonymous because she fears for her safety, reports that "doctors said she had no other option than undergoing the surgery" (in T. Morgan 2019). Since the surgery, she has dealt with depression and bone loss due to hormone deficiencies. She explains, "I have thought about killing myself ... They stole my life, my existence. Just like that they took away my dream" (quoted in T. Morgan 2019). Without a doubt, these procedures did not cure these women of anything or make them "properly" competition-ready. The interventions effectively removed them from competition and gratuitously harmed, traumatized, and disabled them. In addition to possibly being subjected to curative violence, many athletes have seen their identities, athletic achievements, and careers publicly challenged and disparaged. Their lives and dreams have been dashed.

As the specific sex tests changed and attempted to re/stabilize compulsory dyadism, the justification for testing also changed. However, the supposed investment in fairness has remained constant. No longer do sex tests "protect" women athletes from supposedly superior masquerading male athletes, but instead women athletes need to be protected from other women: sex/gender-deceiving trans and intersex women athletes with "unfair" masculine advantages. Due to the belief that men are inherently better at sport because of their testosterone levels, women athletes' spectral "masculine" intersex characteristics must be "discovered" and exorcised because said characteristics give them an unfair advantage over endosex cis women athletes. The idea that women athletes with intersex variations deceive the sports community is a contemporary iteration of the old trope that "hermaphrodites" are "deliberately deceptive or shady" (Reis 2005, 412). Rather than misleading, cheating, or seeking an unfair advantage, these athletes simply want and deserve to compete without violent commentary, humiliating tests, or curative violence to make them "real" women and "fair" competitors.

The concern with inter/sex un/fairness, historically and currently, has been primarily restricted to women who compete in track and field events (Hargreaves 2003; Pieper 2014, 2016).[6] There was a moral panic when women began entering sports arenas in the early twentieth century. The panic was especially intense around track and field because these events were particularly associated with masculinity and masculine achievement. The public, male athletes, male sport organizers, and institutions like the IOC and the IAAF were distressed about women entering this masculine arena. They were also troubled by how women looked when they participated in track and field events. Whereas athletes' (sexed and gendered) physiques are usually more covered up to face the cold climate and/or potential injury in winter sports (e.g., ice hockey, skiing, and snowboarding), athletes' bodies are more readily visible in track and field. Track and field athletes wear less clothing due to the weather and the unique demands of the sport. And due to track and field's physical and clothing requirements, women who participated in the sport looked strong, muscular, capable, dynamic, and therefore supposedly ugly, masculine, and unfeminine (Pieper 2016). Indeed, people where distressed by women's "ugly" noises and by the "unladylike" facial expressions that they made while competing. Women track athletes' noises, expressions, and strong, muscular bodies were not fulfilling or reproducing sexist standards of feminine beauty when they performed such physically demanding sports. They undermined hegemonic feminine ideals about what women should look like and be capable of doing.

Medical professionals worked to legitimize this panic about women entering track and field. Sport sociologist Jennifer Hargreaves (2003, 131) explains, "Because of the intrinsically vigorous nature of running, jumping and throwing events, female athletes [in track and field] were particularly vulnerable to reactionary medical arguments." Many medical professionals rationalized that women should not participate – and encouraged them not to participate – in track and field because doing so would be bad for their health. Pieper (2016, 16) writes that doctors "not only suggested that the sport harmed women's health and damaged the female physique but also specifically described its detrimental effects on reproduction." These were sexist, compulsory reproductive medical standards of femininity and were not scientifically sound. Yet these standards continue to effect women athletes in all sports: many are encouraged to appear "sexy" and heterosexual, to appeal to the hegemonic male gaze, and not to get "too" muscular or manly (Krane 2001).

Historically, women who defiantly entered track and field events faced social and medical scrutiny, opposition, and suspicion. Currently, women who enter track and field face essentially the same scrutiny and must contend with the IAAF and the IOC if they want to participate in "sport megaevents" (Horne 2012, 31) and, in turn, to make a living and/or gain sponsors. The current sex testing policies, outlined below, unequivocally illustrate that this targeted suspicion continues to this day for women track athletes. This history contextualizes why sex testing concerns typically vanish from cultural consciousness when it comes to the Winter Olympics and to most summer sports events (e.g., diving and volleyball) and why track athletes have been and remain the primary target of sex/gender speculation. The current regulations and policies are a continuation of this discriminatory history. The fact that the moral panic around sex testing is primarily a social issue, not a scientific or medical issue, is clear.

Finding and aiming to destroy or level the intersex spectre in the name of fairness is allegedly the central goal of sex testing suspect women. The spectre apparently must be found and exorcised to, as explained by the IAAF (2018, 1), "ensure fair and meaningful competition"; the IAAF will not risk "having unfair competition conditions that deny athletes a fair opportunity to succeed." However, numerous studies and scholars demonstrate that sport has never been, and never could be, a level playing field.[7] As gender, sport, and health studies scholars Cheryl Cooky and Shari L. Dworkin (2013, 107) confirm, "sport as a level playing field is neither an organizational reality nor a possibility, given the historical and contemporary social, economic, and cultural arrangements of sport." There is no concern with fairness when certain athletes in wealthier countries, neighbourhoods, or families have (or have had their entire lives) greater access to expensive training, technology, nourishing food, equipment, and health care. Likewise, sport is never a level playing field because committees do not and cannot police all the "myriad physical advantages that are not available to nor attainable by all athletes" (Cooky and Dworkin 2013, 107). Such physical advantages include extreme tallness (diagnosed as acromegaly), as with retired professional basketball player Kenny George Jr. (b. 1986), and increased hemoglobin levels and oxygen capacity (diagnosed as congenital polycythemia), as with decorated Olympic cross-country skier Eero Mäntyranta (1937–2013). There is no concern with fairness when it comes to these sorts of advantages or "disorders." Concern spikes when assumed advantages come from one's "disordered" or "disabled" sex. That is, concern spikes when there is a challenge to compulsory dyadism and sexist ideals about what women are physically capable of.

This disquiet is evident when one considers the fact that Caster Semenya's assumed intersex advantage is punished, whereas former[8] elite competitive swimmer Michael Phelps's indisputable advantages of a long wingspan, double-jointed ankles and elbows, and low levels of lactic acid production are celebrated (Cooper 2010). Semenya's supposed advantage cannot be proven, yet she is disparaged for seemingly having the perfect body for running. Phelps's "perfect body for swimming" and all of his "physical advantages" are indisputable *and* admired; he is, after all, known as the "Flying Fish" (De Bellefonds 2019). The IOC certainly never tried to level Phelps's embodied advantages in the name of fairness. The fact that sport governing institutions and viewers of sport appear to be invested in fair play only when it comes to supposed disordered or disabled sex suggests that the discourse of fair play functions primarily as a guise for exclusionary and discriminatory policies.

Policies that sought to regulate women athletes' testosterone levels did not go unchallenged. In line with the IOC's and the IAAF's testosterone regulations, Dutee Chand was dropped from the Commonwealth Games in 2014 because she "failed" a sex test. The test became public knowledge, and she was banned from sport. The Indian government appealed to the

Court of Arbitration for Sport (CAS) to contest Chand's exclusion and the hyperandrogenism policies. A long case between Chand and the IAAF ensued. Due to the case, the CAS suspended the hyperandrogenism rules in July 2015. The CAS provided the IAAF with two years to submit scientifically sound evidence to justify the rules that excluded women athletes like Chand. The final date to submit evidence was initially July 24, 2017. The IAAF submitted inconclusive evidence before this date. The date to submit evidence was then extended to September 28, 2017 (Court of Arbitration for Sport 2017). Unless new evidence tabled within this timeframe convinced the court that these athletes have an unfair advantage, "the Hypoandrogenism Regulations [would] be declared void" (Court of Arbitration for Sport 2017). Commenting on the situation, Joanna Harper (quoted in Tucker 2016), an adviser on gender issues to the IOC, reported that the IAAF's lawyers "are working to reverse that verdict. Since I am involved with the case, I will have no further comment on it." Yet, commenting further, Harper revealed, "If the IAAF ultimately loses the case, I believe they will try to come up with some other way to place limits on who gets to compete in women's sport." Not only did Harper express that women athletes with intersex traits should be excluded from participating, but she also disclosed that the IAAF was clearly not invested in sound scientific evidence. If evidence demonstrated that these women should not be barred, the IAAF would work to exclude them anyway.

In relation to the suspended rule, in 2016 *Outsports* obtained a copy of the IOC's new proposed guidelines that would loosen restrictions concerning trans athletes *and* women athletes with hyperandrogenism (Zeigler 2016b). There were two potential changes. First, the new guidelines would not mandate compulsory surgery for trans or intersex athletes. Second, whereas trans men would be able to compete without restriction, trans women and women with hyperandrogenism would be required to maintain testosterone levels below 10 nmol/L for at least twelve months prior to competition. I commend the ruling that trans men would be able to compete without restriction. Yet, given the asymmetry in the policy, the ruling is clearly rooted in cisgenderist ideologies. The ruling suggests that trans men are women and therefore do not really pose an athletic threat to "real" cis men, the idea being that trans men will probably lose anyway. The ruling suggests that trans and intersex women are men or not really women and, therefore, have an unfair "manly" advantage and threaten "real" cis, endosex women; they will supposedly inevitably win.

As the two-year suspension drew near and the possibility of loosened restrictions seemed imminent, a methodologically dubious study was published and used to support the IAAF's hyperandrogenism regulations (Bermon and Garnier 2017). Forty-three track and field events were studied, and the subjects included "athletes competing at the highest level in the different track and field events (of which there are 21 for females and 22 for males)" (Bermon and Garnier 2017, 2). The study's authors, Stéphane Bermon and Pierre-Yves Garnier (2017), conclude that there are five events in which women with higher levels of testosterone have a significant advantage: 400 metres, 400-metre hurdles, 800 metres, hammer throw, and pole vault. The authors propose that women athletes with naturally high levels of testosterone have an unfair advantage. Not only is the study steeped in evident conflicts of interest – it was funded by the IAAF, and one of the authors, Bermon, works for the IAAF – but the study's methodological analysis is also unsound, and the findings, therefore, are invalid (Jordan-Young and Karkazis 2019). As explained by epidemiologist Gideon Meyerowitz-Katz (2017), when Bermon and Garnier ran their statistical analyses, they failed to perform an "adjustment for multiple comparisons" in order to check whether the significance was real or an "artifact of chance":

> There is a good chance that this [i.e., the study's outcome] was just down to luck. So I went through the paper and ran ... a Bonferroni Correction. What this basically does is raise the bar for statistical significance according to the number of tests that had been done. According to these results, none of them are actually significant ... [In the study,] you'll notice that there are 16 insignificant results, many of which had women with *low* levels beating women with high levels. From these results we could just as easily conclude that, for the majority of athletic events, testosterone levels had no impact on performance whatsoever.

Elsewhere, Karkazis and Meyerowitz-Katz (2017) write, "None of these results were statistically significant, but they nevertheless show that 'significant competitive advantage' was not evidenced across the board." Statistician Andrew Gelman (2017) also comments on the study that "the statistical analysis data processing in this paper is such a mess that I can't really figure out what data they are working with, what exactly they are doing, or the connection between some of their analyses and their scientific goals ... The analysis in that paper is so tangled." Given that the statistics contradict Bermon and Garnier's conclusions about unfair advantages, Gelman shrewdly suggests that they should "leave the data analysis to others." Even though the study is highly problematic, it is "ratcheting up what it takes to be a woman athlete" (Orr and Watson 2018, 34).

Not only is the study unsound, but one of the main premises – testosterone determines one's success in sport – is also utterly unfounded. This taken-for-granted belief about testosterone and its link to athleticism is not based on science. "Testosterone is not the master molecule of athleticism. One glaring clue," Jordan-Young and Karkazis (2012) verify, "is that women whose tissues do not respond to testosterone at all are actually overrepresented among elite athletes. As counterintuitive as it might seem, there is no evidence that successful athletes have higher testosterone levels than less successful ones." Indeed, some women athletes – those with the intersex variation partial androgen insensitivity syndrome (PAIS) or complete androgen insensitivity syndrome (CAIS) – have very high levels of testosterone but are partially or completely insensitive to testosterone and, nevertheless, prove to be competitive athletes. In addition, high levels of testosterone could indicate that one's body is not effective at using the testosterone, so the body produces more to compensate (Jordan-Young and Karkazis 2019). In fact, a proper analysis of Bermon and Garnier's study illustrates that women with low testosterone levels often beat women with high levels (Jordan-Young and Karkazis 2019). That said, this aspect of the study clearly did not inform the IAAF's regulations, indicating that fairness and meaningful competition are not the real aim of these regulations.

Despite what the science indicates, some insist that when an athlete's naturally high testosterone levels are lowered and she performs worse, this outcome proves that her testosterone levels gave her an unfair advantage. Addressing this concern, Jordan-Young and Karkazis (2019, 196) explain,

> A woman might perform better with her natural level and perform more poorly if her T levels are artificially lowered, but that isn't grounds for concluding that T levels are responsible for performance differences between women athletes. Among other possibilities, the drop in performance might be attributable to the many side effects and physiological changes that go along with dramatically lowering T.

In other words, correlation does not equal causation. When people's tissues have been habituated to higher testosterone levels since puberty and then their hormonal climate quickly and dramatically is artificially changed, their ability to function like they previously did is radically altered: "It's not the fact that T is low, it's the fact that T dramatically dropped from those individuals' previous hormonal environment" (Jordan-Young and Karkazis 2019, 191). As discussed in previous chapters, altering peoples' hormonal environment can be risky and disabling and can have profound impacts on their body-minds, particularly when they do not want to change – possibly irreversibly change – their body-minds. Ultimately, one's athletic abilities cannot be reduced to one's testosterone levels. There is no evidence to suggest that athletic abilities are purely a matter of, or exclusively extend from, sex (however sex is defined). Ultimately, barring athletes who are trans women and athletes with certain intersex variations from participating in their sport if their physical attributes do not conform to cisgenderist, sexist, and interphobic standards of femininity is not only institutionalized discrimination but also *anti-science*.

By the deadline of September 28, 2017, there had been no public announcement about the IAAF's case nor a definitive ruling. It seemed that the jury remained out as the IAAF waited until it could assert that women with hyperandrogenism are unfairly advantaged. At the time, one could only assume, as Harper predicted, that dates were pushed again because the IAAF was trying to find any way to prevent intersex women athletes from competing. The IOC, however, needed to speak to the policies, as the 2018 Winter Olympics in Pyeongchang were approaching. The IOC (Carr 2017) reported that there would be no regulations because it was still waiting for the Chand case to be resolved. Although concerns about sex testing and fears of intersex-cheating women seemed to vanish from cultural consciousness during the Winter Olympics, this was undoubtedly good news for some of the athletes who participated.

Finally, in late April 2018, the IAAF released the new regulations, which were to take effect on November 1, 2018, if the CAS approved. Like previous policies, the 2018 policy notes that "the IAAF Medical Manager may investigate at any time" so long as this person is "acting in good faith and on reasonable grounds" (IAAF 2018, 4–5). Unlike previous regulations, in order for a woman to be eligible to compete, "she must reduce her blood testosterone level to below five (5) nmol/L for a continuous period of at least six months (e.g., by use of hormonal contraceptives); and ... therefore she must maintain her blood testosterone level below five (5) nmol/L continuously (i.e., whether she is in competition or out of competition) for so long as she wishes to remain eligibile to compete" (IAAF 2018, 3). The IAAF cut the acceptable testosterone level in half. Altering its previous assertions about normal testosterone levels (outlined above), the IAAF asserted that normal women's testosterone levels range from 0.12 to 1.79 nmol/L and that normal men's levels range from 7.7 to 29.4 nmol/L. What remained the same, however, were the fact that claims about "normal" testosterone levels are quite arbitrary, the IAAF's unscientific belief that testosterone dictates one's athletic abilities, and the IAAF's investment in compulsory dyadism.

As in previous policies, not all women track and field athletes are subjected to these regulations. The regulations are clearly targeted. Contrary to Bermon and Garnier's unsound study funded by the IAAF, which claimed that there is an unfair advantage surrounding the 400 metres, 400-metre hurdles, 800 metres, hammer throw, and pole vault, the 2018 policy was restricted to "400m races, 400m hurdles races, 800m races, 1500m races, one mile races, and all other Track Events over distances between 400m and one mile" (IAAF 2018, 3). That is, events that Semenya and all of the aforementioned suspect athletes compete/d in were restricted.

Numerous scholars, activists, social commentators, and even previous IAAF members critiqued these regulations because they lacked sound scientific support and because the policies were used to target women of colour in colonized nations of the Global South (see Cherry 2018; Jordan-Young and Karkazis 2019; Orr and Watson 2018; and Shalala 2018). For example, Steve Cornelius, a professor at the University of Pretoria in the Department of Private Law, publicly resigned from the IAAF's disciplinary tribunal in protest of the discriminatory policy. Gregory Ioannidis, a colleague of Cornelius, tweeted his resignation letter on May 1, 2018, which reads in part,

> I cannot in good conscience continue to associate myself with an organization that insists on ostracizing certain individuals, all of them female, for no reason other than being what they were born to be ... On deep moral grounds I cannot see myself being part of a system in which I may well be called upon to apply regulations which I deem to be fundamentally flawed and most likely unlawful in various jurisdictions across the globe.

Cornelius also explains in the letter that he aims to "expose the warped ideology behind the new regulations." Like Cornelius, Semenya and her legal team sought to expose the warped ideology, and therefore they appealed the case.

The regulations were supposed to take effect on November 1, 2018. However, implementation of the regulations was postponed, as reported by the Associated Press (2018), "until the Court of Arbitration for Sport concludes an appeal case brought by Olympic champion Caster Semenya." The CAS was expected to give a verdict on or before March 26, 2019. It was no coincidence that the verdict date was "six months and two days before the start of the 2019 world championships in Doha, Qatar" (Associated Press 2018). That is, the women athletes who would be impacted by the ruling would have just enough time to begin HRT to become "competition-ready." Despite all the valid criticisms, an IAAF spokesperson (quoted in Associated Press 2018) remarked on the appeal, "The IAAF remains very confident of the legal, scientific, and ethical bases for the regulations, and therefore fully expects the Court of Arbitration for Sport to reject these challenges." Although a successful appeal would indicate a reinvestment in scientific proof, there was, unfortunately, good reason to doubt that the appeal would be positive given the historical precedent for sex testing.

The ruling was delayed to May 1, 2019. A few days before the ruling, the World Medical Association (WMA) (2019) held a council meeting and released a statement. Following the South African Medical Association's suggestions, the WMA demanded that the CAS withdraw the regulations and called on doctors to take no part in implementing the regulations if they were approved. The WMA explained that the regulations discriminate against intersex women athletes, run contrary to international human rights standards and medical ethics, and promote procedures that are not medically necessary and may harm athletes. The statement concluded with a quote from the WMA's president, Leonid Eidelman: "We have strong reservations about the ethical validity of these regulations. They are based on weak evidence from a single study, which is currently being widely debated by the scientific community. They are also contrary to a number of key WMA ethical statements and declarations, and as such we are calling for their immediate withdrawal."

Unfortunately, the CAS did not heed these recommendations. Semenya lost the appeal. The CAS ruled and explicitly stated that the IAAF's policies are discriminatory to intersex athletes, but it claimed that they are a necessary form of discrimination so that athletes with intersex variations do not have an unfair advantage (Dunbar 2019). In other words, as contradictory as it sounds, the CAS ruled that discrimination in sport is legal so long as it is justified (Ingle 2019). Scientists, doctors, scholars, activists, and cultural critics rightly argue that the ruling and regulations are unjustified, unfair, targeted, racist, sexist, interphobic, queerphobic, cisgenderist, and anti-science.[9]

After the ruling, the IAAF's representatives – Angelica Linden Hirschberg, Richard Auchus, and Stéphane Bermon (2019) – penned an open letter responding to the WMA's statement, which questioned the science behind the policy and noted the human rights implications. Despite the lack of science backing the policy, the IAAF's self-assured hubris is clear in the letter; it doubled down, insisting that the policy is rooted in valid science. What troubles me most about the letter are the ways that the authors co-opt seemingly pro-feminist, pro-queer, pro-consent, and care discourses to mask the anti-scientific, discriminatory nature of the policy. This co-opting of seemingly progressive discourses is particularly dangerous because the IAAF strategically positions itself as a caring – not discriminatory – institution and effectively positions its detractors as unreasonable and perhaps even discriminatory.

On behalf of the IAAF, Hirschberg, Auchus, and Bermon (2019) write that women athletes with naturally high levels of testosterone must "[reduce] serum testosterone to female levels by using a contraceptive pill (or other means)." The authors claim that disorders of sex development (DSDs) "are associated with an increased risk of cancer" and note that reducing testosterone levels "is the recognized standard of care ... These medications are gender-affirming." They continue, "If the individual has a female gender identity, a suitable form of treatment is recommended to lower the testosterone level, provided the patient accepts it herself ... In any case, it is the athlete's right to decide (in consultation with their medical team) whether or not to proceed with any assessment and/or treatment."

As explained in Chapter 1, the term "gender-affirming" is typically used by LGBTQIA2 scholars and activists to describe social and medical interactions that affirm and support trans, intersex, genderqueer, and nonbinary people's genders (e.g., gender-affirming surgery). By co-opting this expression, the IAAF positions itself as affirmative, even as it implements discriminatory policies demanding that women athletes, like Semenya, undergo medical interventions that they do not want, that they do not need, and/or that do not affirm their gender expression. Given Semenya's appeal of the policy, the IAAF's policy does not seek to affirm her gender identity but actively undermines it by claiming that she is not woman enough.

The authors also employ pro-consent rhetoric – "the athlete's right to decide" and "provided the patient accepts it" – to mask the fact that the policy creates an environment that does not leave room for one to wholly consent or refuse. An athlete cannot simply refuse an assessment or intervention because, if she does, she cannot compete. And this issue is not simply about athletes being passionate about a sport and not being allowed to participate (on discriminatory grounds), although their love for and dedication to the sport should be recognized and honoured. If one refuses to be invaded and scrutinized with impunity as well as possibly have details of her biology published, discussed, and admonished, she will be prevented from engaging in a sport that likely secures her economic well-being and possibly that of her family. Given that the women athletes of colour targeted for and subjected to sex testing are often from poor, rural regions in the Global South, their ability to fully refuse or consent is already compromised. These athletes have no real choice when their future economic well-being may hang in the balance.

That said, the letter implies that one would be unwise not to consent, noting that intersex variations "are associated with an increased risk of cancer" – the intersex spectre being supposedly a dangerous bringer of deadly disease. As explained at length in Chapter 1, claims of cancer risk are inflated and inconsistent. In fact, taking hormones for extended periods of time increases one's risk of developing certain types of cancer. Reproducing the false claim that intersex variations cause cancer frames the athlete who refuses to be investigated and "treated" as unreasonable. The IAAF implicitly asks why one would not want to exorcise the cancerous intersex spectre. According to the IAAF's logic, athletes who refuse to consent and critics of the IAAF are illogical, not the discriminatory anti-scientific policy.

To reinforce the "need" for these athletes to "consent" to "affirmation" of their gender and to avoid the supposed dangers of cancer, the IAAF tactically uses the word "medications": "These medications are gender-affirming." "Medications" implies a need, a way to heal, get better, and be cured. By using the term "medications," the authors reproduce the ableist intersex-as/is-disability medical model and, in turn, seek to justify invading athletes' body-minds and enforcing curative violence. Again, therefore, athletes who refuse ostensibly curative medications and critics of the IAAF are framed as irrational, whereas the IAAF frames itself as the healer-curer. In reality, the IAAF is the violent, interphobic exorcist.

What medications must one take to apparently become competition-ready and to prevent cancer? As discussed above, Hirschberg, Auchus, and Bermon (2019) note that under the IAAF's (2019) official regulations, athletes who "consent" must "[reduce] serum testosterone to female levels by using a contraceptive pill (or other means)." The fact that the IAAF consistently offers only one example of a means to reduce testosterone and strategically brackets "or other means" functions to de-emphasize the invasive, possibly disabling nature of hormone intervention. The "other means" may include skin patches, topical creams, vaginal suppositories, or injections.

Additionally, failing to mention the possible short- and/or long-term disabling side effects – such as blood clots, stroke, cancer, heart attack, abdominal or back pain, nausea, depression, mood changes, ir/reversible body changes, and interference with other (necessary) medications – frames the intervention as no big deal. In other words, the IAAF neglects to attend to the profound embodied consequences that come with altering one's hormonal environment. Implicitly framing radically altering one's hormone levels as no big deal not only counters confirmed scientific knowledge about doing so but also ignores the fact that the CAS explained in its ruling (see Ingle 2019) that it is concerned with the harmful side effects of mandating hormone manipulation. Despite these concerns, the CAS ruled in favour of jeopardizing athletes' welfare. That being said, once again, unconsenting athletes and critics of the IAAF are constructed as unreasonable. Both the lack of regard for these athletes' well-being and the lack of attention to the impacts of changing one's hormonal environment are unsurprising given the IAAF's apparent reliance on coercion and manipulation: athletes are coerced into fundamentally and irreversibly altering their body-minds, and the public is persuaded to continue ignoring the science and taking for granted compulsory dyadism and intersecting discriminatory beliefs.

Countering the WMA's claim that the policy is not in line with medical ethics, Hirschberg, Auchus, and Bermon (2019) explain that, according to DSD medical guidelines, intervention "is the recognized standard of care." The IAAF's representatives are not wrong. Doctors across the globe pathologize intersex traits, maintaining that intersex people must be surveilled and subjected to curative violence, and all of these interventions are generally accepted as the best course of action. The WMA's position deviates from that of the majority of doctors. However, the course of action deemed appropriate by most medical professionals is not always ethical medical practice. The underlying justification for medical intervention is not rooted in evidence-based medicine but rather in interconnected forms of discrimination and compulsory modes of being.[10] Ultimately, the IAAF's discursive manoeuvres are cunning and misleading. They are also dangerous to athletes' well-being, body-mind autonomy, and futures. As so many people across the globe continue to criticize the IAAF's policies, it is important to also critique the problematic co-opting of seemingly pro-feminist, pro-queer, pro-consent, and care discourses. These discourses mask the anti-scientific, prejudiced nature of the policy and obscure the extent to which women athletes can resist having their body-minds scrutinized, pathologized, invaded, and changed with impunity.

After the ruling, the IAAF also addressed Semenya's situation. The IAAF demanded that Semenya lower her naturally high levels of testosterone if she wanted to continue to compete in her preferred race, the 800 metres. Semenya (quoted in Dunbar 2019) remarks on the case, "I know that the IAAF's regulations have always targeted me specifically ... For a decade the IAAF has tried to slow me down, but this has actually made me stronger. The decision of the CAS will not hold me back. I will once again rise above and continue to inspire young women and athletes in South Africa and around the world." Indeed, her talent and ingenuity were not entirely stifled. Semenya trained for and was set to compete in the unrestricted 3,000-metre event at the Prefontaine Classic at Stanford University (Longman 2019). Since the CAS falls under Swiss legal jurisdiction, Semenya also approached the Swiss Federal Tribunal, Switzerland's supreme court, for assistance in appealing the case (Burfoot 2019). Although she was permitted to switch to the 800-metre event at the Prefontaine Classic as the court reviewed the case, in the end, unfortunately, the court did not think that Semenya had a winning case (Burfoot 2019). Yet again, her athleticism and inventiveness were not completely restrained. In the fall of 2019, Semenya announced that she had traded her track spikes for football cleats, joining the JVW Football Club in South Africa's Sasol League. As reported on JVW's (2019) website, Semenya expressed excitement about being welcomed to the club and about her future in football.

The IAAF legally continues its legacy of perpetuating and institutionalizing anti-scientific and compulsory dyadic policies and the false idea that testosterone is a marker of people's "true" sex (or pathology) as well as their athletic capabilities or, as with women, their potentially unfair capabilities. However, only a part of the discrimination embedded in how this practice is executed can be captured by tracing the historical account of various sex-testing methods, debunking the faulty science that underpins the practice, and examining the current justification for the IAAF's policy. Tracking which women athletes from which nations have been and currently are targeted for sex tests, rendered suspect intersex, and/or subjected to curative violence while taking into account the broader global climate demonstrates that sport sex-testing policies were, and remain, a domain for political battles. Sex testing is a political jackknife that does more than maintain compulsory dyadism, interphobia, sexism, and cisgenderism. Sex testing is also used to maintain or shift inequitable power relations that are colonial, global, and economic as well as gendered, sexed, racialized, and international.

The Shifting Spectre in Sport: Who Has Been and Who Currently Is Targeted for Sex Testing?

Sex testing promotes and relies on interphobic, sexist, cisgenderist, racist, Eurocentric notions of femininity.[11] Sex testing is critiqued because the practice is not uniform, and this lack of uniformity reveals the discriminatory ideologies that underpin it. For instance, only women were tested, and currently only women who appear "too" muscular, manly, or athletically able are tested. In other words, women who excel in sport and do not conform to oppressive standards of compulsory dyadism, femininity, and feminine beauty are presumed to house the phantom and are required to undergo invasive and humiliating procedures in order to "confirm" their sex or possibly exorcise the spectre.

Men athletes never provoke such outrage. Men's sex is never questioned or tested because "all men in sport are assumed to be 'real men' at the outset" (Dworkin and Cooky 2012, 21). Men are expected to be athletically capable, dynamic, and muscular. Hence, sex tests function to maintain "one of the most central and coveted beliefs in sport," namely that men have inherently superior athletic abilities and body-minds compared to women (Dworkin and Cooky 2012, 21). Or, in feminist sport psychologist Vikki Krane's (2001, 115) terms, "the underlying message is that athleticism and femininity are contradictory." Athleticism and femininity are understood to be, and are typically represented as, antithetical. In other words, one's presumed dis/in/abilities are bound up with one's sex/gender.

Nor is sex testing uniform across national borders, citizenship status, or race. This lack of consistency suggests that intersex haunts certain women and places; sex "deceivers" are presumed to come from certain geographical locations (presently, the Global South) and to look a certain way (currently, racialized). The fact that women track athletes of colour in colonized nations of the Global South are currently targeted is well documented; and many argue that the current employment of sex testing is evidently informed by intersecting interphobic, racist, cisgenderist, sexist, and colonial logics.[12]

Sex testing all women athletes, not just suspect women, was instituted in the twentieth century during the Cold War. And, as Pieper (2016, 36) outlines, "the IAAF and IOC grew more concerned about sex/gender transgressions as Cold War tensions developed internationally." Although all women were subjected to humiliating sex tests during this time, in line with established anxieties about women athletes who participate in track and field events, track and field women athletes from the Soviet Union were overwhelming slandered in the media and humiliated at events. These Soviet women athletes – most notably sprinter Ewa Kłobukowska (b. 1946) – were not just accused of doping but were also inter/sex- and gender-suspect. The fact that Soviet women excelled in track and field events at that time made these accusations seem credible. These athletes, including Kłobukowska, were often publicly disqualified from competitions, information about their anatomies was leaked to the media, and as a result, these women were disparaged by the press as well as by their fellow competitors and colleagues.[13] Soviet women athletes were presented as doping, masculine cheats and gender-deceiving freaks – steroid "Übermenschen" and "ball-bearing females" (Beamish and Ritchie 2007, 11). And "suddenly they were not women any more, nor were they considered men" (Martínez-Patiño et al. 2010, 315). They were "in-between," freakish, manly, communist deceivers.

In addition to confronting Cold War anxieties, America was still dealing with postwar sex/gender anxieties. For example, the ideal of the white masculine breadwinner was threatened by women refusing to leave the workforce after the Second World War, traditional conceptions of femininity were threatened by working women, men were struggling to embody traditional archetypes of manhood, and the gay rights and women's movements were threatening heteropatriarchal ideals (see Kimmel 1996; and Loftin 2007). The apparent threat to the boundaries of femininity and masculinity was, in essence, a "threat to the security of the nation" (Cuordileone 2000, 516).

The American media placed the phantasm "over there" in Soviet women. They exploited (inter)sex/gender speculation to disparage communism and Soviet conceptions of femininity that did not reflect America's investment in capitalism and American notions of femininity, namely the idea that women belong in the domestic sphere and are innately quieter, weaker, smaller, and less muscular than men (Cole 2000; Pieper 2014, 2016). That is, sex testing and the scrutinizing of Soviet women's athleticism and physiologies were used as a political multi-tool of war to stoke anxieties about communism and to naturalize traditional Western sex and gender roles. Sex testing alleged ball-bearing Soviet women bolstered American images "of normalized gender and sex roles ..., centering heterosexuality, the nuclear family, and 'gender-appropriate,' 'biologically natural' behaviour" (Beamish and Ritchie 2007, 11). America's "super-heterosexualized Cold War family ideal was used as a 'psychological fortress' against the fear of communist aggression" (Beamish and Ritchie 2007, 19). Implying that the spectre of intersex was a communist threat and targeting Soviet women were means to protect and strengthen the psychological strongholds around traditional American gender roles and anti-communist ideals.

After the collapse of the Soviet Union, similar to Soviet women athletes, women athletes of the People's Republic of China excelled in international track and field and became suspect. As Pieper (2014, 1560) attests, these women were deemed fraudulent and unnatural:

> With the collapse of the Soviet Union in 1991, the divisions between Cold-War-East and Cold-War-West somewhat dissipated. The People's Republic of China, however, emerged as a new global enterprise that challenged countries of the geographic-West. China's increased economic authority and improved international influence created new political and geographic tensions. This threat extended into sport as Chinese teams achieved un-precedented success and dominated international competition. Tellingly, the Chinese female athletes emerged in the 1990s as the new "other."

China's growing economic power threatened the West (Xuetong 2006), and since it was a communist nation, China was easily rendered suspect in the Western imagination. As the intersex phantasm was now imagined to reside in a new geographical location, Chinese women athletes became suspect. The sex testing of supposedly gender-deceiving Chinese women athletes was a way that Western forces could exploit communist anxieties in the attempt to destabilize China's emerging economic power while also restabilizing the sex and gender dyads. The destabilizing project succeeded in establishing Chinese women athletes "as the racial and gendered 'other' in the realm of sport" (Pieper 2016, 168). Put simply, the intersex spectre was presented as residing in a specifically Eastern nation soon after the Soviet collapse because of the economic and political threat that the East posed.

Beginning in the early 2000s, sex/gender anxieties expanded as women of other countries began to dominate the track. The spectre appeared to move across borders again. Racialized women of colonized nations in the Global South excelled on the track and became inter/sex-suspect. In particular, women of colour in India and in various countries of Africa have been tar-geted, rendered intersex-suspect, subjected to sex testing, and/or publicly libelled: Semenya of South Africa, Negesa of Uganda, Niyonsaba of Burundi, Soundarajan of India, Margaret Wambui of Kenya, and Chand of India. Sport sociologist and athletes' rights advocate Payoshni Mitra (2014b) con-firms that "athletes from developing nations are targeted" for sex testing.

Furthermore, it is worth nothing that the Intersex Rights Movement was gaining considerable ground and a remarkable amount of mainstream press in the early 2000s (see G. Davis 2015). Just as the gay and feminist movements threated traditional, Western gender roles in the twentieth century, the Intersex Rights Movement was destabilizing conservative conceptions of sex and gender. Compulsory dyadism, therefore, needed to be reaffirmed. Hence, testing these athletes served several political purposes, including the effort to restabilize sex and gender binaries threatened by activist forces and the desire to punish or undermine non-Western nations and athletes who succeeded on the track.

Why are women of colour targeted? Or why are they easily targeted? In addition to the fact that women of colour from the Global South are still dominating the track, feminist sociologist and critical race studies scholar Patricia Hill Collins's insights are instructive. Speaking specifically of Black women – hence, the reader can keep Semenya in mind here – Collins (2004, 199) explains that Black women, "by definition, cannot achieve the idealized feminine ideal because the fact of Blackness excludes them." Idealized or hegemonic femininity is white. Embodying hegemonic femininity is not merely about not looking or acting masculine but also about looking, being, or passing as white.[14] Because Black women, and women of colour in general, do not and cannot achieve idealized femininity or be read as "real" women, they become suspect women or are not understood or recognized as women at all. Given these ideologies, Semenya's Blackness already renders her not quite a woman or a suspect woman. Moreover, her "manly" muscular physicality and athletic abilities, supposed "unfeminine" gender presentation, and lesbian sexuality render her double, triple, and quadruple suspect. Her body-mind and way of being in the world, and what she does with her body-mind, challenge and threaten views about what "real" women look like, desire (i.e., men), and are capable of doing. Consequently, questioning Semenya's femininity and subjecting her to sex testing are means to restabilize hegemonic white femininity, dyadism, and heterosexuality, as well as to re-emphasize the notion that Black women are not and cannot be real women.

In the *Sowetan,* one of South Africa's largest newspapers, Len Anderson has drawn attention to the racism in current sport sex-testing practices and hegemonic femininity. Speaking of Semenya, Anderson (2009) states, "It is very clear that the IAAF used Western stereotypes of what a woman should look like as probable cause [for sex testing] and that is racist and sexist." Anderson continues, "Those making the determination [about sex testing] are fat and ugly European men." Although the comment "fat and ugly" is problematic, Anderson is correct that mostly white European, Western men of the Global North decide who is properly feminine. Informed by oppressive ideologies, they decide who might be hiding the spectre of intersex and haunting sport; they decide where the phantom resides and which body-minds to investigate.

Although all of the women athletes mentioned thus far have been and are integral to countering discriminatory sex testing policies, Semenya has garnered the most international attention in scholarship and the media, and although she is a contested figure, she has become a household name. I suspect that Semenya's sex-testing case has become such a focus because slandering her as a sex-deceiver is much easier than slandering, for example, Dutee Chand, who is a rather small person, standing 5 feet and 4 inches, and does not read as "manly." Moreover, there was less fodder for those wanting to undermine Chand's femininity given that her lesbian sexuality remained publicly unknown until 2019, long after her highly publicized court battles.[15] Semenya, in contrast, is an evidently muscular woman, standing 5 feet and 10 inches, and her sexuality has been quite clear for several years – at least since she got engaged to and married Violet Raseboya in 2015. Slandering Semenya as "manly" due to her embodiment and sexuality while alleging that she hides the spectre is not as difficult to do simply because of the optics. And, unsurprisingly, Semenya's physical attributes and sexuality figure prominently in many conversations about her.

For example, in an article written for *Christian Voice*, Stephen Green (2016) calls Semenya's sex/gender into question by misgendering her and drawing attention to her relationship with Raseboya:

> The story gets murkier ... Semenya 'married' a woman ... Semenya and her/his long-time girlfriend, Violet Raseboya, held a ceremony in Ga-Dikgale in the Capricorn district of Limpopo ... Semenya, 24, sent her parents to Raseboya's family in Polokwane to negotiate lobola (dowry). An insider revealed at the time both families were happy to negotiate lobola, with Semenya's family paying R25,000 ... Dowry in Africa is paid by the man's family to the women's. That fits, because sadly, Caster Semenya, you are not a woman.

According to Green's reasoning, Semenya's apparent innate masculinity or intersex anatomy is confirmed by her lesbian relationship and wedding negotiations. In a *Sports Illustrated* article that deploys similar logics, Tim

Layden (2016) emphasizes Semenya's supposed unfeminine characteristics to "prove" that it would be unfair if she competed in the 2016 Olympics in Rio de Janeiro: "She is 5'10" and weighs 161 pounds, with muscular arms, broad shoulders and narrow hips. She has a severe jawline, hard and strong, and a competitor's unflinching eyes." Layden implies that these characteristics are antithetical to femininity and women athletes. Apparently, according to Layden, an elite track athlete who is a woman should not have the essential qualities – muscular, fit, strong, hard, and a competitive disposition – that enable her to perform at elite levels.

Even though there have been shifts in who and which nations have been targeted most throughout the decades, Western European colonizers have been placing the spectre of intersex "over there" in racialized women – or intersexualizing the Other – for centuries. John Horne (2012, 31) speaks of "the four Cs" needed to analyze sports mega-events like the Olympics: capitalism, connections, citizenship, and contradictions. However, taking another "C" into account is clearly vital: colonialism. Doing so helps us to acknowledge and address how colonialism shaped and shapes sporting events and policies as well as the participating nations and citizens.[16] Taking colonialism into account reveals that sex testing is a colonial, imperial practice given that it imposes and "promotes Western notions of biology, gender and race" (Pieper 2016, 1558). Abolishing sport sex-testing practices and, by extension, questioning sex-segregated sport (as I do in the next chapter) are decolonizing projects that aim to make sport more fair and to bolster many marginalized athletes, nations, identities, and citizenships.

More specifically, as explored in Chapter 4, representing African women, particularly South African women like Semenya, as sexually ambiguous, in-between, hermaphrodite, or unnaturally masculine is not new. There is a long Western, colonial, imperial, and scientific history of labelling African women's genitals ambiguous, primitive, and abnormal. Starting in the seventeenth century, sometimes citing Western, European, male colonizers' travelling texts and tales of "discovery," European, American, and South African medical texts maintained that "malformed or ambiguous genitalia ... were particularly common among women of African descent" (Magubane 2014, 769). Due to this belief, an African woman "becomes her genitalia" (Gilman 1985, 121); she is reduced to her alleged ambiguous physical characteristics. We have witnessed this violent process happen to Semenya, who has been reduced to her sex through the scrutiny of her supposed sex traits in news stories with headlines like "Caster Semenya 'Is a Hermaphrodite,' Tests

Show" (Hart 2009), "Caster Semenya Has Male Sex Organs and No Womb or Ovaries" (Hurst 2009), and "Semenya, Forced to Take Gender Test, Is a Woman ... and a Man" (Yaniv 2009). These sorts of headlines reproduce the colonial practice of othering racialized, non-Western women by inter-sexualizing them, which renders them sexually deviant, threatening, abnormal, or ambiguous.[17]

Recounting this brief historical account alongside Semenya's sex-testing controversy draws attention to the way that the spectre of supposed degenerate genital and sexual ambiguity was, and remains to be, imagined and constructed by colonial and imperial forces across gender, racial, national, and geographical lines. The spectre of intersex has been and continues to be used as a colonial and imperial tool with which to classify racialized women and nations as suspicious, threatening Others in order to justify various forms of violence. Addressing the history of the construction of genital "ambiguity" underscores the fact that race and nation play a significant role in determining which body-minds are labelled sexually "ambiguous" or disordered, where the spectre supposedly haunts, and how citizenship statuses and nations are admonished (Magubane 2014). This history reveals how various forms of oppression literally and symbolically converge on and shape certain people's body-minds and nations. It contextualizes the violence enacted on Semenya – and other Black women athletes – and demonstrates that the institutionalized violence that these athletes endured, and continue to endure, must be read as a contemporary iteration of the "ambiguously" sexed African woman (Munro 2010).

In the face of this Western imposition, South African media outlets, politicians, family members, and fellow citizens supported and continue to support Semenya. Whereas Western media outlets slandered and questioned Semenya and assumed that she was a man, not a real woman, intersex, disordered, or a hermaphrodite, South Africans defended Semenya's identity, claim to womanhood, and right to body-mind autonomy.[18] Many of the arguments defending Semenya were rooted in nationalist, anti-imperialist discourses that were largely lost on Western viewers and critics (Magubane 2014; Orr and Watson 2018). Defending Semenya's female identity and right to body-mind integrity was a means to oppose imperial forces that seek to define and name South Africans. Although some Western commentators and scholars claim that Semenya's, her family's, and her nation's rejection of the labels intersex and DSD is interphobic, backwards, or anti-science, this claim neglects the colonial, imperial context (Magubane 2014; Munro 2010;

Orr and Watson 2018). Such a claim reproduces the historical dismissal of Black women's narratives of their body-minds and identities as well as the historical dismissal of colonized nations' own narratives. Moreover, as I and Amanda D. Watson (Orr and Watson 2018, 31) explain, such a claim, at least in part, overlooks the fact that Semenya's status and her nation's support for her "expand the strict confines of femininity and challenge the dominant ethos that authentic femininity is frail, unmuscular, less able or athletic than men, and white." Semenya explicitly speaks to this challenge in the television documentary *Too Fast to Be a Woman? The Story of Caster Semenya* (Ginnane 2011), where she asks and answers, "What makes a lady? Does it mean if you're wearing skirts and dresses you're a lady? No. What kind of a lady is that? Yeah I'm a lady. There's nothing I can say, yes, I'm a lady. I have those cards of being a lady." Much like the late American abolitionist and women's rights activist Sojourner Truth's (1851) famous address, Semenya is essentially asking, "Ain't I a Woman?"[19] And she passionately declares that indeed she is.

Indian women athletes, most notably Dutee Chand and Santhi Soundarajan, have also been targeted as inter/sex-suspect and slandered in the media. Hence, I turn my attention to India. Around the same time as Indian athletes were rendered sex-suspect in the early 2000s, anxieties about India's growing global power increased. In 2000, American diplomat and political scientist Condoleezza Rice (2000, 55) stated in a *Foreign Affairs* article, "India is not a great power yet, but it has the potential to emerge as one." Hence, according to Rice, America must combat this power and protect its own interests. Only a few years later, exaggerated claims that India threatened the livelihoods of Americans began to emerge. For example, political commentator and author Thomas L. Friedman (2005) argues that, due to globalization, India has created more economic competition and, therefore, now threatens American jobs and American people's ability to prosper. Friedman subsequently encourages his children to study hard because Indian children are also studying hard and may compete with them for jobs. Smacking of American and white entitlement, Friedman's arguments imply that these hypothetical jobs belong to Americans and that Indians will steal them. Although "India's economy has accelerated sharply since the late 1980s" (Binswanger-Mkhize 2013, 5), Friedman's American-centric work has been criticized time and again for exaggerating and falsifying the trends that he observes and analyzes.[20] Despite the valid criticism of claims made by individuals like Friedman, American anxieties about India's supposed threat have grown. This is the global climate in which Indian women track athletes like Chand and Soundarajan have been defamed in the media and sex-tested.

These twenty-first-century anxieties about India's economic growth and global position, as well as the slandering and literal invasion of Indian women athletes' body-minds via sex testing, must be read alongside the much longer (and ongoing) colonial, imperial, and orientalist history. Doing so illustrates even more troubling implications for how sport sex testing has been deployed in the twenty-first-century. Drawing from extensive historical literature, Mitra (2014a, 389) explains that "the binary sex model was not as integral to the cultures of traditional Indian societies"; the notion that "bodies are naturally completely one sex or another" was not prominent in traditional Indian societies. Western, colonial, orientalist, and imperial forces decimated these traditional cultural systems.[21] Imposing strict, dyadic Western biological categories and ideologies through sex testing is a colonial act that delegitimizes people's identities, subjectivities, and experiences. Imposing Western conceptions of dyadic sex and gender contributes to the erasure of many culturally specific identities and social formations that do not institutionalize compulsory dyadism or reproduce the belief that people are always completely one of two possible sexes/genders.

Various Indian cultures have long recognized a "third sex/gender," such as that of hijras or kinnars.[22] "Hijra" appears to be the general term used to name a person aligned with any of these various identities and groups. At the current moment, hijra is a marginalized, yet institutionalized, sex in India. Sociologist Tara Atluri (2012, 727) notes, "Hijras have been labeled as trans, India's lady boys, India's third sex, drag queens, and a whole host of other English terms," including intersex, by people in the Global North. Yet, Atluri affirms that these English descriptors are insufficient. They do not capture the cultural contexts, identities, citizenship status, or unique marginalization that hijras experience. These terms do not reflect the body-mind or cultural diversity of the communities. Moreover, the contexts in which these English terms are typically used often erase the complexity of colonial history. In "backwards" India, these terms also function to impose Western, dyadic ideas of sex and gender, Western discourses about DSD, intersex, and gender identity disorder, and/or supposedly liberal, progressive Western notions of LGBTQIA2 liberation and rights (Atluri 2012). Colonization, imperialism, and orientalism have delegitimized and pathologized hijra identities, practices, expressions, and communities. Western views about sex and gender binaries are imposed and institutionalized in India. As feminist and political science studies scholar Nivedita Menon

(2011) explains, some nationalist elites throughout the nineteenth and twentieth centuries embraced "colonial modernity," including dyadic notions of sex and gender.

Considering this context, while remaining cognizant of the fact that Soundarajan and Chand have always identified as women, we can see that both suspecting Indian women athletes and imposing Western understandings of sex, gender, intersex, pathology, and DSD through sport sex testing not only undermine fundamental aspects of these athletes' identities as women but also continue the colonial work of erasing, renaming, and pathologizing hijras. The impacts of this work are tragic and have been tragically effective. Consider, specifically, Soundarajan's case. Soundarajan was tested in 2006 after winning silver at the Doha Asian Games. Her medal was subsequently taken away from her and remains withheld. The fact that she "failed" a sex test became public knowledge. After information about her anatomy was leaked to the public, she was objectified, disparaged, and reduced to her sex characteristics in the media. She then attempted suicide. Soundarajan suffered from violent and invasive treatment and inter/national rejection.[23] There was a "sense of national shame," Mitra (2014a, 387) writes. Indian news outlets, sports officials, federations, and politicians "deserted her" and "discussed her case[,] calling it 'mysterious' or 'strange'" (Mitra 2014a, 387). That is, in an effort to resist being othered and shamed, powerful people in India distanced themselves from Soundarajan and the apparent spectre. In this effort, however, colonial ideologies regarding the sex dyad are confirmed and maintained. The rejection of athletes like Soundarajan by important news outlets and Indian figures mirrors the ways that some Indian elites throughout the nineteenth and twentieth centuries embraced dyadic notions of sex and gender and rejected traditional Indian conceptions of sex and gender in the name of colonial modernity.

That said, supporting and defending these athletes can appear counterintuitive, even illogical, if one believes in the "objective" discourses of science and fairness that are used by sport governing bodies. Discourses of fairness, scientific progress, and scientific objectivity are strategically deployed to impose Western iterations of sex/gender through sport. This practice ultimately continues the colonial process of limiting and controlling colonized nations' sexual citizenship. In other words, this practice is a problem of who has the power to name body-mind characteristics and to erode culturally specific identities. Indeed, women, intersex, intersex-as/is-disabled, racialized, and colonized peoples alike have struggled, and continue to struggle, to gain the right to name and control their body-minds, identities, and modes of being in the world on their own terms.

Coining the phrase "intersex citizenship," law professor Emily Grabham (2007, 29) demonstrates that folks with intersex anatomy are not treated as proper citizens because their body-minds are presumed to be out of control, abnormal, and disordered. However, as the experiences of suspect intersex athletes demonstrate, people need not be medically confirmed as having a DSD before being treated as intersex citizens. Suspicion is enough. Having a body-mind, sex, gender, race, and nationality deemed suspicious by Western, colonial ideologies and institutions was enough for Semenya, Chand, and Soundarajan, among others, to be stripped of their autonomy, career opportunities, income, and hard-won titles. Suspicion is built into the guidelines that govern sport sex testing. Semenya illustrates this reality in the documentary *Too Fast to Be a Woman?* (Ginnane 2011): "I don't have rights. Let's put it this way: in athletics, I don't have rights. I'm just a competitor." Being a competitor with suspect or supposedly incongruous characteristics should not and need not involve exclusion or the denial of rights, privacy, and self-determination. Yet Semenya is not *just* a competitor, as she states in the above quotation. None of the athletes discussed thus far are just competitors. By institutionalizing compulsory dyadism and enforcing Western ideas about body-minds, sport governing bodies render such athletes (potential) vehicles for these ideals to be further entrenched in their nations and across the globe.

Mapping which athletes (by and large women track athletes) and which nations have been targeted and maligned demonstrates that athletes who dominate the track, athletes who undermine Western traditional notions of femininity, and/or nations that are perceived to threaten or undermine Western ideals or global positioning become intersex-suspect. And said athletes may be or are subjected to invasive sex testing and curative violence in the name of fair play and science. The intersex spectre has shifted through time and space, and currently women track athletes of colour in colonized nations of the Global South are targeted for testing. This fact illustrates that all sport mega-events were, and remain, a domain for old and new political battles. Sex testing is a political multi-tool that aims to maintain and advance intersecting forms of oppression. By exploiting and imposing Western notions of sex, gender, femininity, masculinity, pathology, and DSD, sport sex testing is used as a tool with which to limit, control, and impose sexual citizenship, intersex citizenship, or, if intersex is understood to be a disability, disability citizenship. Analyzing how the phantom is currently imagined to reside in women athletes of colour in colonized nations of the Global South also reveals that sex testing is used as a racist, colonial, imperial tool. And, it must be noted, this violent tool has always been used on already marginalized people: intersex, trans, racialized, queer, and colonized individuals and women. The fact that sex testing needs to be abolished is clear. Doing so would constitute a necessary decolonizing and anti-discriminatory undertaking. I endorse immediately scrapping all sex-testing policies and creating new policies that reject future sex-testing proposals and protect athletes from intersecting forms of discrimination.

Unfairly Advantaged Yet Disordered Intersex Athletes

What can a disability studies lens bring to the sport sex-testing controversy? What would it look like to crip sport sex testing? Analyzing sex testing through a disability lens may seem like an unusual inclination. World-class athletes are not typically construed as or imagined to be disabled, and suspect intersex athletes are presumed to have an unfair advantage. In addition, the optics – the remarkable strength, musculature, and achievements of (suspect) intersex athletes like Semenya – seem at odds with traditional conceptions of what disability looks like or means. Moreover, disability seems at odds with the presumed athletic hyperabilities of racialized people, specifically Black people.[24] Seemingly contradictory optics, however, cannot impede analyses. Given that intersex is construed as a (racialized) disability, disorder, or disease, we must crip analyses of sport sex testing. Given their remarkable athleticism, women athletes with ostensible disordered or disabled intersex anatomy complicate the assumed distinction between ability and disability as well as between feminine and masculine abilities. Ultimately, the assumed hyperability of intersex athletes and racialized people, coupled with the presumed in/abilities of women and pathologized people, sheds light on how intersex is constructed differently depending on where one is born, what one looks like, and when and where one performs. A disability perspective on sex testing reveals the contradictory narratives about the presumed effects of having "disabling" intersex characteristics and, in turn, the il/logic of dichotomous thinking.

Cripping sport sex testing uncovers a troubling discrepancy: intersex is pathologized, defined as a disability, disorder, or disease, and represented as an inherent, degenerate, and disabling lack by medical professionals in and outside of sport contexts, but in the context of sport, intersex traits are represented as (unfair) advantages. Cripping this site of compulsory dyad-ism provides us with the tools to identify the il/logic that sport governing bodies employ to uphold sex testing and curative violence. That is to say, adding colonialism to Horne's list of "Cs" needed to analyze sporting events – capitalism, connections, citizenship, and contradictions – is not enough. Dis/ability is required if we are to analyze sport sex testing – indeed, sport organization as a whole.

Consider the comments of IAAF spokesperson Nick Davies (in Ginnane 2011) about Semenya "suffering" from a medical disorder. His commentary points to the tension between ability, hyperability, and disability while repro-ducing the "rhetoric of tragedy" (Fausto-Sterling 2000, 47) or the "tragedy of disability" (Peers 2009, 653) discourse. This narrative justifies inter-phobic sex testing and curative violence through ableist discourses. As documented in *Too Fast to Be a Woman?* (Ginnane 2011), Davies unoffi-cially outed Semenya in 2009 and remarked that her intersex variation is "a medical condition. That's a point to stress. It's clearly not her fault. It's who she is physically." In a pejoratively titled news piece penned by Alastair Jamieson (2009) – "Caster Semenya Gender Row: What Is a Hermaphro-dite?" – Davies is quoted as saying that Semenya "suffer[s] from a genetic disorder." This rhetoric of tragedy, or medical discourse of suffering *from* an intersex disorder, often centres in conversations about intersex traits de-spite the fact that the vast majority of medical issues and disabilities that many intersex people experience come from the socio-medical response to their intersex traits and curative violence, not from the traits themselves. This rhetoric functions to elicit ableist pity from (temporarily) endosex and enabled individuals and implies that there is a need for medical intervention and surveillance. If Semenya is determined to be "suffering," the root of said suffering – the intersex spectre – must be exorcised. In other words, curative violence is narrated as a necessary medical aid.

The idea that Semenya suffers from her physicality is difficult to come to terms with. Her supposed intersex trait does not cause her evident pain or distress. Rather than suffering from her assumed intersex anatomy, she clearly suffers from the violent socio-medical reaction to her physical morphology, athleticism, gender performance, race, and sexuality. This suf-fering is clear given that in 2009, as she was navigating interphobic sport policies and being subjected to invasive sex testing, Semenya (in Ginnane 2011) bluntly stated, "I don't give a shit about athletics anymore." Sound-arajan, found in the same situation a few years before Semenya, attempted suicide because she was suffering from violent and invasive treatment and inter/national rejection, not from her apparent intersex trait. The narrative of suffering masks the fact that, according to dominant ideologies about gender, sex, race, and dis/ability, these athletes have, to borrow Anne Fausto-Sterling's (2000, 8) term, "unruly" body-minds, not inherent medical problems. The proposal that Semenya suffers from an intersex disability is also difficult to reconcile when we consider that she is, by most standards – indeed, by those of the IOC, the IAAF, and the International Paralympic Committee – not disabled. She would not qualify as a disabled athlete or Paralympian. Rather, she is read as able-bodied, hyperable, and unfairly advantaged. Hence, in addition to exploiting the ableist rhetoric of tragedy, which claims that Semenya is pitiably disordered and must be fixed, critics of Semenya simultaneously frame her as unfairly advantaged and, in turn, as someone who ought to be excluded from sport until the advantage is levelled through gratuitously disabling curative violence. The narrative that frames Semenya as unfairly advantaged justifies discriminatory exclusion and medical intervention.

The media have consistently wielded the narrative of unfair advantage. For example, after Semenya won the gold medal in the 800-metre event at the 2016 Olympics, Cyd Zeigler (2016a) took note, drawing attention to Layden's (2016) article in *Sports Illustrated:* "Layden lays about a bunch of nonsensical fear-mongering from people about Semenya, allowing one person to say her advantage is so huge and so unfair that it's like watching the Super Bowl when one team is so much better, you already know the winner." The title of Ben Bloom's (2016) article in the *Telegraph* echoes Layden: "Caster Semenya Destroys Rest of the Field to Claim Easy Gold in Women's 800m Final – Can Anyone Beat Her?" Bloom suggests that Semenya was so unfairly advantaged that her win was easy to achieve; she had to exert "minimum effort." Acknowledging that athletes have beat Semenya, Bloom presumptuously rationalizes that she did not break a world record at the Olympics because "she prioritized gold over records." Her incredible achievements, steadfast training, numerous sacrifices, and dedication to the sport are effectively delegitimized. Unlike endosex athletes' achievements, Semenya's achievements are not recognized or valued as legitimate.

Often, both narratives – Semenya is pitiably disordered *and* unfairly advantaged – are employed simultaneously, which unintentionally undermines ableist logics. Owen Bowcott (2011), in an article for the *Guardian*, explains that Semenya has an "intersex disorder" and, quoting consultant gynecologist Peter Bowen-Simpkins, states that she has "an advantage" over other (apparently "real" endosex) women. As a consequence, albeit unintended, of employing both narratives, this article – undeniably misinformed and discriminatory – undermines the notion that disabled or disordered people are inherently and always disadvantaged and less able. Bowcott inadvertently points to a contradiction. On the one hand, the medical community – alongside institutions like the IAAF and the IOC that rely on medical authority – pathologizes intersex traits and construes them as disordered, disabled, diseased, and disadvantaged. On the other hand, in the context of sport, intersex characteristics are construed as rendering one inherently powerful, hyperable, and advantaged. Narrating a person as disordered *and* advantaged counters dominant, ableist understandings of the embodied effects of pathologized morphologies and reveals the failings of binary thinking. This apparent contradiction reveals the logical shortcomings of Western dichotomous thinking about sex, gender, dis/order, and dis/ability. Claiming that Semenya is both better *and* worse for supposedly having intersex anatomy draws attention to the il/logic that powerful institutions appeal to in order to justify, uphold, and re/institutionalize discriminatory ideologies and practices. Ironically, since the logic cannot hold, the supposed hyperable, disordered intersex athlete undermines the intersecting interphobic and ableist assumption that the embodied effects of disorders, disabilities, and/or intersex traits are always undesirable, painful, insufferable, and disadvantaging.

To expand, although the response to intersex traits – curative violence – remains the same in and outside of sport, the claim that intersex is an embodied disadvantage changes depending on which people are marked as intersex, what they do with their body-minds, where they perform, and what they achieve. If intersex is attached to an infant, child, adolescent, or adult who is not, or could not (yet) be, an elite athlete, this person is deemed unfortunately disabled and must undergo curative violence. If intersex is attached to or is suspected of haunting a woman athlete, this athlete is assumed to be hyperable, her achievements are admonished and delegitimized, and she must undergo curative violence to level the advantage. If intersex is attached to a racialized, Black, or Black African woman athlete who is often already construed as unfairly advantaged due to persistent biological racist claims that racialized (particularly Black) people have essential biological attributes that predispose them to be better in sport, this athlete is assumed to be hyperable and exceedingly unfairly advantaged, her achievements are not recognized as valid, and she must undergo curative violence.

These views are evident in several news media pieces and in the comments of Poland's Joanna Jóźwik after the 800-metre race at the 2016 Olympics (see Blatchford 2016; and Parker 2016). Semenya of South Africa won gold, Francine Niyonsaba of Burundi won silver, Margaret Wambui of Kenya won bronze, Melissa Bishop of Canada placed fourth, Lynsey Sharp of Great Britain placed fifth, and Jóźwik finished sixth. Semenya's, Niyonsaba's, and Wambui's claims to womanhood and their achievements were called into question. Implying that Semenya's, Niyonsaba's, and Wambui's gruelling training and dedication to the sport, improvement over the years, and performances should not be accepted and rewarded, Jóźwik (quoted in Critchley 2016) stated, "The three athletes who were on the podium raise a lot of controversy ... These colleagues have very high testosterone levels, similar to a male's, which is why they look how they look and run like they run." In an attempt to repudiate these athletes' achievements and to deny what many supportive commentators named their "Black excellence" (see Essack 2016; Klein 2016; and Phala 2016), Jóźwik assumes to know intimate details of these athletes' biologies by simply looking at them, and she reproduces essentializing interphobic, sexist, and racist narratives.[25] After the race, Jóźwik (quoted in Karkazis 2016a) asserted, "I'm glad I'm the first European, the second white." Jóźwik (quoted in Critchley 2016) claimed, "I feel like a silver medalist ... I saw Melissa Bishop who was very disappointed, she improved her personal best and was 4th. It's sad, and I think she should be the gold medalist." Jóźwik's comments are, Karkazis (2016a) remarks, "unsporting behaviour." Additionally, Karkazis (2016a) reports, one cannot help but notice "the optics of this controversy – the three Black women of sub-Saharan Africa ebullient on the podium and the three white women of the Global North feeling that they should be there instead." Plainly put, Jóźwik's remarks are interphobic, sexist, and racist, and they smack of white entitlement.

There are many accounts of Jóźwik and Sharp publicly expressing this racist, entitled, unsporting behaviour and stating the the 800-metre event was unfair.[26] However, contrary to Karkazis's suggestion, Bishop did not publicly voice the same concerns or disparage the three medalists. Bishop (quoted in Parker 2016) was accepting and collegial: "Me missing the podium is because I didn't run fast enough, not because of who was in the race. The only thing I can do is keep competing and keep doing what I love."

Rather than adding to the discriminatory chorus, using the controversy around Semenya as a scapegoat for her loss, or stoking the burgeoning skepticism about Niyonsaba's and Wambui's biologies, Bishop recognized her loss and these women's wins. This is the kind of sporting behaviour that is needed. Ultimately, however, the overwhelming discrimination and suspicion levelled at Semenya, as well as Niyonsaba and Wambui, surprisingly challenges ableist assumptions that having a pathologized embodiment is always a disadvantage.

Institutions and people invested in the colonial imposition of compulsory dyadism, in the pathologization of intersex traits, and in curative violence benefit from these logical inconsistencies. And, given the re/institutionalization of hyperandrogenism policies, these institutions and people do not face enough pushback or scrutiny. Drawing from Giorgio Agamben's (2005) notion of "a state of exception," Georgiann Davis (2015, 23) posits, "Medical professionals who frame intersex as an emergency are creating a state of exception that allows them to abandon medical ethics that warn against performing medically unnecessary surgery on children." According to Davis, by establishing a state of exception, medical professionals can endorse medical malpractice to impose curative violence and to maintain compulsory dyadism. In line with Davis's reasoning, I argue that with the help of sensationalist media and misrepresentative medico-scientific knowledge, sport governing bodies establish a similar state of exception and, in turn, disavow medico-scientific knowledge, abandon medical ethics, and ultimately institutionalize unethical, discriminatory sport practices. When a woman athlete is accused of being intersex, she might be prevented from competing until invasive tests are done and analyzed. She might also be stripped of her titles, publicly slandered for being a gender-deceiving freak, coercively subjected to curative violence, and/or pushed out of sport. Semenya's former competitor, Madeleine Pape (2016), who once scorned Semenya but now publicly supports her, describes this state of exception as "nothing short of a modern-day witch-hunt," a comparison that is eerily apt and reminiscent of the haunting analogy that runs throughout this book: people with (potential) intersex traits are treated as though they house a spectre that must be found and killed, cast out, or exorcised (see also Pape 2019).

When this state of exception is created, evidence proving that sex is neither binary nor an objective, identifiable category is abandoned. The fact that evidence cannot support the claim that athletes with intersex anatomy are unfairly advantaged in sport is ignored. The fact that there is no evidence to suggest that athletic abilities are purely a matter of, or exclusively extend from, sex (however sex is defined) is disregarded. And, although coercive policies regarding the medical interventions required to re/enter competition will continue to be debated, people in positions of power are still fighting for coercive, unethical, and medically unnecessary policies that re/solidify compulsory modes of being and justify myriad forms of discrimination.

Nevertheless, sex testing and coercive policies are narrated as ethical, fair, and logical. Sport governing bodies that abandon medical ethics are construed as acting ethically because these tests and practices are in the name of fairness. They abandon medical ethics and, as in the case of the IAAF (2015, C2.17, C3.19), their own *Code of Ethics:* "There shall be no discrimination in Athletics on the basis of race, sex, ethnic origin, colour, culture, religion, political opinion, marital status, sexual orientation or any other unfair or other irrelevant factor," and "all forms of harassment in Athletics, be it physical, verbal, mental or sexual, are prohibited." The code clearly prohibits discrimination, but athletes with intersex-as/is-disabled traits, women athletes, athletes of colour, trans athletes, and athletes of colonized nations continue to be discriminated against, harassed, and subjected to violence in the name of fair play.

Conclusion

The intersex spectre haunts all people and is not bound by racial or geographical borders. However, past and present sport sex-testing policies, the implementation of said policies, and the media response to sex testing controversies reveal the ways that the imaginary spectre is constructed and shifts due to Western, colonial forces. Sex testing is not backed by sound scientific evidence. Past and present sex testing illustrates that it is a dangerous, discriminatory political jackknife: it maintains compulsory dyadism, interphobia, sexism, and cisgenderism; and it is used to conserve or shift inequitable power relations that are colonial, global, and economic as well as gendered, sexed, racial, and international. The fact that sport sex testing needs to be abolished is abundantly clear.

However, if we abolish sex testing and openly acknowledge that the sex binary is a farce, should sport be sex-desegregated? If sport policies do not attempt to police the boundaries of sex, what good purpose does this segregation serve? Moreover, if intersex is construed as a disability, disorder, or disease, should not intersex athletes be relegated to disability sporting events like the Paralympics? Intersex athletes should prompt us to reconsider not simply sex testing and sex segregation but also dis/ability sport segregation. In other words, cripping sport sex testing by analyzing all of the competing and contradictory discourses about (the effects of) intersex-as/is-disability proves that sport is not and cannot be sex- or dis/ability-segregated. Women athletes with (suspect) intersex traits threaten the sex and gender binaries, sexist and ableist beliefs about women and patholo-gized individuals, *and* the divide between abled and disabled, normal and abnormal, natural and unnatural, and Olympian and Paralympian. Out-lawing sport sex testing clearly is not enough. We need more radical visions of equitable, anti-discriminatory sporting organizations and arenas. In the next chapter, I seek to address these concerns.

6

Sport Sex and Dis/ability De/segregation

In 2012, double-amputee athlete Oscar Pistorius (b. 1986), nicknamed "Blade Runner," competed at the 2012 Olympics in London. Many claimed that, similar to (suspect) intersex athletes like Caster Semenya, Pistorius was an unfairly advantaged cyborg and should not compete against "natural" athletes. Unlike Semenya, who must cyborgize herself by synthetically reducing her natural testosterone levels to become a "natural" woman in order to "fairly" compete, Pistorius was deemed an unnatural cyborg who cannot become "natural" enough to fairly compete with "natural" enabled athletes. Additionally, contrary to taken-for-granted ableist ideas that athletes with disabilities are innately disadvantaged and ought to be segregated from enabled athletes for their own good – disabled athletes are presumed to inevitably lose – Pistorius's disability was deemed an unfair advantage. The fact that Pistorius competed at the Olympics blurred the supposedly distinct boundary between Paralympian and Olympian. In turn, he called into question sport dis/ability segregation. Pistorius is not the only athlete to call into question the strict line between disabled and enabled, Paralympian and Olympian. Athletes like Semenya blur this line even further when one considers the ways that pathologization, disorder, disability, and disease figure in conversations about intersex variations. If intersex is interpreted as a disability, disorder, or disease, should not intersex athletes be relegated to disability sporting events like the Paralympics? This chapter considers this query and ultimately contests the supposed need to police disabilities, including intersex-as/is-disability, and to segregate sport by (perceived) sex and dis/ability binaries.

Sport is not as sex- *or* dis/ability-segregated as it is presumed to be. In fact, sport never could be successfully sex- or dis/ability-segregated. All of the competing and contradictory discourses about (the effects of) intersex and disability prove that sport is not and cannot be sex-, dis/ability-, or non/cyborg-segregated. That is, in the context of sport, women athletes with (suspect) intersex traits do not just threaten the sex and gender binaries but also threaten the deeply rooted sexist and ableist beliefs about the in/abilities of women *and* threaten the divide between abled and disabled, natural and unnatural, noncyborg and cyborg, and Olympian and Paralympian. When narrated as medically disordered or understood as falling under the category of disability, intersex traits call us to reconsider what qualifies one as a dis/abled athlete – as a Paralympian or Olympian – and to rethink how sport ought to be organized. Pathologized intersex traits challenge what we assume athletes with disabilities look like – what Olympians and Paralympians may look like. Considering the exorcising response of the International Olympic Committee (IOC) and the International Association of Athletics Federations (IAAF) to the intersex spectre alongside feminist, queer, crip theorist Alison Kafer's (2013) analysis of the cyborg disabled athlete draws attention to the fact that cyborgs are not always (legible) Paralympians. It is clear, however, that unless the tools of disability studies are employed – without the cripping of sport segregation – the il/logic and contradictory narratives used to justify sex testing as well as sex and dis/ability segregation remain obscure.

Not only does the unscientific nature of sex testing and the sex binary prompt me to consider the desegregatation of sport by sex, but the difficultly that (prospective) Paralympians face when trying to qualify as a Paralympian and to prove that they are "disabled enough" prompts me to question the strict line between disabled and enabled, Paralympian and Olympian. Teasing out how disability and disorder centre in conversations about (suspect) intersex athletes allows me to place the maltreatment and (attempted) exclusion of athletes like Semenya and Pistorius on the same continuum. Theorizing intersex and disability together in this context provides us with the opportunity to reimagine sport policies and the organization of sport by complicating the relationship between disability and inter/sex, further blurring the line between Olympian and Paralympian.

This chapter begins by exploring the necessity of approaching sport mega-events through a disability studies lens. Although there are some exceptions, too often Paralympians and the Paralympics are ignored, both in terms of sport studies scholarship and in terms of media representation, coverage, and engagement.[1] Indeed, Paralympians are frequently reduced to inspirational objects that benefit enabled viewers and reproduce ableism. Additionally, their achievements are not valued nearly as much as those of their Olympic counterparts. Paying more attention to disability, pathologization, and narratives of dis/abilities, hyper/abilities, or in/abilities in sport enables us not only to unpack these sorts of issues but also to challenge and reimagine sex and dis/ability sport segregation. Sex and dis/ability segregation, after all, is rooted in intersecting sexist, ableist, and interphobic beliefs.

Moving on, I outline the supposed science behind sport sex segregation, which posits that women are inherently inferior at sport and must be segregated from men for their own good. I illustrate that the reasoning deployed to justify sex segregation does not hold water. Rather than being innately inferior athletes, women are prevented from achieving what they are capable of by forces that tell women athletes to "stay small," exclusionary policies (e.g., sex testing) that mandate certain embodiments and physiological makeups, intersecting sexist and ableist ideologies about women's in/abilities, sexist representations of women athletes, as well as inequitable training, pay, and exposure. The problem is not some homogenized, yet correct, conception of women's innate embodiments and in/abilities; rather, the problem is systemic ableist and sexist understandings of women. In addition, if sex testing is outlawed – as it ought to be – the boundaries between men's and women's sport become increasingly blurrier. Hence, I ask, would maintaining sex-segregated sport even be possible or desirable? To answer this question, I consider the impacts of the sex desegregation of sport. I posit that sport should *not* be segregated by sex. I worry, however, that the sex desegregation of sport would result in the re/marginalization of women. I suspect that many women would be pushed out of sport if sex segregation was eradicated tomorrow. So, before sport is sex-desegregated, many other policies must be instituted.

Extending this line of reasoning, I then explore the pervious boundaries between ability and disability in sport organization. As briefly noted above, disabled and intersex-as/is-disabled athletes like Pistorius and Semenya and the il/logic deployed to justify their exclusion blur the apparently clear boundaries between abled and disabled athletes. They complicate and undermine the ableist underpinnings of dis/ability sport segregation. In line with the Paralympians and disability sports studies scholars who propose integrating the Paralympics and Olympics, I argue that sport should not be segregated in terms of dis/ability. As with my concerns about sex-desegregated sport, many other policies must be instituted to ensure that disabled athletes are not remarginalized in the sport world. Not only do things like media representation need to change in order to ensure that desegregation is successful, but we also need to envision different and new ways of competing, playing, organizing, and rewarding achievement that will benefit all athletes and prevent the remarginalization of all devalued and maligned athletes.

To conclude the chapter, I propose reimaging sport beyond desegregation and binary thinking about sex and dis/ability. Thinking of new ways to organize competitions and to reward athletic achievement, I offer up pragmatic means to change the organization of sport for the better and to change masculinist sport culture that prizes victory over all. I emphasize that even though restructuring sport culture and organization is a massive undertaking, it is not impossible. There are many inspirations and current sport organization to draw from.

Dis/Ability and Sport

Scholars and activists who analyze sport through a disability lens have proven that athletes with disabilities and Paralympians are too often rendered invisible, are reduced to inspirational objects, and are treated as an addendum to sporting events for enabled athletes.[2] Consider, for example, Brazilian *Vogue*'s campaign for the 2016 Paralympics, which featured images of able-bodied models Cleo Pires and Paulo Vilhena photoshopped to look like disabled Paralympians, namely table tennis player Bruna Alexandre and sitting volleyball player Renato Leite. The BBC (2016) reports that British former Paralympic swimmer and medalist Rachael Latham stated of the campaign, "The Paralympics is about showcasing disabled athletes who have trained to be the best person they can be. Allow them to do that by using actual Paralympians, not able-bodied models." The situation is particularly shocking because Paralympians who deserved to be represented, namely Alexandre and Leite, were at the photo shoot. But instead, they functioned as inspirational objects for Pires and Vilhena. "The campaign," Fernando Carneiro (2016) remarks, "is even more outrageous because the magazine had two actual Parathletes at the photo shoot 'as inspiration,' but [they] were not the subject of the campaign." It is also shocking because

Pires and Vilhena, who are ambassadors for the Brazilian Paralympic Committee, presumed that Paralympians could be best represented by them, not by Paralympians themselves. Their photo appeared under the headline "We Are All Paralympians." No, we are not all Paralympians. Suggesting that we all are Paralympians undermines these athletes' elite athletic status and achievements. Implying that we all are or can become Paralympians via photo-shopping is highly offensive.

In addition, although there is evidence that Paralympic media representation is increasing (Martin 2017), there is not nearly as much media coverage of the Paralympics as the Olympics (Affleck 2016; Dembe 2018; Tynedal and Wolbring 2013). Indeed, the Paralympics is an afterthought, an addendum. The Paralympics take place *after* the "main event," the Olympics, and sell far fewer tickets. As a result, British Paralympic gold medalist Ryan Raghoo (quoted in Heilpern 2016) notes that "the same value is not given to the same achievement." Indeed, Paralympians who are world record holders and medalists are not household names like many of their Olympian counterparts. The fact that Paralympians' achievements are not given the same value is clear when *Vogue* suggests, "We Are All Paralympians." Canadian Paralympic gold medalist Rick Hansen (quoted in Migneault 2016) echoes Raghoo, acknowledging that athletes with disabilities are not provided with the same opportunities as enabled athletes. Just as Paralympians' achievements are not given the same value as the achievements of Olympians, intersex-as/is-disabled athletes' and trans women's achievements are not given the same value as the achievements of endosex and cis athletes.

When there is coverage of disabled athletes, the "tragedy of disability" is often emphasized (Peers 2009, 653). The athletes are frequently represented as passive and pitiable. According to sport sociologist Jennifer Hargreaves (2000, 199), having "heroic images" of athletes with disabilities can "change public consciousness and overturn ableism." Perhaps heroic representations can counter the swath of narratives and representations that frame disabled people as tragic and tragically inferior. Nevertheless, as explained in more detail below, seemingly positive heroic images often reproduce what disability studies scholar Eli Clare (2009, 3) terms the "supercrip" trope or what the late journalist, comedian, and disability activist Stella Young (2012, 2014) called "inspiration porn." A supercrip is someone who heroically "overcomes" a disability in ways that are inspiring primarily to enabled people. Likewise, inspiration porn is a feel-good tool that misrepresents the reality of living with disabilities and aims to inspire and cater to enabled viewers. For example, in contrast to passive, pitiable, tragic representations, British television network Channel 4's (2016) trailer for the 2016 Paralympics, "We're the Superhumans," reproduces this inspirational supercrip porn. A blogger known as crippledscholar (2016) writes of the trailer, "It's ironic how closely the term Superhuman is to the term Super crip." The irony is even more palpable given that media outlets were cautioned against overusing terms like "superhuman," "brave," and "heroic" in Paralympic coverage and reporting because the terms are contentious among and offensive to some Paralympians and members of disability communities (Connelly 2016).

In the trailer, none of the athletes' names are stated or represented visually. Paralympic athletes cannot become household names and cannot be interpreted beyond objects of inspiration if they are not named. In a *Guardian* article praising the trailer penned by Homa Khaleeli (2016), some of the featured Paralympians' and other individuals' names are noted. In the article, the athletes' names are accompanied by a list of some of their accomplishments and also often by a brief "origin story"[3] of how they acquired their disabilities or, as pejoratively explained in one story, "deformities." The article lists Alvin Law, Canadian drummer; Bartek Ostalowski, Polish racing driver; Jessica Cox, American pilot, dancer, and taekwondo black belt; Ellie Simmonds, British Paralympic swimmer, medalist, and world record holder; Natalie Blake, British Paralympic powerlifter; Hannah Cockroft, British Paralympic wheelchair racer, world record holder, and medalist; Matthew Phillips, British rock climber; Aaron "Wheelz" Fotheringham, American wheelchair stuntman and motocross athlete; Evan Ruggiero, American tap dancer; and Tony Dee, Australian singer.

Dee sings the Sammy Davis Jr. track "Yes I Can" throughout the trailer, giving new meaning to the song's lyrics "'Gee, I'm afraid to go on,' has turned into, 'Yes I can.'" These athletes, or so the narrative insinuates, were "afraid to go on" because of the tragedy of disability. However, they overcame their fearful, defeatist attitudes. They declared, "Yes I can." And, subsequently, they overcame their disabilities to become superhumans. The athletes, as well as the other talented individuals featured in the video, are framed as overcoming their disabilities via a change in attitude. Like so many ableist neoliberal success stories, they are presumed to have independently overcome their disabilities by working hard and having a positive attitude. One cannot deny that these athletes work tremendously hard and, at times, may have positive attitudes. However, this narrative effectively erases the institutionalized ableism that these people face. It also erases the interpersonal circumstances, the possible medical care and technologies, and the labour that helped these people to reach such elite levels.[4] In addition, this representation ignores the fact that many disabled people do not view their disabilities as something to overcome or defeat but rather experience them as an integral part of their identity and sense of self (Martin 2017). Although the athletes in the trailer are shown actively performing their sports, they are essentially nameless objects of inspiration. They become "in-spite-of" stories that reproduce the narrative that people can independently overcome their disabilities if they just shift their perspective – "Yes I can!"

This trailer is an example of "inspiration porn" (Young 2014); it is "supercrip crap" (Clare 2009, 3). Young (2014) explained that inspiration porn comprises images of people with disabilities – often doing sports – accompanied by motivational rhetoric like "Yes I can," "The only disability in life is a bad attitude," "Before you quit, try," and "Your excuse is invalid." These representations, Young (2014) clarified, "objectify disabled people for the benefit of non-disabled people." They provide enabled people with the opportunity to think, "Well, however bad my life is, it could be worse. I could be that [disabled] person" (Young 2014). Young (2014) then asked, "But what if you are that person?" She suggested that such a person feels reduced and dehumanized. At the objectifying expense of disabled people, enabled viewers are inspired and ultimately end up pitying disabled people.

Inspiration porn like the "We're the Superhumans" trailer also "create[s] unrealistically high expectations of what *all* disabled people should accomplish" and, subsequently, "serve[s] to justify the vilification of particular disabled people who do not manage to overcome, often writing them off as stubborn or lazy and therefore deserving of the poverty or lack of care that they may experience" (Peers 2015, 332). Put differently, inspiration porn and supercrip crap erase ableism and compulsory able-bodiedness, invalidate the difficulties that people with disabilities experience, ignore the fact that some of the tools (e.g., blades, wheelchairs, training, and medication) that some disabled folks need to perform certain activities – in this instance, elite athletics – are unattainable and expensive, erase how economic, legal, and health care systems fail people with disabilities, and function to simply inspire enabled people.

To explain further, Young (2014) states,

That quote, "The only disability in life is a bad attitude," the reason that that's bullshit is because it's just not true ... No amount of smiling at a flight of stairs has ever made it turn into a ramp. Never. Smiling at a television screen isn't going to make closed captions appear for people who are deaf. No amount of standing in the middle of a bookshelf and radiating a positive attitude is going to turn all those books into braille.

No amount of singing "Yes I can" will turn stairs into ramps, magically provide people with the economic and medical services that they need, make one into an elite athlete, or provide one with the expensive resources required to pursue an athletic career as a Paralympian. To borrow from Samantha King's (2010, 286) analyses regarding the commodification and representation of breast cancer, inspiration porn is infused with and relies on "the tyranny of cheerfulness." Disabled people are expected – demanded – to radiate positivity. Yet a positive outlook cannot erase ableist systems and compulsory able-bodiedness. Promoting the idea that all people with disabilities can overcome their "undesirable" disabilities, be happy, perhaps even transform stairs into ramps, and become elite athletes if they shift their attitudes – if they just declare, "Yes I can," or if they just "draw on their own inherent energy and power" (McWhorter 1999, 155) – encourages enabled individuals to think of disability as a personal problem or choice, not an instituted problem that they influence. Inspiration porn and supercrip crap, therefore, allow enabled people to remain complicit in reproducing ableist structures.

There is evidence that the narrative of the inspirational supercrip does not always dominate conversations about or representations of Paralympians (Martin 2017). However, it clearly still governs and informs many viewers' perceptions of disabilities, Paralympians, and people with disabilities in general. This is clear given that the "We're the Superhumans" trailer has been viewed over 10 million times and has been praised by numerous high-profile media and news outlets. That said, as disability and sport studies researchers Liam French and Jill M. Le Clair (2018, 99) explain, the proliferation of social media platforms (e.g., Twitter) has the potential to radically contest "the established gate-keeping role of professional sports broadcasters and journalists," subsequently aiding in the spread of alternative narratives and representations and changing the ways that people engage with the Paralympics. Ensuring that Paralympians represent themselves, diversifying representations of Paralympians, and moving away from stereotypical tragedy, inspirational representations, and supercrip crap at all levels of sport and (social) media are vital to countering ableist, reductive, and objectifying representations of both athletes with disabilities and people with disabilities in general.

In the introduction to Kim Q. Hall's (2011, 3) edited collection *Feminist Disability Studies,* Hall considers whether Semenya could be read as a supercrip, despite the fact that Semenya "neither self-identifies as nor is widely perceived to be disabled." Given that Semenya is pathologized, her remarkable athletic abilities and accomplishments may exemplify the narrative of the overcoming supercrip; Semenya heroically "overcame" her intersex-as/is-disability and, perhaps, qualifies as a "superhuman." One could also note that, like athletes with disabilities, Semenya has been and is consistently objectified by the medical gaze. However, unlike Paralympians and other disabled or pathologized athletes, Semenya – indeed, any athlete with (suspect) intersex traits – is not represented as a supercrip. She is represented as a threat to fairness and women's sport. If she were represented as a supercrip, rather than a threat, maintaining sex testing would be quite difficult. That is, a disability studies lens is imperative when considering sex testing. In fact, paying more attention to disability, pathologization, and narratives of dis/abilities, hyper/abilities, or in/abilities in sport enables us to unpack sex testing and, in turn, to reimagine sex and dis/ability sport segregation. Ultimately, sex and dis/ability segregation are rooted in intersecting sexist and ableist ideologies and must therefore be contested.

Sex Sport Segregation

As demonstrated in the previous chapter, the fact that sex testing needs to be abolished is unquestionably clear. Doing so would constitute a necessary decolonizing and anti-discriminatory undertaking. I endorse immediately scrapping all sex-testing policies and creating policies that reject future sex-testing proposals and protect athletes with intersex traits from curative violence and intersecting forms of discrimination. Deinstitutionalizing sex testing, however, leaves us with a conundrum. Sex testing and sex segregation, Shari L. Dworkin and Cheryl Cooky (2012, 21, 22) explain, cannot be "disentangled"; they are "mutually constitutive" policies. Without sex testing, how can sex segregation be enforced? If sex testing was abolished and the fact that the sex binary is a farce was openly acknowledged, we would have to wonder whether sport ought to be sex-desegregated. If sport policies do not attempt to police the porous boundaries of sex, what good purpose does sport sex segregation serve? Given that the sex binary is untenable, sport never was and never could be successfully segregated by sex. Sex desegregation seems like the reasonable solution. That said, would abolishing sex segregation at this time contribute to creating a more equitable sport system?

Sport sex segregation is presumed to be a de facto necessary kindness because, so the sexist logic goes, women are too delicate and weak to compete alongside or against men. Consequently, women must be protected from competing against men, trans women (who are presumed to be men by sport organizations), and "masculinized" intersex women. This "protectionist discourse" serves to justify sex segregation, sex testing, and the development of supposedly inferior women-specific sports. Rather than accepting this "protectionist discourse," Dworkin and Cooky (2012, 22) point to the fact that sex segregation in sport was

> put forward historically when women outperformed men at athletic performances. For example, Jackie Mitchell, the first woman to sign a professional baseball contract, struck out both Babe Ruth and Lou Gehrig in 1936 ... The commissioner of baseball was so perturbed that he banned women from professional baseball and they have been banned from the sport ever since. Softball, which is perceived as inferior due to the larger, slower ball, was then further developed as a sport specifically for women.

According to Dworkin and Cooky, sex segregation, subsequent sex testing, and "subordinate" sports for women were not established to reflect innate gendered physical in/abilities but to preserve male supremacy and, I add, the interconnected logics of sexism and ableism.

Rejecting male supremacy and sex/ist sport segregation, sociologist and anthropologist Ann Travers (2008, 90) argues that institutional powers should "entirely eliminate sex as an organizational category in sport":

> Queer postmodern feminism's deconstruction of the two sex system as ideological rather than natural (Fausto-Sterling, 2000, 1992; Haraway, 1997, 1991; Butler, 2004) supports an argument for the elimination of sex segregated sport. This argument can be summed up as follows: First, differences in men's and women's athletic performances can be attributed to social, political, economic, and psychological discrimination rather than biological factors ... Second, sport is implicated in translating the ideology of the two sex system into the material reality of bodies that conform to sexist expectations ... Third, the very separation of the girls from boys and women from men constitutes gender injustice.

Travers's arguments are convincing. But we must ask, as Travers does, what desegregation means for women's sport. Would women be positively or negatively impacted by desegregation? Travers (2008, 92) suggests that, if sport was sex-desegregated without considerable cultural and ideological renovations, women would be discouraged from participating because they would inevitably "be subjected to sexist and masculinist sporting cultures." Rather than creating an equitable sporting environment, sex desegregation would likely cause women's participation to drastically decrease. And, Travers (2008, 92) notes, the marginal women athletes who remained and "flourish[ed] under such a restructuring would be so distanced from the majority as to be viewed as abnormal." The few remaining women athletes would be construed as anomalous – possibly pathological, intersex, trans, or "manly" – outliers. Rather than achieving equitable sporting arenas and broadening ideas of what it means to be a woman and what women can do, sex desegregation would likely reinforce intersecting interphobic, sexist, ableist, cisgenderist, and racist ideologies.

In addition to sexist and masculinist sporting cultures that would likely drive women athletes out of sporting competitions, medical geneticist Eric Vilain (2012) notes in a *New York Times* article that if sport was sex-desegregated, "female athletes would lose most, if not all, elite competitions. For all the brouhaha around Semenya's eligibility as a female athlete and perceived advantage, one should remember that her time in the 800 meters at the [2009] world championships – 1 minute 55.45 seconds – would not have even qualified for the men's final." Many would lose because of, as Travers (2008) notes, the social, political, economic, and psychological discrimination that women athletes have faced for decades. Additionally, some athletes with intersex traits may not even be able to compete because of the body-mind disabilities acquired via past sex testing and curative violence. It seems like sport sex desegregation would ultimately help men to continue dominating the sports world and would further marginalize women. As a result, Rebecca Jordan-Young and Katrina Karkazis (2012) seem skeptical of desegregating sport: "Sex segregation is probably a good idea in some sports, at some levels and at some moments."

Although Joanna Harper (quoted in Bennett 2016), an adviser on gender issues to the International Olympic Committee, would likely never support sex-desegregated sport or outlawing sex testing, she remarks that permitting intersex athletes to compete in women's sport without reducing their natural testosterone levels "threatens the very fabric of women's sport." Harper's views are undeniably discriminatory. The concern for women's sport, however, is valid. Women athletes, their coaches, and their supporters have long fought for women's place in the sport world, their unique sport culture, and the same recognition as men athletes. This history and culture must not be erased, forgotten, or conquered by masculinist sport culture as we consider the impacts of sex desegregation. Subsequently, we must not conceptualize sport sex desegregation as women entering men's sport, the destruction of women's sport, or the active erasure of women's sport. Sport sex desegregation is about imagining and creating an equitable sport world so that women can thrive alongside men and people of all genders. Desegregating sport does not have to result in the remarginalization of women athletes. Desegregating sport need not be antithetical to maintaining the fabric of women's sport. Rather, if done right, sex desegregation can add to the fabric of women sporting history, as well as sporting history as a whole.

In addition to the radical ideological and cultural shifts required to ensure that sex desegregation is successful and constructive (Travers 2008), policies must be in place to ensure "gender equity through access to opportunity" (Jordan-Young and Karkazis 2012), such as equitable pay, funding and sponsorship opportunities, access to training facilities, and media coverage. These are feasible goals and promising stepping stones to future legislative changes concerning sport organization, including sex desegregation. As Jordan-Young and Karkazis (2012) write, "It is time to refocus policy discussions at every level [of sport] so that sex segregation is one means to achieve fairness, not the ultimate goal." Sex segregation should not be the ultimate goal. It marginalizes women (especially intersex and trans women), fuels sexist, ableist, and racist conceptions about women/femininity, reproduces compulsory dyadism, justifies sex testing and curative violence, erases nonbinary and genderqueer athletes, and stifles our ability to imagine otherwise. Ultimately, the sex binary is a farce. Consequently, sport could never successfully be segregated by sex. Rather than restructuring intersex and trans people's body-minds to fit them into an imaginary sex binary and devaluing women's sport, sport can and should be restructured so that it reflects and acknowledges the complex reality of sex/gender diversity and women's abilities.

Dis/ability Sport Segregation

Comparable to the protectionist logics used to justify sport sex segregation and, by extension, sex testing and curative violence, sport is segregated by dis/ability because athletes with disabilities presumably need to be "protected" from able-bodied athletes. Able-bodied athletes will inevitably win in a competition against disabled athletes, so the ableist logic goes. Dis/ability sport segregation is a paternalistic, organizational measure ostensibly enacted for disabled athletes' own good. However, the activism and achievements of Para-lympians, the work of scholars in disability sport studies, and the patholo-gization of intersex-as/is-disabled athletes call into question and complicate the dis/ability binary and the presumed necessity of dis/ability segregation. That is, intersex-as/is-disabled athletes complicate not only the sex binary and sex segregation but also the boundaries between ability and disability.

According to the International Paralympic Committee's (IPC) (n.d.) web-page concerning the Paralympic Movement, although organized sport for people with disabilities can be traced back to well over a hundred years ago, sport for disabled folks was not popularized until after the Second World War (see also Bailey 2008). Intended to abet and rehabilitate, sport was or-ganized for the large numbers of war veterans and civilians who were dis-abled by the war. Named after the British hospital that opened a centre to treat spinal cord injuries and that encouraged rehabilitation sport, the Stoke Mandeville Games took place on the hospital grounds on the same day as the opening ceremony of the 1948 Olympics in London. The Stoke Mande-ville Games took place in the same city as the Olympics – Rome, Italy – for the first time in 1960. Those games, although not called the Paralympics at the time, are generally deemed the first Paralympics. "Paralympics" is a portmanteau that combines "paraplegic" and "Olympics."

Reflecting the subsequent inclusion of athletes with many other types of disabilities, "para" now refers to "parallel" (Goggin and Newell 2000, 74). "Para" implies that the Olympics and the Paralympics are not divided but occur in tandem, together. However, as disability studies scholars Gerard Goggin and Christopher Newell (2000, 71) note, they do not really occur together: "The Paralympics are very much a separate event held almost three weeks after the Olympics finish." There are a few notable exceptions, but this separation – this ableist dis/ability segregation – "is not questioned" (Goggin and Newell 2000, 71).[5] Dis/ability segregation is understood as natural because there are many circumstances (e.g., education, sports, and institutionalization) in which folks with disabilities have long been segre-gated. Underpinning systemic dis/ability segregation is the assumption that disabilities render people inherently worse, less capable, and undesirable. Although the segregation of Olympic and Paralympic athletes is presumed natural because of the apparent body-mind differences and dis/abilities of Paralympians, a closer examination of the discourses that surround Olym-pians and Paralympians demonstrates that the segregation is narrated as being needed, logical, and just.

Similar to the narratives around sport sex segregation, underpinning the assumption that dis/ability segregation is necessary and fair – separate but equal – is the ableist idea that enabled people's abilities and body-minds are inherently better than disabled people's abilities and body-minds. Hence, segregation is apparently necessary for Paralympians' own good since they will inevitably lose against Olympians. In addition, comparable to women-specific sports (e.g., softball), disabled-specific sporting events (e.g., wheelchair basketball, sitting volleyball, and wheelchair tennis) are presumed to be inferior, to require less skill, and/or to be less exciting to watch. These ableist assumptions are evidently categorically false to anyone who has watched the Paralympics or engaged in parasports. Rather than requiring fewer skills, parasports may require different skills. The assumption that it is less exciting to watch disabled people – including elite disabled athletes – is rooted in ableist assumptions and expectations. In addition, Paralympians consistently challenge the ableist, protectionist discourse, and Paralympians can and do outperform Olympians (Wolbring 2012). Oscar Pistorius is one such example. This fact should prompt us to question who benefits from segregation, who is really being protected, and whether the logic that disabled athletes need to be protected holds up to scrutiny.

Kafer (2013) critiques the supposed need for and fairness of dis/ability segregation by analyzing the media response to Pistorius's attempt to compete as an Olympian at the 2008 Olympics in Beijing and the media response to his successful bid to compete at the 2012 Olympics in London. Kafer observes that Pistorius's disability and Olympian status complicate the taken-for-granted distinction between enabled and disabled athletes. However, "Blade Runner" Pistorius was represented as a cyborg by mainstream media, which functioned to resolidify the dis/abled and un/natural binaries and the idea that enabled and disabled athletes must remain segregated. Kafer (2013, 108–9) states,

> With his gleaming high-tech prosthetics, Pistorius perfectly embodied the cultural understanding of a cyborg; he was one with his machine ... What I want to highlight here is the way in which news writers presented Pistorius as a definitive cyborg and, therefore, almost of a different species than his fellow runners. Anna Salleh [2010], writing for an Australian news outlet, described the Pistorius case as one involving "the competing rights of cyborgs and non-cyborgs." Bloggers from both sports and technology sites described the case in terms of the arrival of the "cyborg athlete" ... Not only

was Pistorius's cyborgization taken for granted in these stories, but so, too – and relatedly – was his difference. As Swartz and Watermeyer [2008, 188] note, doping can also be seen as cyborg technology, but athletes accused of doping are not described in those terms; physical disability and its attendant technologies render one cyborgian in a way nothing else can.

The cyborg/noncyborg distinction points to a problematic assumption underlying popular conceptions of the cyborg. Although Haraway intended the figure to critique dualistic understandings of nature and culture or of humans and machine, too often it serves only to reify such binary logic. In these news stories, "cyborg" represents the melding of pure body and pure machine; there is an original purity that, thanks to the assistive technology, has only now been mixed, hybridized, blurred. To return to the Pistorius case, the athlete is simply a body; when it gets mixed with the prosthetic machine, it becomes impure, mixed, cyborg. A nondisabled runner, in other words, is natural, unmixed, unadultered ... The "cyborg" concept thus serves to perpetuate binaries of pure/impure, natural/unnatural, and natural/technological; rather than breaking down binaries, it buttresses them.

Presenting Pistorius as a cyborg naturalizes the un/natural dichotomy and justifies Paralympian-Olympian segregation. Competition can be fair, the narrative proposes, only if Paralympians and Olympians, cyborgs and noncyborgs, are segregated. Akin to representing Pistorius as an impure cyborg, naming the 2016 Paralympians "superhumans" – unnatural, unbelievable, and cyborgian – in Channel 4's (2016) trailer also functions to reinforce the "naturalness" of Paralympian-Olympian segregation.

Like intersex-as/is-disabled athletes' characterization as unfairly advantaged, Pistorius was represented not simply as a tainted cyborg but also as an unfairly advantaged cyborg. This representation challenges ableist assumptions that having a disability or pathologized embodiment is always a disadvantage. In turn, dis/ability segregation is contested. For example, Rose Eveleth's (2012) article for *Smithsonian Magazine* posits that Pistorius has an unfair advantage: "Science shows that Pistorius uses less energy than his competitors, raising questions about whether or not he should be allowed to compete" as an Olympian. Like (suspect) intersex athletes, in the context of sport, Pistorius's disabled and allegedly inherently disadvantaged morphology becomes an unfair advantage. The seeming illogic – Pistorius is disabled *and* advantaged – undermines the ableist narrative that people with disabilities are always and already disadvantaged, less capable, or incapable. This contradiction also challenges the protectionist narrative that athletes with disabilities must be segregated for their own good.

The similarity in contradictory, dichotomous discourses used to justify excluding both Pistorius (from competing as an Olympian) and Semenya (from competing unless she undergoes curative violence) prompts me to think of Pistorius and Semenya on the same continuum even though (suspect) intersex athletes are not necessarily legibly disabled, disordered, or cyborgian. In other words, the discriminatory treatment of athletes with disabilities and athletes with (suspect) intersex-as/is-disabled traits cannot be regarded or treated as distinct academic, social, sport, and human rights issues. If we place intersex and disability on the same continuum when evaluating sport segregation and sex testing, the seemingly justified segregation between men and women, Paralympians and Olympians, and cyborgs and noncyborgs blurs.

The response to disabled and intersex athletes reveals that sport governing bodies and troubled sport fans are not genuinely invested in keeping cyborgs and noncyborgs separate in the name of fairness. In order for intersex athletes to become supposedly proper, natural women, they must cyborgize by ingesting synthetic hormones to alter their hormonal environment. At the same time, many argue that Pistorius must compete as a Paralympian precisely because he is a cyborg. It is clear that narratives used to justify exclusion and segregation are selectively chosen and deployed to maintain discriminatory ideologies and sex and dis/ability segregation.

Moreover, the concern with sport fairness spikes when one's assumed advantages come from one's "disordered" or "disabled" (sex) characteristics. Concern spikes when compulsory dyadism as well as sexist and ableist ideals about what women are physically capable of are challenged; concern spikes when one's assumed advantage comes from one's disability or disorder. The fact that sport governing institutions and viewers of sport appear to be worried about fair play only when it comes to disorders or disabilities – not, for example, embodied advantages like tallness, increased hemoglobin levels, and double-joints or economic disparities between competitors, teams, and countries – suggests that the discourse of fair play and equality functions primarily as a guise for exclusionary and discriminatory ideologies and policies.

Before Pistorius challenged what being a Paralympian and Olympian means in mainstream conversation, the criteria regarding who can be classified as disabled and can therefore compete as a Paralympian had been challenged and had shifted within the IPC:

> Although this group [i.e., Paralympians] was initially restricted to those
> with spinal cord injuries, it later came to include athletes with cerebral
> palsy, amputations, restricted sight and various other medicalized physical
> conditions listed under the umbrella term *les autres* [the other]. Athletes
> with intellectual disabilities did compete for medals in one Paralympic
> Games (2000), but were disqualified from further competition shortly
> thereafter. (Peers 2009, 662)

People with intellectual disabilities were eligible to compete again several
years later and did so. Ultimately, however, certain medicalized and medically classifiable disabled and disordered athletes – although not those with
intersex characteristics – can compete as Paralympians (see IPC 2015,
2016). And there have been shifts in who is eligible and who qualifies to
compete because creating a definitive classification system to determine
who is disabled "enough" or disabled in the "right" way is impossible.
Stephanie Dixon (quoted in C. Brown and Corday 2016), a CBC Paralympic
commentator and former Paralympian, explains that "it's really difficult to
draw the line"; hence, there is a level of arbitrariness involved in classifying
athletes with disabilities.

The disabilities of all prospective Paralympians are assessed to determine
whether they are "properly" disabled. The fact that people's disabilities may
manifest differently through time and space presents challenges for these
athletes on assessment day. For example, Amy Burk (quoted in C. Brown
and Corday 2016), a Team Canada goalball player with a visual impairment,
has been excluded from competitions because her impairment on various
occasions was not "severe enough to qualify her as a disabled athlete." Burk
explains that her vision varies from day to day and that lighting in a room,
for example, can influence her vision. As a result, some days she might be
classified as disabled enough to compete, whereas other days she might not.

Drawing from their own experiences as a former Paralympic wheelchair
basketball athlete, disability, queer, and crip theorist Danielle Peers (2012)
notes that getting re/classified as a Paralympian is a long, difficult, objectifying,
and invasive process that re/creates the category of disability. Re/classifying
as a Paralympian requires these athletes to repeatedly demonstrate that they
have a definitively medically diagnosable disability and certain body-mind
in/capacities. They must do so via various performances that include, but
are not limited to, displaying medical documents, retelling origin stories
(e.g., about an accident or about being born a certain way), and performing
physical movements that highlight the disability but do not jeopardize one's

supercrip status, movements that satisfy enabled onlookers, and movements that satisfy fellow athletes. Drawing from Michel Foucault's analyses of self-/ surveillance, Peers (2015, 332, 335) describes enacting complicated performances as a properly disabled, supercrip Paralympian before becoming, in their words, a "revolting gimp," one "who either cannot or will not inspirationally overcome disabling circumstances":

> I meticulously trained myself out of every possible sign of "gimpy" fatigue or pain that would call into question the legitimacy of my supercrip status. I simultaneously trained myself out of leg movement and other signs of ability that would call into question the legitimacy of my disabled status. Strangers, too, actively policed my inspiration disabled status insofar as their inspired looks often changed to looks of disapproval – which were sometimes even accompanied by angry accusations that I was a "faker" – if and when I moved my legs, stood up from my wheelchair, or switched from my wheelchair to my crutches, and vice versa. I came to learn that the capacity to inspire is linked to the capacity to act *as if* I were a stereotypical disabled subject with a complete spinal cord injury.

Diagnosed with a progressive genetic myopathy, Peers's disability and re/ classifiable status as a Paralympian shifted throughout their athletic career depending on how they policed themself, who was looking, how they behaved, what origin story they told and when they told it, and what they were presumably in/capable of doing. Through enough successful performances, they *became* disabled (enough); they *became* a supercrip. Comparable to (inter)sex classifications in sport that "*construct* sex difference" (McDonagh and Pappano 2008, 15), "disability stories produce disabled subjects," Peers (2012, 186) notes. Who is classifiable as properly disabled in sport is not as clear-cut as one might assume. These binaries are fragile and therefore require constant maintenance and self-/surveillance.

Just as I reject sex segregation, I maintain that sport should not be dis/ ability-segregated, but there are some valid concerns with desegregation. My rejection of dis/ability segregation, at least in part, echoes Goggin and Newell's (2000, 75) observation that, for some people with disabilities,

> the notion of a Paralympics is ethically unacceptable, even if in the real world it does give some people with disability the opportunity to achieve in sport. For these, the existence of a special event for people identified as having disability is a painful reminder of inequity and injustice, and its

presence perpetuates the discourse of "special needs" and "special events" – excluded from the moral community. It occurs in a world where oppression and segregation have been the collective experience of people with disabilities ... It is certainly remarkable that the claims of people with disability for participation in mainstream society stand in stark and unremarkable contrast to a sporting event where a select few medically defined disability types are organised into yet another special or separate event.

Segregation and "special" events are normalized and deemed necessary, but they are heavily critiqued by disability studies scholars and activists for being patronizing and exclusionary.[6] Supporting Goggin and Newell's statement that some people with disabilities deem the Paralympics unacceptable, a survey conducted by ComRes on behalf of Scope (2011), a British-based disability equity organization, suggests that this view is perhaps widespread. Of the 386 people with disabilities who were polled, 65 percent of participants supported jettisoning the Paralympics entirely and, instead, allowing athletes with disabilities to compete in the Olympics. Likewise, Rick Hansen (2010) proposes that the Olympics and the Paralympics be merged.

Recognizing the numerous logistical problems with merging the Olympics and Paralympics, namely accommodating thousands more athletes in the same space and at the same time, a former president of the IPC, Sir Philip Craven (quoted in D. Rose 2012), notes that the IPC is "very keen" at the prospect; the IPC hopes that a merger is possible in the 2020s and has stated that it "would maintain the number of athletes." The IPC would ensure that the number of athletes with disabilities did not shrink with a merger. For a merger to work successfully, the best approach would not likely be to try to fit all athletes into the same place at the same time, which would require the host city to build many more facilities and would likely decimate environments and people's communities. A better alternative would be to have athletes come and leave in waves while ensuring that the waves were a mix of disabled and enabled athletes as well as sports. I am aware that this proposal means that many athletes would miss the much-anticipated opening and closing ceremonies. However, this sacrifice is needed given that environmental destruction occurs and communities are routinely torn down and displaced to make room for the Olympics and Paralympics. Host countries should actively work to prevent such psychological, physical, economic, and environmental trauma.

Similar to Harper (quoted in Bennett 2016), who is concerned for "the very fabric of women's sport," former Paralympian Baroness Tanni Grey-Thompson (quoted in D. Rose 2012) worries that, with a merger, the Paralympics would "disappear off the face of the earth." Disabled athletes would likely be pushed out of most competitions, and the rich history and culture of the Paralympics could be erased. This is a valid concern. Nevertheless, it is time to start imagining sport organization differently, centring marginalized athletes' voices in the process. In doing so, we can ensure that merging the Olympics and the Paralympics does not involve pushing out Paralympians or erasing history. Before we proceed with dis/ability desegregation, we need to institute initiatives to ensure that, to add to Jordan-Young and Karkazis's (2012) proposal, gender, sex, racial, national, *and* disability equity is instituted through, for instance, equal access to opportunity, resources, health care, and training, as well as via equitable and anti-discriminatory media coverage, funding redistribution, and rethinking the ways that athletes are re/classified. And these initiatives are needed at all levels of sport – youth to elite – so that the change is radical and enduring.

We can start this change by entertaining the idea of holding the Paralympics before the Olympics and ensuring equitable, anti-discriminatory media coverage. These sorts of initiatives are needed. Consider that after the 2016 Olympics in Rio de Janeiro, yet before the Paralympics took place, not only were ticket sales terribly low, but there were also economic cuts to venues, the workforce, and transportation; there were also delays in travel-grant payments that jeopardized the ability of ten countries' athletes to arrive and participate (Heilpern 2016; Owen 2016). Some even conjectured that the 2016 Paralympics might be cancelled entirely (Springer 2016). Holding the Paralympics before the Olympics would ensure that the Paralympics were not an afterthought and that Paralympic competition was not placed in peril. Foregrounding Paralympians' athleticism and achievements and ensuring equitable, anti-ableist promotion and media coverage would help to change – and crip – sporting culture for the better. Paralympians can become celebrated household names only if we witness them perform, ensure that they represent themselves, and avoid ableist tropes. We can collectively start to question who really benefits from sport segregation only if we witness their brilliance.

Thinking through the supposed need to sex-test athletes as well as to segregate sport by sex and dis/ability alongside each other makes it clear that the discriminatory treatment of disabled athletes and the discriminatory treatment of athletes with (suspect) intersex-as/is-disabled traits cannot be regarded or confronted as distinct issues. Placing intersex and disability on the same continuum when evaluating sport sex segregation and sex testing blurs the seemingly justified segregation between men and women, Paralympians and Olympians, and cyborgs and noncyborgs. Cripping sport segregation reveals the fact that these binary distinctions are rooted in Western, colonial, imperial ideologies about body-mind morphologies. This theorizing productively draws links between intersex studies and movements and disability studies and movements while pointing to a location where the studies and movements of both, in addition to anti-colonial and anti-racist studies and movements, can effectively align to contest systemic, intersecting oppressive policies.

I like to envision creative, inventive sports arenas where all sorts of non/cyborgian, dis/abled, dis/ordered, inter/sexed, and gendered people of all races and nations come together to reimagine how we play, move, compete, and reward athleticism. I like to imagine a future in which sports arenas actually strive to and fulfill the modern Olympic and Paralympic goals of cultivating and promoting peace, uniting people across countries and continents, building bridges across differences, and treating all people as equals.[7] If the goal is to create unity and equality and to build figurative and possibly literal bridges, reinforcing barriers by segregating sport and actively discriminating against marginalized people's embodiments prevents this goal from manifesting. Not only does buttressing barriers impact specific individual athletes, but doing so is also a colonial practice that impacts numerous nations, cultures, and communities. Sex and dis/ability binaries and segregated sports represent a very specific cultural approach, namely a Western, colonial, binary approach to classifying, organizing, thinking about, and treating people. Not only is this approach inapplicable in the context of sport because it does not reflect the diversity of body-minds or numerous communities and countries, but it also naturalizes and institutionalizes myriad forms of violence. Sex- and dis/ability-segregated sport is ethically intolerable.

Conclusion: Reimaging Sport beyond Desegregation

Anti-ableist, anti-colonial, anti-sexist, anti-cisgenderist, and anti-interphobic analyses show us that sport segregation is not the only organizational model. Decolonizing and cripping sport should not be limited to ensuring that disabled athletes and countries in the Global South have access to events and, as outlined in the previous chapter, prohibiting sex testing.[8] We must radically rethink and do away with binary models. There are other ways of thinking about dis/ability, body-mind diversity, sex, race, nationality, gender, and awarding athletic accomplishments. Various scholars and cultures offer up less oppressive and less pathologizing alternatives. For example, one can look toward many Indigenous, Aboriginal, First Nations, Inuit, and Métis communities and nations across the globe that, historically and/or currently, recognize numerous gender and/or sex categories because they acknowledge and structure their lives around more expansive understandings of gender, sex, sexual anatomies, and sexualities.[9] The Western two-sex dyad is not inevitable. Therefore, sport sex segregation is not inevitable. To quote Cheryl Cooky, Ranissa Dycus, and Shari L. Dworkin (2013, 50–51), we have "the potential to extend beyond the sex/gender binary in sport" and, I add, the dis/ability binary in sport, which could lead to "the eradication of sex, gender, race, and sexuality," as well as the end of disability injustice. Equally, we have the potential and the tools to decolonize and crip sport in a way that extends beyond the desegregation of sport to the eradication of myriad forms of discrimination, the creation of new possible sporting arenas, and the development of new modes of rewarding athletic achievement.

That said, current organizations and the people in power cannot merely look toward or draw from different models, cultures, and communities. As Ryan Raghoo (quoted in Heilpern 2016) states, whether the Paralympics and the Olympics merge, or the Paralympics are held before the Olympics, or the Paralympics and/or the Olympics are dissolved, "the athletes [with disabilities] have to be at the very centre of whatever decision is made." However sport is reorganized, athletes from all participating nations, athletes of colour, and athletes who are women, intersex, queer, or trans must be central to the reorganization process. Additionally, countries and communities in which sport mega-events may be held must be central to conversations about the possible physical, psychological, economic, colonial, and environmental impacts of holding such large events.

As noted above, if sport were sex- and dis/ability-desegregated, women and disabled athletes would likely be pushed out. This is the case not because of inherent deficits and not simply because of the social, political, economic, and psychological discrimination that women and disabled athletes are subjected to, but also because sport is not organized in a way that wholly recognizes, plans for, or celebrates human body-mind diversity or rewards alternative achievements. My suggestion to desegregate sport does not mean that all human morphologies, abilities, and required technologies for various sports are the same. Human biological diversity, dis/abilities, and cyborg embodiments should be recognized and celebrated, not downplayed or ignored. As a result, it is imperative to think beyond desegregating sport;

we need to think of new ways to organize sporting events that attend to non/cyborg and body-mind diversity.

We can think in terms of, for instance, height, weight, dis/ability, and what technologies are used to do the sport. That is, we can draw inspiration from the ways that the Paralympics, Olympics, and other sporting competitions currently organize events based on people's body-mind variations and capacities. Jonathan Migneault (2016) reports on his conversation with Rick Hansen: "Some sports, like boxing, ... segregate athletes based on their size and weight ... Hansen said it would not be a big jump to acknowledge the differences between able-bodied athletes, and those with physical disabilities, in the same games." In a similar vein, disability, technology, and bioethics scholar Gregor Wolbring (2012, 260) argues, "Given what the future holds for the ability modification of humans, the prudent way forward seems to be to have one big Olympics and no separate -lympics. That would very likely in the future also entail events where 'disabled' and 'non-disabled' athletes perform in the same event based on some external tools such as everyone in a wheelchair or exoskeleton." Thinking about these possibilities can open up new ways to play, participate, and compete. Doing so will allow us to focus on "being enthralled by people trying to achieve their best within their framework without judging one framework superior to another" (Wolbring 2012, 261).

We also need to think beyond the dichotomous, masculinist, win-lose, competitive mentality. To do so, we can and should reward and recognize other athletic achievements, not simply the feat of placing first, second, or third. This proposal is not a new concept. We already have, for example, awards for most improved, most valued, rookie of the year, hustle, and participation from youth to elite levels of sport. That said, the value placed on these types of awards is not nearly as high as the value placed on winning. Colleen English (2018, 109–10), a professor of kinesiology, rethinks youth sports, participation awards, and rewarding athletes' successes, arguing that young athletes

> should be given opportunities for earning awards beyond mere victory. This is because a variety of values, such as symbolic meaning, challenge and risk, aesthetics, and high-quality relationships with teammates and opponents, deserve reward as well ... An excessive focus on competition can be harmful to athletes. By emphasizing hypercompetitive, win-at-all costs attitudes, organizations and coaches weaken other values. When young athletes are only rewarded for winning, they receive the message that

the only and most worthwhile value of sport is victory ... Tokens of achievement can be given for meeting, or striving to meet, a variety of alternate sport values.

English writes in terms of youth athletics, but her ideas can extend to elite athletics. Furthermore, although English does not note that most of these devalued sporting ideals – symbolic meaning, aesthetics, and relationship building – are feminized, taking stock of this fact reveals the sexist underpinnings of resisting efforts to widen what is worth rewarding. Is sport really depreciated if it is "feminized"? Is there something inherently wrong with supposedly feminizing sport by widening what achievements are celebrated? It seems to me that broadening cultural conceptions of athletic achievement threatens masculinist, sexist, ableist, capitalistic, neoliberal ideologies – both in the sporting world and beyond.

I suspect that my proposal and endorsement of English's argument will be met with suspicion by some folks. Perhaps it will be construed as an overly sentimental, entitled, millennial impulse to give everyone a participation trophy. As a result, I am compelled to address the decades-long debate involving sports writers and commentators, cultural critics, sports fans, athletes, and parents concerning participation trophies. Those who reject participation awards claim that they breed entitlement and teach people that they do not need to earn "real" accomplishments (Nguyen 2018). This belief is expressed by James Harrison, an American former football player. Upon learning that his sons had received participation trophies, Harrison (quoted in English 2018, 110) stated, "These trophies will be given back until they EARN a real trophy. I'm sorry I'm not sorry for believing that everything in life should be earned and I'm not about to raise two boys to be men by making them believe that they are entitled to something just because they tried their best ... cause sometimes your best is not enough." English (2018, 110) wonders, "Are participation trophies really that bad?" Will they set up children to have unrealistic expectations? Have these trophies set up all millennials to be entitled adults? Are these awards really that powerful?

The idea that participation awards have fuelled a sense of entitlement that has fundamentally distorted millennials' expectations and made us all feel privileged is not grounded in evidence. The myth that millennials are a monolithic group of people who feel entitled to things – including awards for showing up – has been thoroughly debunked (Cairns 2017). On a personal note, reflecting on my own experiences growing up as a millennial who swam and ran, I did not value the participation awards that I received, and I was not deluded into thinking that I had won first, second, or third place. I had internalized the idea that the only "worthwhile value of sport is victory" (English 2018, 110). However, as a very mediocre adult runner, I have revelled in receiving tokens for half- and full-marathon participation. They remind me how emotionally, physically, and athletically challenging and interpersonally fulfilling it is to train for and participate in a race.[10] That is, after all, the reason why youth and elite sport events (e.g., the Olympics) give out participation tokens. Ultimately, thinking of new or devalued ways to reward athletic achievement and involvement is not some extension of deluded millennial entitlement.

The idea that children's grasp on reality will weaken or warp if they receive participation awards underestimates children's intelligence by denying their ability to decipher the difference between a participation award and a victory award. It is untenable to claim that children, despite the very different look, colour, and size of awards as well as the very different ways that awards are presented, are unable to discern the difference in the cultural value placed on each award. Additionally, the idea that children's grasp on reality is warped by these awards underestimates how quickly children internalize dominant cultural values. Children internalize dominant cultural ideologies at a very young age. Considering young boys, for example, psychologist Ronald F. Levant (2005, 161) explicates, "By the time a boy enters school, he has learned to hide and feel ashamed of two important sets of emotions: those that express vulnerability in one way or another (fear, sadness, loneliness, hurt, shame, and disappointment) and those that express neediness, caring, or connection to others."[11] It makes sense to conclude that when Harrison's young sons lose, they understand that their claim to masculinity is challenged and therefore feel disappointed. It is reasonable to suspect that they understand that masculinity and "feminized" participation awards are contradictory, especially given their father's response. Further, it stands to reason, given the masculinist sporting culture, that people (including children) understand that any nonvictory award is given less cultural value.

If participation awards threaten the masculinist, sexist, neoliberal, capitalistic, win-at-all-costs mentality and the belief that the only thing that is valuable is winning, said awards do not seem that bad to me. In other words, rejecting participation awards or awards that acknowledge devalued, feminized sporting values maintains these discriminatory and inequitable cultural ideologies in the sporting world and beyond. If these awards undermine the "reality" or "inevitability" of these ideologies, I am not opposed to this reality warp. I asked above whether these awards are really that powerful. It appears that they have disruptive potential, but there are some lingering concerns. Participation awards do not necessarily or inevitably threaten ableism.

Approaching this debate through a disability studies lens complicates the cultural distain or support for participation awards. Debates about whether or not participants should be given said awards always revolve around able-bodied sports, typically youth sports. I have not come across one person who mocks participation awards when they are given to disabled athletes at any level. Perhaps these people refrain from disparaging such awards when they are given to disabled athletes because they presume that disabled people's lives are so miserable that they need awards for "bravely" existing, showing up, and trying to "overcome" their disability. Or perhaps they assume that disabled people are incapable of discerning the cultural value placed on various awards. These assumptions are guided by infantilizing ableist logics. The late Stella Young (2014), who coined the term "inspiration porn" and was a wheelchair user, recounted some of her experiences, including a time when a community member wanted to nominate her for an award:

When I was 15, a member of my local community approached my parents and wanted to nominate me for a community achievement award. And my parents said, "Hm, that's really nice, but there's kind of one glaring problem with that. She hasn't actually achieved anything." And they were right, you know. I went to school, I got good marks, I had a very low-key after school job in my mum's hairdressing salon, and I spent a lot of time watching *Buffy the Vampire Slayer* and *Dawson's Creek*. Yeah, I know. What a contradiction. But they were right, you know. I wasn't doing anything that was out of the ordinary at all. I wasn't doing anything that could be considered an achievement if you took disability out of the equation ... We have been lied to about disability. Yeah, we've been sold the lie that disability is a Bad Thing, capital B, capital T. It's a bad thing, and to live with a disability makes you exceptional. It's not a bad thing, and it doesn't make you exceptional ... I've lost count of the number of times that I've been approached by strangers wanting to tell me that they think I'm brave or inspirational ... They were just kind of congratulating me for managing to get up in the morning and remember my own name.

Young was not specifically discussing sports, but her analysis can be applied to the lack of commentary about disabled athletes and participation awards. Her insights draw attention to the fact that enabled people and disabled people are held to different standards and are "rewarded" in different ways because of ableism. People with disabilities are presumed to be exceptional or brave and worthy of awards for watching *Buffy the Vampire Slayer*, going to work, getting up in the morning, or participating in sports – for simply existing – whereas enabled people are not. Disability and the capacity to achieve something great (typically by ableist standards) are construed as contradictory (Kafer 2013). This is likely the reason why there is a vacuum of silence about disabled athletes when participation awards are discussed.

When applied to sport, Young's insights call into question the idea that participation awards are de facto beneficial or positively culturally disruptive. Hence, like English, I do not think that participation awards are always the best course of action. Indeed, despite the fact that these awards have been around for decades, they have not dramatically unsettled masculinist sporting culture and organization in the ways that we need. However, instituting and valuing awards at all levels of sport that extend beyond mere victory can radically undermine noxious sport culture. In addition to English's examples of which sporting qualities we should consider valuing and rewarding, we can also think of alternative awards beyond mere victory that honour remarkable athleticism. For example, consider figure skating. A figure skater may flawlessly execute the most difficult and complex movement of all the other athletes but finish with an overall score that does not result in a win. Awarding this remarkable athletic achievement is worthwhile. Instituting awards like this one for a particular movement could result in composing teams differently so that they can achieve in a way that goes beyond the traditional win-lose mentality. I am not suggesting that victory in the traditional sense should no longer be esteemed but rather that striving for other athletic accomplishments as well as for "a variety of values," including victory, "is worthwhile and meaningful" and should be revered just as much (English 2018, 118). Appreciating and rewarding other athletic triumphs as well as "feminized" sporting values – weaving these values so thoroughly into sport culture that they constituted an essential element of sport – would have positive impacts on sport culture and organization. Doing so could free athletes to strive differently without compromising their ability to collectively work toward a victory.

PART 3

NEW EUGENICS: PREIMPLANTATION GENETIC DIAGNOSIS AND COMPULSORY DYADISM

7

Intersex, PGD, and the Eugenics Agenda

Preimplantation genetic diagnosis (PGD) is a reproductive technology that can accompany in vitro fertilization (IVF). PGD screens the genetic material of possible implantable embryos. Originally developed to circumvent life-threatening genetic diseases (e.g., Tay-Sachs)[1] (Behrmann and Ravitsky 2013), PGD can be and is now used to test for hundreds of culturally devalued characteristics, like Down syndrome, deafness, blindness, and a variety of intersex variations (Amato 2016; Kaposy 2018). PGD can enact a prenatal exorcism of sorts to ensure that a potentially pregnant person does not house and gestate a supposed unviable, queer, crip, disabled, or intersex spectral monstrosity.

This use of PGD concerns intersex activists and scholars. At the "Public Consultation on Protection against Violence and Discrimination Based on Sexual Orientation and Gender Identity" (United Nations Human Rights 2017), intersex activist and co-founder of OII Europe Miriam van der Have stated, "Intersex is an undesirable outcome of pregnancy and is visible in medical technologies such as PGD," whose use "may lead to the erasure of intersex in society." In other words, intersex variations are presumed to be so innately objectionable, unviable, and disabling that technologies like PGD are developed and deployed to prevent the gestation of embryos and the birth of fetuses with intersex traits. The proliferation of PGD, van der Have notes, has the ability to decimate the intersex population. Despite this concern, bioethicist and proponent of anti-intersex selection Robert

Sparrow (2013, 30) notes that there is "little written" on this issue. Sparrow is correct that, compared to other intersex bioethical matters, such as intersex genital mutilation (IGM), there is not a significant amount of literature about PGD and intersex. In addition to a smattering of academic and activist articles that focus on intersex and reproductive technologies and/or that mention PGD,[2] *The American Journal of Bioethics* (volume 13, number 10) devoted a large portion of one 2013 issue to PGD and anti-intersex selection.[3]

Most troubling about using PGD to select against intersex are the possible eugenic implications. Consequently, this chapter asks whether this practice constitutes eugenics. The desire to develop and use technologies and policies in order to prevent the gestation or birth of fetuses with intersex traits is not new. Intersex – or, as expressed by eugenics advocate Karl Pearson (1857–1936) (quoted in Kevles 1985, 39), "hermaphroditism" – has always been on the eugenics agenda. Even though people often presume that eugenics is a horrific relic of the past, disability studies scholars demonstrate that eugenic initiatives, ideologies, and policies never went away; rather, they were transformed from "old" to "new" eugenics.[4] And, as this transformation took place, intersex remained on the agenda.

Disability studies scholars' and activists' knowledges are vital to unpacking anti-intersex PGD deployment not only because intersex is a disability issue but also because for decades they have been engaged in debates concerning reproductive technologies – amniocentesis and chorionic villus sampling (CVS), MaterniT21,[5] sterilization, ultrasound, abortion, PGD, and contraception – and their eugenic implications.[6] Ronald J. Berger (2013, 14) explains that in "reject[ing] approaches to disability that seek to eradicate it," disability studies scholars and activists have outlined the history of (ableist) eugenics, examined current usages of reproductive technologies as new forms of eugenics, analyzed discourses about reproductive technologies that extol able-bodiedness, and critiqued reproductive policies for excluding the perspectives of people with disabilities. Essentially, these scholars and activists challenge the ableist idea that a disabled person has "no good future" (Kafer 2013, 3). It is assumed that, for their own good, people with disabilities – including people with intersex-is/as-disabled variations – should not be born because they will have an insufferably low quality of life.

Nevertheless, employing reproductive technologies to prevent the implantation, gestation, or birth of embryos, fetuses, or people with disabilities, disorders, or diseases remains intuitively benevolent to many bioethicists, medical professionals, genetic counsellors, and the general public.[7]

Additionally, it is assumed that people with disabilities should not reproduce because they may pass along their "defective" genes to offspring and/or because they will be incapable of adequately caring for children. Eugenic policies and practices, such as forced sterilization, have been institutionalized in various ways through time and space to ensure that people with disabilities, disorders, or diseases as well as racialized, poor, and LGBTQIA2 people do not reproduce and cannot, therefore, exercise their right to bodily autonomy and cannot shape their (reproductive) futures. Given the belief that intersex traits are innate disabilities, disorders, or diseases, disability studies scholars' analyses are integral to combatting assumptions, practices, and technologies that seek to "benevolently" eradicate intersex (futures).

This chapter has three main aims. First, I offer some details about PGD, namely which intersex traits it can detect and how widespread PGD use is. PGD usage is not particularly common given that it is rarely covered by insurance plans and is costly. However, the PGD market is growing. The future ubiquitous use of PGD cannot be underestimated. Therefore, second, I ask whether anti-intersex selection via PGD constitutes eugenics. Drawing primarily from disability studies scholars' expertise on past and present eugenic ideologies, initiatives, and polices, I demonstrate that it is indeed eugenics. Deploying PGD to detect and prevent the implantation of embryos with intersex traits continues the eugenics legacy in and outside of Canada. Third, primarily drawing from the authors featured in the 2013 issue of *The American Journal of Bioethics* (volume 13, number 10) that is largely devoted to PGD and anti-intersex selection, I outline and critique the main justifications and consequentialist logics employed to defend anti-intersex selection. I argue that the proposed reasons for claiming that selecting against intersex is good are not grounded in evidence. Further, I posit that the consequentialist reasoning used to justify anti-intersex selection problematically relies on dichotomous thinking and fails to acknowledge that people's lives, value, and be(com)ing in the world cannot be reduced to such unintersectional and reductive calculations.

PGD: Confronting, Exorcising, and Eliminating Intersex

"Confronted with the spectre of intersex," Sparrow (2013, 29) contends, "modern medicine makes choices available to parents and physicians" who want to exorcise the spectre. For example, in addition to surgery and hormone replacement therapy (HRT), one of the "choices" presented to (prospective) parents is PGD. PGD can prevent the potentially pregnant person from housing, gestating, and birthing such a spectre. As noted above, PGD can test for hundreds of genetic variations that are deemed "undesirable simply because they fall outside the scope of what is considered by some to be 'normal'" (Behrmann and Ravitsky 2013, 39). Society allegedly cannot invest its "reproductive futurism" (Edelman 2004, 3) in non-normate, spectral body-minds; such morphologies are not wanted in the future since "the value of a disability-free future is seen as self-evident" (Kafer 2013, 3). The intersex traits or genetic variations that PGD is used to detect include, for instance, congenital adrenal hyperplasia (CAH), Klinefelter syndrome (or 47,XXY), androgen insensitivity syndrome (AIS), and Turner syndrome (or 45,XO) (Amato 2016; Carpenter 2014). PGD cannot detect all intersex characteristics because not all intersex traits are genetic. Intersex is too spontaneous – spectral. Many intersex variations arise extemporaneously and are influenced by in utero environmental conditions (Gupta and Freeman 2013). Therefore, the possibility of employing PGD to select against intersex depends on the intersex variation in question and on its etiology.

Although the cost of PGD varies depending on one's location and private or public insurance coverage, PGD is expensive (Couture et al. 2013; Jain and Hornstein 2005). The cost of PGD also depends on, for instance, the types of variations that will be detected, the number of embryos that will be tested, the number of PGD cycles, and whether the patient is local or from abroad (Geraedts et al. 2001). According to the Government of Canada's (2013) website, one of the "disadvantages of PGD" is the expense. Costs vary, but let us look at a couple of specific examples. According to Ottawa Fertility Centre's (n.d.) "Fees" webpage, as of 2020, an embryo biopsy for PGD cost $1,800. This amount excluded embryo freezing ($1,000), frozen embryo transfer ($2,500), unfunded IVF ($7,500 to $12,100), and other possible additional fees (e.g., physician and nursing services). Mount Sinai Fertility (2019), which has clinics in Toronto, North York, Vaughan, and Mississauga, charges $2,500 for an embryo biopsy. This coast excludes things like genetic counselling ($250), thawing of embryos for biopsy ($400), and so on. Given the high costs, the technology is accessed by relatively few people, typically by affluent, highly educated, white people. Hence, it is reasonable to assume that using PGD to select against intersex traits is currently relatively rare.[8]

Nevertheless, we cannot underestimate the future ubiquitous use of PGD. There are studies emerging that consider the dis/advantages and trade-offs of PGD coverage (e.g., see Goh et al. 2019). Whether or not PGD is (ever) covered by private or public health insurance, it is clear that genetics counsellors endorse and want to provide PGD and possible coverage. As I discuss below, this endorsement is rooted in eugenic ideologies. It is also economically motivated given that reproductive technologies are "big business" (Kaposy 2014). As reported by Transparency Market Research (2016), the global PGD market in 2013 was US\$77.2 million, and it has continued to rise since then. Grand View Research (2016) estimates that the market for noninvasive prenatal testing (which includes PGD) will be worth US\$5.5 billion by 2025. The global COVID-19 pandemic undoubtedly is impacting and will continue to impact this market for the foreseeable future. However, according to a research report on the pharmaceuticals market by Transparency Market Research (2020), "the growing demand for genetically testing [embryos] and rising knowledge of genetics" are "promising driver[s] for growth of the preimplantation genetic testing market ... The new technologies made available due to preimplantation genetic testing [are] expected to witness a robust future as economies of scale drive down costs." As costs go down, more people will engage with PGD.

Although access to PGD is relatively uncommon at the moment, it is conceivable that PGD could become standard practice in the near future. Reflecting on PGD and intersex, bioethicists Jason Behrmann and Vardit Ravitsky (2013, 39) claim that "PGD may soon become an integral part of in vitro fertilization."[9] Indeed, many reproductive technologies that were previously available to only wealthy people are now more readily – although not universally – accessible, including contraceptives, ultrasounds, amniocentesis, and IVF. For instance, more Canadians in Ontario than ever before are seeking out IVF because in 2015 the Ontario Health Insurance Plan (OHIP) began covering one round of IVF services for all Ontarians under the age of forty-three with fertility issues, "regardless of sex, gender, sexual orientation or family status" (Government of Ontario 2015; see also Blackwell 2016; and Church 2015).[10] Many Ontarians are learning about and are confronted with PGD as they research and take advantage of the this IVF coverage. In addition to the recently expanded IVF coverage, OHIP has covered one complete and one limited ultrasound for "normal" or "low-risk" pregnancies for decades, and more ultrasounds are made available for "abnormal" or "high-risk" pregnancies (Ontario Ministry of Health and Long-Term Care 1998). Although PGD is not typically covered by health care plans in and outside of Canada, future PGD coverage is in the realm of possibility. Looking south, we see that American insurance providers also rarely cover PGD. That said, one can easily access online forums or the websites of fertility clinics to learn about strategies regarding how to persuade insurance providers to cover PGD costs (see Sherbahn n.d.).

According to medical ethicists Diana Aurenque and Hans-Jörg Ehni (2013, 55), a bioethical analysis of anti-intersex PGD selection is necessary because "demand for it appears to be primarily cosmetic rather than medical." A bioethical analysis of PGD, anti-intersex selection, *and* the eugenic implications of PGD usage is crucial. Since PGD is promoted, wildly profitable, and/or under/unregulated in various countries, including the United States, Canada, Australia, and the United Kingdom, this bioethical, eugenics concern may be more pressing than initially assumed. In fact, recognizing the eugenic implications, countries like Germany, Austria, Italy, France, and Switzerland highly regulate PGD and/or have banned using PGD to detect variations that are not fatal (Hyder 2011; S. O'Neill and Blackmer 2015). In fact, the National Ethics Committee in France has proposed outlawing PGD because the technology may be used for nonmedical, cosmetic reasons (S. O'Neill and Blackmer 2015). One cannot underestimate the future ubiquitous use of PGD and its broader eugenic implications. So does PGD usage constitute eugenics?

The Eugenic Implications of PGD

Intersex activists Curtis E. Hinkle and Hida Viloria (2012) write, "Surgical 'normalization' of intersex bodies is an attempt, *like eugenics,* to remove differences which some people have decided are undesirable" (emphasis added). However, "eugenics" was not and *is* not just a simile. Pearson (quoted in Kevles 1985, 39), a leading figure of the eugenics movement in the early twentieth century, published data regarding assumed undesirable, inheritable characteristics, including "hermaphroditism, hemophilia, cleft palate, harelip, tuberculosis, diabetes, deaf-mutism, polydactyly (more than five fingers) or brachydactyly (stub fingers), insanity, and mental deficiency." "Hermaphroditism" was deemed a degenerate state of being that should be eliminated by eugenic policies and practices. Intersex – "hermaphroditism" – has always been on the eugenics agenda. The agenda has always been racist, classist, queerphobic, ableist, *and* interphobic.

Typically associated with the Nazis and the Holocaust, "old-style" eugenics was popularized in the United Kingdom in the early twentieth century.[11] Drawing from Charles Darwin's theory of evolution, Darwin's half-cousin Sir Francis Galton (2015, 321) coined the term "eugenics" and defined it as "the study of agencies under social control that may improve or impair the racial qualities of future generations, either physically or mentally." Positioning disabled and racialized people as well as other "unviable" individuals (e.g., hermaphrodites, perverts, morons, and criminals) "along the wayside as evolutionary defectives," Galton and his advocates believed that the social body could and ought to be improved by ridding the population of these people (L.J. Davis 2013, 3). State-sanctioned interventions – such as propaganda initiatives, strict immigration policies, strategic family planning, and involuntary sterilization of people with disabilities, criminals, and women who were Indigenous or racialized – supported this aim to enhance the social body by controlling "problem populations" (Baker 2002, 672).

Galton's old-style eugenics "enjoy[ed] wide currency," quickly spreading to Canada and America (Hansen and King 2001, 240). Eugenic beliefs were not fringe but rather endorsed by numerous influential people. After hearing Galton deliver a paper titled "Eugenics: Its Definition, Scope and Aims," famous playwright and cultural critic George Bernard Shaw (quoted in Saleeby 1911, 178) wrote, "I agree with the paper, and go so far as to say that there is now no reasonable excuse for refusing to face the fact that nothing but eugenic religion can save our civilisation from the fate that has overtaken all previous civilisations." Anarchist political activist and writer Emma Goldman (quoted in L.J. Davis 2013, 6), seemingly contrary to her anarchist politics, expressed similar sentiments, arguing that unless eugenic birth control policies were espoused, the state would in essence "legally encourage the increase of paupers, syphilitics, epileptics, dipsomaniacs, cripples, criminals, and degenerates."

Eugenic sentiments and policies were not specific to Nazi Germany and were not eradicated after the Second World War. As a result, we must view eugenics as "a complicated and heterogeneous series of discourses that have transmogrified into a variety of assumptions and practices" that still enjoy wide currency today (Baker 2002, 664). Old-style eugenics, characterized by state-institutionalized racial and national "improvement," shifted after the war to become a "new" eugenics that was narrated through the seemingly apolitical and objective medical rhetoric of ill/health, welfare, and ab/normality. To clarify, according to old eugenics discourses, the state ought to ensure that people with unviable body-minds do not pollute the quality of the social body and spread their inferior genes. According to new eugenics discourses, for the baby's welfare, people ought to use reproductive technologies to select for, in Sparrow's (2013, 32) words, "species-typical functioning" and to select against defects, abnormalities, and disabilities. In line with neoliberal ideologies, there was an identifiable shift from state welfare to individual welfare and from state responsibility to individual responsibility.

Responsibility for ensuring that supposed pollutants (or future spectral noncitizens) are not born shifted from the state to individual parents. Or, as expressed by Christine Crowe (2000, 176), new eugenics is "operationalised by appeals to individual responsibility for the health of future offspring. The site of intervention in this case is ... the management of fertility, of conception, such that 'viable' embryos of choice, will be implanted." Although there have been shifts from old to new eugenics, the focus on quality control remains the same. Just like old eugenics, new eugenics aims "to eliminate the birthing of bodies marked as 'disabled' or, in the event of their/our postnatal 'existence', to engage in 'perfecting' technologies that morph ableism and enshrine a particular understanding of ableist normativity and (real) human subjectivity" (Campbell 2000, 308). Examples of such "perfecting" or "curative" technologies include IGM and HRT, which can violently disable and even sterilize people with intersex variations – perhaps, in part, to ensure that they do not give birth to other "defectives."

Nevertheless, even though surgical procedures have resulted in the sterilization of numerous intersex individuals, the claim that sterilizing intersex people and that practising anti-intersex selection via PGD are eugenic may not be self-evident. However, viewing eugenics as an ever-shifting discourse, rather than a definitive political movement, demonstrates that technologies that often render intersex people infertile and that prevent intersex bodyminds from being born because they are deemed defective are contemporary forms of eugenics. These procedures are new eugenic practices that apotheosize normative understandings of body-minds. Using PGD to select against intersex variations is a new eugenic practice and will thus be referred to as such throughout the rest of this book to emphasize the political stakes.

Arguments For and Against PGD Intersex Eugenics

The 2013 issue of *The American Journal of Bioethics* (volume 13, number 10) is the only publication that is largely devoted to, as the first article is titled, "Critically Appraising Prenatal Genetic Diagnosis to Prevent Disorders of Sexual Development: An Opportunity Missed" (McCullough 2013, 1). This collection is noteworthy not simply because it is the only one but also because the contributing authors come from a variety of academic fields: gender, sexuality, and feminist studies; sociology and intersex studies; medical ethics and health policy; philosophy; bioethics and medicine; reproductive genetics and science; neuroscience; and psychology. This volume offers diverse, interdisciplinary perspectives. Interestingly, as I flesh out in the next chapter, disability and disability studies analyses are scarcely critically analyzed despite the fact that intersex is deemed a disability, disorder, or disease.

Some of the main concerns guiding the debate in this collection will be addressed in the remainder of this chapter. First, I ask whether PGD is an alternative to "normalizing" surgery. Sparrow (2013) believes that PGD is a favourable alternative. Clinician and researarcher Jeff Nisker (2013), on the other hand, provides compelling opposing arguments. Second, I ask whether using PGD for intersex eugenics is an ethical means to prevent the medical and social harms associated with intersex traits? Sparrow (2013) and psychologist David Trafimow (2013) maintain that PGD will prevent harms, not exacerbate them. Intersex studies scholar and activist Georgiann Davis (2013), among others, demonstrates that medical issues attributed to intersex are overstated and that discrimination will not be resolved by eliminating intersex body-minds. Third, I ask whether this practice negatively impacts societal diversity and the intersex community. Some argue that there is no evident intersex community and, therefore, that diversity would not be harmed. Other scholars point to local and transnational intersex communities and movements.

Is PGD an Alternative to Surgery?
The first concern, as noted above, is whether or not PGD is an auspicious alternative to "normailizing" surgery – in other words, curative violence and disabling mutilation. Sparrow (2013, 29, 34) posits, "PGD for those [intersex] conditions that involve serious medical risks for those born with them is morally permissible," "perhaps even morally required." "PGD for other 'cosmetic' variations in sexual anatomy," Sparrow (2013, 29) continues, "is more defensible than it might first appear." According to Sparrow (2013, 31), intersex eugenics[12] is morally permissible, perhaps required, because the harm caused by "corrective" surgery is avoided: "PGD has several advantages over 'corrective' surgery if parents are concerned to raise a child with normal sexual anatomy ... Questions about the possibility of surgical and/or psychological harms to the individual being 'treated,' which loom so large in the context of the debate about surgery for intersex conditions, do not arise in the context of genetic selection." For Sparrow, (potential) parents can avoid considering surgery and the anxiety associated with raising a child with "abnormal" sexual anatomy. No one need be harmed by curative violence if the newborn does not have intersex characteristics.

Sparrow's position troubles Nisker because it privileges parents' anxieties about sex differences. The assumed advantages of PGD, in this view, "are to the potential parents rather than the potential child" (Nisker 2013, 48). Nisker echoes many other intersex studies scholars and activists who critique medical intervention meant to abate parents' anxieties about (perceived) body-mind disabilities and abnormalities. Rather than attempting to avoid (potential) parents' anxieties, the focus should be on the potential child's welfare – on "the future well-being of their offspring" (Behrmann and Ravitsky 2013, 39). The focus should be on combatting curative violence and medical malpractice and on providing parents "with information showing the reality of intersex people leading fulfilled lives, as well as the existence of clinical and social biases against diversity in sex, gender, and sexual orientation" (Nisker 2013, 39). Providing parents with this information could lessen (potential) parents' concerns and alter their decision making. Preventing culturally problematic, spectral, or anxiety-inducing embryos from being implanted and possibly gestated and born does not solve the problems of mutilation, discrimination, medical malpractice, and curative violence. Doing so avoids the necessary labour involved in combatting compulsory dyadism.

Does PGD Prevent Medical and Social Harms?

Sparrow (2013, 36, 34) proposes that, out of "concern for the well-being of the child," intersex eugenics protects potential intersex people from the "serious medical risks" that stem from intersex anatomy and from the "hostile social environment" that people with intersex traits confront. Addressing Sparrow's concern about medical risks, Georgiann Davis (2013) notes that there is no unanimity about the medical issues that stem from intersex traits themselves. In fact, as demonstrated at length in Chapter 1, many of the claims about the presumed medical issues that stem directly from intersex traits are typically based on overestimates, are incorrect, or are misinformed. Even so, people who experience medical issues throughout their lives – that is, all people to varying degrees – do not have wholly or fundamentally insufferable, unlivable lives.

Refusing to work within the dichotomous medical-social framework, Davis (2013, 53) emphasizes the interconnectedness of medical and social environments: "If one wishes to use the social and psychological harm argument to justify PGD to select against intersex traits, it is important to acknowledge that it is largely, albeit perhaps not exclusively, the medical field – not the intersex trait itself – that causes such stigmatization and creates the 'hostile social environment'" that Sparrow notes. Although some people with intersex characteristics may deal with health problems that extend from their intersex traits, the social stigma against intersex variations more often than not extends from the medicalization of said traits. To elaborate, "because the medical profession, not the intersex trait itself, is a major source of the social and psychological harm that perpetuates intersex stigmatization ..., justifying PGD by pointing to such negative outcomes is ill-advised and a circular logic" (G. Davis 2013, 52). There is a cyclical, blurry, or overlapping relationship between the institution of medicine and society; medicine is an aspect of society and culture. As suggested by philosopher and gender studies scholar Chelsea Haramia (2013, 42), rather than endorsing intersex eugenics so that potential people do not experience compulsory dyadism – rather than "perpetuating social injustices" – we need to work toward creating a more inclusive and less dichotomous social climate that truly privileges intersex people's well-being. And this anti-interphobic work is performed every day, whether in classrooms; at conferences, meetings, and consultations; through artistic, testimonial, and educational projects; or via numerous intersex rights organizations and initiatives.

Does PGD Negatively Impact Societal Diversity and the Intersex Community?

Failing to acknowledge the intersex community and the anti-interphobic work done by people engaged with the Intersex Rights Movement, Sparrow reasons that using PGD for intersex eugenics would not harm social diversity. For Sparrow, there are so few intersex people that the community is invisible or nonexistent, and therefore social diversity would not be harmed if fewer intersex people were born. Additionally, he claims that intersex people have no role models to look up to and that their life prospects are hindered for this reason. Sparrow (2013, 34) begins his argument by comparing the use of PGD to select against queer, racialized, and intersex embodiments/experiences:

> The conclusion that it is immoral to select on the basis of race or same-sex attractedness out of concern for the future well-being of one's child is less well-founded than might first appear ... Each couple has only a limited power to combat the racism and homophobia that are likely to [have an] impact on their child's welfare ... The reproductive choice that parents face is whether *their* child should suffer reduced welfare as a result of social injustices. It is far from clear that it would be morally blameworthy for

parents to decide to prevent this. Indeed, arguing that parents should choose a child that is likely to suffer as a result of injustice, for the sake of the political project of combating such injustices, seems to demand that parents should sacrifice the interests of their children for the sake of the larger good ... Pending a convincing account of parental obligations in reproductive decisions in the context of injustice, ... we might still hold that parents have good reasons to select against genes for intersex conditions.

Presenting an argument characteristic of new eugenics discourses, Sparrow implies that selecting against culturally devalued characteristics – queer, racialized, and intersex – or, perhaps, not reproducing at all for the sake of the potential child is benevolent. Ignoring the fact that parents need not engage with PGD and need not choose between one embryo or another at all, Sparrow sets up a false dichotomy and creates a moral imperative to select against culturally devalued characteristics. According to Sparrow, on the one hand, there are parents who select against devalued traits. He presents this selection as apolitical (or at least less political than selecting for said traits) by emphasizing that these (potential) parents are magnanimously concerned for their future child's welfare. On the other hand, there are parents who select *for* queerness, racialized characteristics, or intersex variations. These parents are explicitly politicized. Reproducing negative stereotypes about activists, Sparrow depicts these parents as militant, irrational, sanctimonious political protesters who view their potential children as sacrificial lambs.[13] In doing so, Sparrow praises people who engage with new eugenics discourses and new eugenic technologies and villainizes those who value stigmatized traits.

To be clear, both choices are political. Judgments about the un/viability or prospective suffering of a possible human being are necessarily the outcome of politically fraught analyses with potentially eugenic ends. And, of course, claiming that culturally devalued embodiments and ways of being are viable, valuable, and beautiful is indeed political. Consider the political rallying cries "Lame is sexy" (Clare 2010), "Nothing About Us Without Us" (Charlton 1998), "Black is beautiful" (Hraba and Grant 1970; Taylor 2016), "We are intersexy" (Wall et al. 2015), "Intersexy fat" (G. Davis 2016), "Gay is good" (Darsey 1991; Dunn 2016), and "The personal is political" (Hanisch 2000). That said, valuing such characteristics and having concern for a child's welfare are not mutually exclusive. Regardless, the parental binary presented by Sparrow creates a moral imperative for people to select against stigmatized traits and to collude with systems of oppression. Focusing on potential individual children – rather than locating the problem in the systems, discourses, and ideologies that mandate certain ways of being and that uphold discrimination – masks the eugenic implications of (choosing) PGD.

Remarkably, in an article published before the piece in question, Sparrow articulates the same critique that I am attempting to express. Critiquing philosopher and bioethicist Julian Savulescu's (2001) position that parents have a moral obligation to select for the "best" child possible, Sparrow (2007, 43) writes: "Savulescu's argument ... requires parents to become complicit with racism and homophobia (and other forms of oppression), which is yet another reason to reject it." In this article, Sparrow goes as far as to suggest that Savulescu endorses eugenics. Yet, in his paper about intersex and PGD, Sparrow does not recognize that his position, just like Savulescu's argument, also requires parents to become complicit with various forms of oppression and eugenics.

After comparing and endorsing racist, queerphobic, and interphobic eugenics, Sparrow notes a problem with his comparison. Racialized and queer individuals have positive communities, role models, and a distinct way of life, whereas intersex people, apparently, do not. Sparrow (2013, 34–35) therefore infers that intersex eugenics via PGD will not harm cultural diversity or a distinctive intersex community:

The relative infrequency of intersex conditions differentiates them from race and sexual preference, and the ability of many intersex individuals to "pass" as one or the other of the conventional genders also differentiates intersex from race. For both these reasons, it is more plausible to divorce decisions about intersex conditions from the concerns about culture and identity that dominate discussions of these other cases. A child born with dark skin may suffer as a result of racism but also has the opportunity to gain strength from the identification as black, from the example of other black role models, and from participation in the black community. Being black opens some doors even if others are closed due to racism. Similarly, persons who are same-sex-attracted will usually have access to a community of other same-sex-attracted persons. These communities defined by race or sexual preference may then sustain and transmit a distinct set of cultural (or subcultural) ideas and values. Except in very large cities, persons born intersex are likely to be one of only very few individuals with their particular form of embodiment.[14] Even in large cities, intersexed persons may be effectively invisible to each other as well as to the larger community. It is therefore much less plausible to object to a reduction in the number of children born intersex, as a result of PGD, on the grounds that this would jeopardize a distinctive "way of life" or "culture."

Conflating racialization, Blackness, dark skin, and Black identity, while also assuming that race and sexuality are always evidently and unproblematically read off people's physical characteristics, Sparrow posits that selecting against intersex is different from, perhaps less (obviously) eugenic than, selecting against Blackness and queerness. Black and queer people have access to supportive communities and role models, Sparrow reports. These communities and role models apparently outweigh the negativity of institutionalized racism and queerphobia. Intersex people supposedly cannot find each other and do not have a community or role models. As a result, according to Sparrow, the interphobia that intersex people experience is not offset or balanced out by positive forces or life experiences. And, since there is apparently no intersex community, intersex eugenics will not impact a specific community or cultural diversity.

However, as Georgiann Davis (2013, 51) caustically and succinctly observes, "the intersex community is only 'invisible' (Sparrow 2013) to those who choose to ignore it." Although this community is perhaps smaller than other marginalized communities, there are numerous transnational intersex organizations, communities, conferences, and meetings with extraordinary contributing role models whom anyone, intersex or not, can look to. In fact, we know that the Intersex Rights Movement has been underway for decades. Moreover, with assistance from the Internet, intersex people form bonds with other intersex folks all over the world and perform activist work online and offline, community building, and labour that is healing and restorative. The growing mainstream media representation of intersex people and intersex experiences is also increasing visibility. In addition to countless anti-interphobic mainstream news articles about and authored by intersex people, there are many celebrated television series, films, and documentaries featuring intersex characters, actors, and people, such as *Ponyboi* (Joseph and Gallo 2019), *Transparent* (Soloway and Sperling 2014–19), *Faking It* (Covington 2014–16), and *Intersexion* (Lahood 2012). This increased mainstream representation of intersex people, characters, and narratives prompted one *Advocate* contributor to ask, "Are We Witnessing the Birth of TV's Intersex Liberation?" (Anderson-Minshall 2016). There is much work to be done, but "Sparrow's exclusively negative portrayal of intersex people as being inherently deficient in opportunities, isolated without role models, is misleading if not completely inaccurate" (Behrmann and Ravitsky 2013, 40). Sparrow's assertion that intersex people and communities are invisible or nonexistent is indisputably false.

Even so, the size of a population ought to be irrelevant when considering whether people should acknowledge and respect another group of people. Unfortunately, the "minority" status and population of a given group are often deemed relevant and sometimes used to justify re/marginalizing a group of people, as Sparrow attempts to do. The intersex activist community may be small, but it is growing by the day. That said, the intersex population is not nearly as small as Sparrow claims. As I outline in Chapter 4, intersex variations are quite common. Cary Gabriel Costello (2012a) explains that a "conservative estimate is that more than 1 in 150 people are born with intersex bodies." Contrary to Sparrow's claim, folks with intersex traits are not anomalous and, therefore, should not be treated as such.

Entering this conversation, Trafimow counters Sparrow and his critics and suggests that the negative medical issues and social stigma that intersex people experience outweigh any positive diversity and creativity that intersex people bring to society. In writing that is peppered with ableist language, Trafimow (2013, 54) asserts:

> It seems like a fragile leg to stand on, to argue that society as a whole will have more creative ideas as a result of increasing the number of intersex children who are born. In addition, a defender of this conclusion would have to further argue that this gain in the totality of creative ideas in society would be so large as to make up for the negative consequences that ... tend to happen to intersex individuals.

Trafimow (2013, 55) is unsure that the "expected value" of increased creativity and diversity "would be sufficiently impressive so as to outweigh the potential for harm to [intersex] individuals." Trafimow reasons that when one weighs the potential benefits of intersex people's contributions to society against their inevitable suffering, one discerns that the suffering endured by intersex people is far too great to justify their contributions. One will not be adequately "[impressed]," to use Trafimow's (2013, 55) term. Since I address the concern for intersex people's medical and social issues above, at this juncture, I am more troubled by the equations that Trafimow and Sparrow attempt to make. Their arguments hinge on pleasure-harm and positive-negative calculations to justify intersex eugenics. They take the liberty of judging intersex individuals' quality of life (and, as with Sparrow, that of racialized and queer individuals as well) to determine the social utility of intersex people. This analytical tool or mode of analysis, known as consequentialism or utilitarianism, problematically relies on dichotomous thinking and fails to acknowledge that people's lives, value, and be(com)ing in the world cannot be reduced to such an unintersectional and reductive calculation.

Consequentialism and Justifying Intersex Eugenics

Sparrow's and Trafimow's arguments for intersex eugenics rely on consequentialist logic.[15] Because this tool for evaluating ethical decisions and behaviours is problematically rooted in "impartiality" and binary thinking, it misrepresents body-minds, embodied be(com)ing, and people's subjectivities. Since the nineteenth century, consequentialism has been a dominant method for unpacking ethical conundrums. With roots in Western, male-dominated philosophical traditions, consequentialism attempts to impartially identify and calculate possible good-bad, pleasure-suffering outcomes.[16] When the outcomes are analyzed and identified, one apparently discovers the universal ethical standard, "the right thing," or the course of action "with the best consequences" and least amount of harm (Mulgan 2001, 3). In addition to Trafimow and Sparrow, many other traditional bio/ethicists and philosophers concerned with the ethics of reproductive technologies still appeal to this logic while trying to discern the quality of particular lives and which potential children are the "best" or "healthiest."[17] In fact, the objection that an argument is "unconvincing in consequentialist terms" is taken quite seriously in certain bio/ethical and philosophical circles (Sandel 2007, 92).

For decades, feminist philosophers and bio/ethicists have been troubled by the demand for objectivity and by the notion of a universal ethical standard. Acknowledging people's affective relations and material concerns, Patricia Hill Collins, Donna Haraway, and Nancy Hartsock, among many others,[18] demonstrate that the consequentialist demand to remain objective is unfeasible. All people come from particular standpoints and cannot objectively weigh possible outcomes or experiences. Since ethics is always partisan, the idea of a universal ethical standard is absurd. In rejecting consequentialist methods, many feminist philosophers have contributed to the development of standpoint theory. Standpoint theory takes into account people's, particularly marginalized people's, unique standpoints and "situated knowledges" (Haraway 1988, 575). In addition, feminist scholars have developed an "ethic of care" (Gilligan 1982). Critiquing enlightenment philosopher David Hume's distaste for sentimentalism and his utilitarian ethic, which is intended to avoid sentimentalism and partiality, feminist philosopher Nel Noddings (1984) demonstrates that care, affect, and emotions are integral to ethical decisions. Instead of idealizing the idea(l) of impartiality, our systems and language ought to reflect the partisan nature of ethical decision making.

Disability and gender studies scholar Margrit Shildrick (2005, 3) posits that traditional consequentialist bioethics, "with its confidence in a determinable calculus of harms and benefits," lacks awareness of the complexities of experience and embodiment. Consequentialism is, Shildrick (2005, 1–2) writes,

> out of touch with bodies themselves, in the phenomenological sense in which the being, or rather the becoming, of the self is always intricately interwoven with the fabric of the body; it is out of touch with the developments in and impact of postmodernist theory as it problematizes the hitherto unchallenged certainty of binary thinking; and it is out of touch with the postmodern culture in which bioscience itself forces us to question what is meant by the notion of the human self.

Bioethical concerns sieved through a consequentialist framework do not engage with the bodies of scholarship – postmodern, phenomenology, trans, intersex, disability, crip, feminist, queer, anti-racist, and anti-colonial – that demonstrate that dichotomies misrepresent body-minds, be(com)ing, and people's lived realities. Binary thinking always fails us. Consequentialism fails us. No one has objective authority to make pleasure-harm calculations about other people's experiences.

Sparrow assumes authority over all intersex, racialized, and queer people's experiences and weighs the positive and negative aspects of said experiences to determine whether there is more or less happiness versus suffering and whether there is more or less diversity. Recall the quotation cited above:

> A child born with dark skin may suffer as a result of racism but also has the opportunity to gain strength from the identification as black, from the example of other black role models, and from participation in the black community ... Similarly, persons who are same-sex-attracted will usually

have access to a community of other same-sex-attracted persons ... Even in
large cities, intersexed persons may be effectively invisible to each other as
well as to the larger community. (Sparrow 2013, 35)

Sparrow assumes an objective position and reasons that there are not
enough positive elements in intersex people's lives to outweigh the negative.
Hence, according to this logic, it is for their own good that intersex people
need not be born; their futures are "no good" (Kafer 2013, 3). Further, it is
proposed that society will also not suffer a loss with fewer intersex people in
the world because they are already invisible to the larger endosex community. This consequentialist mode of analysis enables Sparrow to claim jurisdiction over countless people's lives and reduces these lives to an equation
that is a simplistic, unintersectional iteration of systemic oppression, compulsory ways of being, identity formation, subjectivity, and life experiences.

The facile nature of this equation is evident in Sparrow's conflation of
racialization, dark skin, Blackness, and Black community or identity. The
problematic, unintersectional nature of Sparrow's analysis is further pronounced by the fact that there is no singular Black, dark-skin, queer, or
intersex experience. Not only are these subjectivities, communities, identities, and the related forms of oppression experienced individually, but they
are also not mutually exclusive. They have never been, nor will they ever be,
discursively or literally distinct. Recall the racist historical construction of
sexual "ambiguity" and how this construction maintains compulsory dyadism and spans over centuries. Recall the queerphobic, sexist, and racist
historical motivations to "cure" intersex and the current conflation of pathological queerness and intersex. Recall Sean Saifa M. Wall's (2016) assertion
"I am not just intersex. I am Black and I am queer." Wall's identities, what
his body-mind characteristics signify, and his experiences of oppression cannot be separated, as Sparrow's analysis incorrectly implies. It is *not*, employing Sparrow's (2013, 34) phrase, "plausible to divorce" intersex, race,
and queerness.

Employing the same unnuanced consequentialist logic, Trafimow assumes objective authority over intersex people's life experiences. He determines that all intersex individuals endure too much medical and social
suffering to justify their creative, diverse contributions to society, which is
to say that intersex people should not exist for their own good and, possibly, for society's good, as they do not have much to offer. The fact that
intersex people have offered so much creatively and intellectually is hard
to dispute. Many films, television shows, musical works, artworks, articles,

books, conferences, and so on are created by intersex people or clearly rely on, come about because of, or draw from intersex people's creative, diverse, intellectual ideas.[19] That being said, intersex people's lives cannot be reduced to such a dichotomous equation. Furthermore, intersex people – or any devalued or supposedly unviable group of people – do not exist to meet some quota of neoliberal diversity, creativity, capitalistic productivity, or utility. Lives "lived with and through difference" have "inherent value" (Holmes 2008b, 175).

Given that consequentialist arguments rely on dichotomous reasoning, the idea that there is an objective truth regarding ab/normal, un/healthy, dis/ordered, and dis/abled morphologies is privileged.[20] Consider Sparrow's (2013, 32, 31) proposal that intersex people deviate from "species-typical functioning" and do not have "normal sexual anatomy." Many scholars and activists prefer the term "typical" over "normal" because the former has fewer negative and pathologizing associations. However, in an online comment dated April 1, 2013, intersex activist and biological anthropologist Claudia Astorino (2012) notes that a/typical discourses have the potential to reinforce the idea that intersex is abnormal and pathological because a/typical is often conflated with ab/normal: "Typical totally doesn't have the same connotation as 'normal' or something, but I think that people would still say, 'Oh, you're sex-ATYPICAL...' and not think of the distinction between a/typical as more/less frequent but less/more weird." Sparrow's interchangeable use of a/typical and ab/normal discourses is concerning. He conflates atypicality with abnormality and, in turn, with undesirable pathology.

Aurenque and Ehni (2013, 55) observe, "This is not the first time Sparrow has defended the normative significance for medicine of the 'normal human body.'" Notwithstanding Sparrow's (2010, 10, 9) insistence elsewhere that he, in his own words, is "not inclined to conservatism," he "believe[s] that sexual dimorphism is a deep and valuable feature of the human condition." I do not necessarily disagree. Sexual dimorphism and compulsory dyadism have long been fundamental to and deeply valued by Western culture and colonial forces. But the fact that a Western cultural ideology is valued does not mean that it should be valued. That said, according to this logic, characteristics that defy compulsory dyadism are not valuable. They are pathologically abnormal; they violate and haunt the deified Western dyadic state of being.[21] Hence, by employing the ab/normal binary as an epistemological foundation, Sparrow can more easily justify intersex eugenics. Despite Sparrow's efforts, "the normative meaning of 'normal' sexual anatomy remains keenly disputed" (Aurenque and Ehni 2013, 55).

Normal and abnormal are not objective, identifiable states; they are ideological constructs. This fact is particularly clear when we examine Sparrow's (2013, 32) proposal that, unlike intersex people, Black people and queer folks fall under the "normal range of human variation." Since these types of people are supposedly deemed normal variants, selecting against Blackness or queerness (although Sparrow sympathizes with doing so) is more obviously eugenic. Aurenque and Ehni (2013, 56) respond to this claim:

> When Sparrow argues that "same-sex attractedness and dark skin color are part of the normal range of human variation" he is white-washing the long, frequently brutal historical struggle to establish the normality of those features of human phenotype and behavior. The normality of homosexuality in modern Western societies, like the unacceptability of treating individuals differently based on their skin tone, has only recently come to be a broadly accepted notion ... Indeed, it is exactly because of the flexibility of the concept of "normal health" that the intersex community hopes for a society that someday will understand the condition as within the normal bounds of human sexual diversity.

The category "normal" has only recently expanded to *sometimes*, arguably rarely, include people of colour and queer individuals. Sparrow (2005, 139), in part, acknowledges this fact in another article: "For much of the history of Western culture the 'normal' person was white," and people of colour "were thought to be inferior examples of the human form." Furthermore, as many studies and analyses demonstrate, legal, ideological, and institutional discrimination against racialized and queer folks is far from being entirely abolished.[22] Since the boundaries of "the normal" expand and contract through time and space for political reasons, we cannot work under the assumption that there are objectively normal or species-typical states of being.

The above considerations demonstrate that consequentialism, with its investment in the notion of innate ab/normality, is a flawed and outdated analytical tool. Hence, it is very troubling that consequentialism appears integral to new eugenics discourses and new eugenic practices. In order to justify new eugenics, an ethical analysis (i.e., consequentialism) that supposedly can prove that certain lives are not worth living is required. Without an ethical framework that enables one to assume impartiality, calculate pleasure and suffering, and identify ab/normal body-minds, one cannot claim that a group of people's lives are so insufferable or abnormal that they should not exist for their own good. Consequentialist logics support and are intimately entangled with new eugenics discourses and new eugenic practices. In other words, without the justification provided by consequentialist reasoning, new eugenics would immediately appear ethically reprehensible and intolerable. If we started from an ethic that recognized "the inherent value in a life lived with and through difference," the ethical imperative to determine whether a life is worth living or whether a body-mind or mode of be(com)ing is ab/normal would not be central or necessary to discussions at all (Holmes 2008b, 175).

Rather than being addressed with consequentialism, as Shildrick (2005, 4) demonstrates, bioethical issues "would be better addressed by a post-conventional or postmodernist approach that specifically seeks to break down such binary categories as those of the normal and abnormal, of health and illness, of self and other." In a similar vein, disability studies scholars Anne Kerr and Tom Shakespeare (2002) posit that traditional bioethics is too top-down. It is too invested in and focused on making normative prescriptions, both ideological and medical. Due to this top-down approach, contemporary bioethics has not satisfactorily engaged with people's ethical concerns about eugenics, old and new. Bioethics, therefore, ought to be more bottom-up and reliant on marginalized people's knowledges as well as on the social sciences and humanities. These debates ought to centre the perspectives of the people in question: intersex, disabled, queer, and racialized people. And these debates ought to rely on fields like queer, disability, crip, feminist, intersex, and critical race studies that do not take for granted normative prescriptions and ideologies – fields that are invested in social equity and in resisting white supremacy, colonialism, and culturally mandated ways of be(com)ing.

Conclusion

This chapter demonstrates that deploying PGD to detect and prevent the implantation of embryos with intersex traits continues the eugenics legacy in and outside of Canada. The main justifications employed to defend intersex eugenics are not grounded in sound evidence. Moreover, the consequentialist reasoning used to justify said eugenics problematically relies on dichotomous thinking and fails to acknowledge that people's lives, value, and be(com)ing in the world cannot be reduced to such an unintersectional and reductive calculation. In addition, the fact that the future ubiquitous use of PGD cannot be underestimated is clear. The current cost of PGD is high. However, the PGD market is growing every day, costs may decrease, and technologies can disseminate very quickly.

The relationship between intersex, PGD, and eugenics deserves immediate attention not only for the reasons noted above but also because, as intersex activist Morgan Carpenter (2016) observes, there is a troubling trend toward fertility clinics now paradoxically sponsoring and speaking at LGBTQIA2 events in Australia. For example, Carpenter notes, a representative of Australian-based City Fertility spoke at the "LBQ Women's Health and Wellbeing Conference" in 2016, held by the Victorian AIDS Council. The representative, Carpenter explains, endorsed using PGD to screen out "genetic abnormalities" such as Klinefelter syndrome (47,XXY), an intersex trait. Carpenter also notes that Rainbow Fertility "sponsored a conference on 'LGBTIQ' inclusion in higher education at the University of Western Sydney in June [2016]. Rainbow Fertility provides services for 'the LGBTI community' ... The organisation also supports or provides 'preimplantation genetic diagnosis' to eliminate 'severe genetic disorders' including Turner Syndrome ... Turner Syndrome is a chromosomal [intersex] variation." Put simply, fertility clinics that sponsor, support, and speak at LGBTQIA2 events promote and provide a technology that can select against the "I" in LGBTQIA2.

This practice is not unique to Australia. For instance, using PGD to detect ostensibly undesirable intersex traits is promoted in Canada because PGD is profitable, legal, and "remains unregulated" (S. O'Neill and Blackmer 2015, 10). Further, many of the fertility clinics that provide PGD in Canada promote themselves as LGBTQIA2 friendly. Many of these clinics are found and endorsed in Sherbourne Health's (n.d.) online resources for LGBT2SQ parents and families. This paradoxical promotion is especially concerning in Ontario given that, as noted above, OHIP covers one round of IVF services for all Ontarians under the age of forty-three with fertility issues. Many Ontarians are learning about and are confronted with PGD as they research and take advantage of this IVF coverage. Even though not all people who engage with IVF will opt for PGD, providing more IVF access to Ontarians, particularly (some) LGBTQIA2 Ontarians, is ironic when juxtaposed with the interphobic and eugenic logics of using PGD to select against intersex traits. The legacy of eugenics in and outside of Canada continues; it is just cloaked in a rainbow flag of "benevolence."

8

A Crip Intersex Approach to PGD

Using preimplantation genetic diagnosis (PGD) to select against intersex variations is a new eugenic practice. However, what sort of eugenic practice is it? Is it "Gender Eugenics?" Robert Sparrow (2013) inquires. If so, Vincent Couture and colleagues (2013, 59) ask, "which gender would be the target?" Avoiding the common conflation of sex and gender, Couture and colleagues note that PGD detects (inter)*sex* characteristics, not gender identity or performance. Drawing the same distinction, Georgiann Davis (2013, 51) concludes, "This is sex (not 'gender') eugenics." Interestingly, rather than explicitly arguing that the practice is intersex or interphobic eugenics, Davis implies that since the technology detects and can be used to select against traits typically deemed *sex*, this practice is sex eugenics.[1] Taking liberties with this argument, one may be compelled to posit further that this practice is sex*ist* eugenics. Framing said practice as sexist could be productive in legal circumstances. Opposing sexism by prohibiting sex selection because XY "males" will be favoured is widely supported in mainstream culture and reflected in various national policies (e.g., Canada and the United Kingdom) (S. O'Neill and Blackmer 2015). If people are troubled by the idea of selecting against XX "females" (with "normal" sex characteristics) because doing so is sexist, selecting against another embryo or fetus because of the un/expected intersex anatomy could be similarly explained as sexist.

Thinking of the Canadian context, for example, using the discourse of sexism points to contradictions in Canadian policy. In Canada, sex selection is prohibited because "it contravenes the dignity of human beings" and "may lead to gender discrimination and inequality" (S. O'Neill and Blackmer 2015, 10). However, there is a caveat in this policy: "Selection for the purpose of preventing, diagnosing, or treating sex-linked disorders or diseases is permitted in Canada" (S. O'Neill and Blackmer 2015, 10). According to medico-scientific definitions of "sex-linked disorders or diseases," these disorders or diseases include any "abnormality" inherited through sex chromosomes (X or Y). For example, hemophilia is a "sex-linked disorder or disease," and some intersex variations also fall under this umbrella. Positioning interphobic PGD employment as sex or sexist selection could enable one to argue that sex/ist selection, like eugenics, is in fact legal in Canada. Nevertheless, there are serious dangers in conflating sexism with interphobia and compulsory dyadism. The political, social, and legal discrimination that trans, cis, and endosex women (and femme folks) experience due to sexism does, at times, overlap with the forms of discrimination that intersex people experience. Conflating sexism with interphobia, however, misrepresents both forms of interlocking systems of oppression.

So what kind of eugenics is this? In order to answer this query, this chapter analyzes the discriminatory logics that underpin intersex eugenic selection via PGD. Using the language of intersectionality, I demonstrate that interphobic eugenics is situated at a complicated juncture where queerphobia, ableism, racism, and interphobia meet and cannot be rendered distinct. Even though intersex studies scholars, activists, and bioethicists are concerned with this eugenic PGD deployment, too few scholars approach this matter through a disability or anti-ableist lens. This chapter, therefore, analyzes and synthesizes pertinent bioethical, governmental, and reproductive clinic literatures through a feminist disability and crip framework. Some feminist intersex studies scholars critique this eugenic PGD practice by drawing attention to the fact that queerphobia and compulsory heterosexuality intersect with interphobia and, consequently, underpin the desire to eradicate intersex via reproductive technologies. My own analyses support these claims. However, disability does not figure prominently in this literature despite the fact that intersex is discursively constructed as a disability. I identify the ableist narratives that fuel intersex new eugenics. Claims that intersex traits are inherently unhealthy, diseased, disabled, disordered, unnatural, or deformed saturate bioethics articles that endorse intersex eugenics, fertility clinic documents and guidelines, and governmental policies concerning access to and regulation of PGD and reproductive technologies more generally. In this case, intersex is effectively integrated into conventional, ableist notions of disability to validate pre-emptive exorcisms and intersex eradication. I also draw readers' attention to the fact that although racism intersects with intersex eugenics, this fact is entirely ignored. As discussed in previous chapters, race and racism have been central to the construction of sexual "ambiguity" and continue to inform decisions regarding who ought to be subjected to curative violence.

I propose that ableist narratives figure prominently in discriminatory literature and conversations about PGD because harnessing ableist logics is more culturally admissible than explicitly employing queerphobic and racist rhetoric. Unlike queerphobia and racism, ableism is typically undetected or perceived to be natural and a matter of common sense. As a result, ableist logics are liberally mobilized. Since ableism is so central to promoting this new eugenic application of PGD, I suggest that anti-ableist discourses and disability analyses of reproduction, eugenics, and reproductive "choice" and "freedom" are vital as intersex studies scholars and activists continue to critique and combat this new eugenic practice. Cripping intersex in this context is a pragmatic means to successfully combat anti-intersex eugenics.

Interphobia and Queerphobia

It is well documented that queerphobia and compulsory heterosexuality underpin interphobia and curative violence. For example, curative violence is a way that compulsory heterosexuality and dyadism (and, as I discuss below, able-bodiedness) are enforced, surveilled, and literally carved or integrated into intersexualized body-minds. To borrow from Judith Butler (2006, 24), curative violence is a "regulatory practice that can be identified as compulsory heterosexuality" and, I add, compulsory dyadism. Therefore, technological interventions like PGD that prevent the implantation of embryos, gestation of fetuses, and birth of people with intersex traits must also be underpinned by these intersecting ideologies. Indeed, intersex eugenics is another way that compulsory heterosexuality and dyadism are enforced and literally constructed and implanted into (potentially) pregnant people's body-minds. That is, the reach of compulsory dyadism extends beyond people diagnosed with intersex traits or people presumed to have intersex traits. (Potentially) pregnant people, embryos, and fetuses are also apparently at a pathological risk of propagating or embodying the spectre of intersex; hence, they must embody and reproduce compulsory dyadism and heterosexuality. Emphasizing that queerphobia and compulsory heterosexuality contribute to the new eugenic, interphobic discourses and practices that call (potentially) pregnant individuals to reproduce heteronormative logics, fetuses, and people is imperative to undermining interphobic eugenics.

As sociologist Katrina Roen (2005, 260) explains, unnecessary medical interventions are performed not only to "straighten out" the intersex child's "deviant" body-mind but also to ensure "straightness" or heterosexuality – "to set everything straight." The desire for straightness is evident in surgeons' assessments that "the ability to engage in penis-vagina intercourse is considered to be the mark of successful surgery" (Roen 2005, 266). Compulsory heterosexuality and dyadism are also illustrated in testimonies made by intersex people who have been socio-medically assigned female. Many of these people explain that medical professionals ask about, speak of, and encourage heterosexual engagement with (potential) boyfriends and husbands following curative violence.[2] For example, Daniela Truffer (2015, 112) reports, "My endocrinologist always told me I couldn't have a boyfriend without a proper vagina ... After surgery, I was bleeding and in pain, but I had to dilate my vaginal opening to prevent stenosis. It was humiliating. The doctors said, I 'best get a boyfriend soon.'" Some preoperative intersex patients have been told that "curative" surgery is vital so that they can have "normal" heterosexual sex in the future. For instance, as noted in Chapter 1, Laura Inter (pseud.) (2015, 96) recalls, "One doctor explained that after the surgery I would have to use dilators and then I would be ready to 'have sex normally, with your husband, when you get married.' What the doctors didn't know ... was that since I was very young I had been attracted to women." These sorts of testimonies illustrate the coercion and shaming that often take place in medical contexts. They also highlight that heterosexuality and dyadism are not merely assumed but also enforced and literally carved onto people's physiologies. When intersex people do not adhere to or embody legible heterosexuality, some medical professionals deem the treatment a failure or maintain that lesbian, gay, bisexual, or queer intersex subjects were assigned the wrong gender even if intersex people's stories and identities cannot corroborate such claims (Chase 2006; G. Davis 2015; Karkazis 2008).

Parents of intersex children also express queerphobic and heteronormative ideologies, beliefs that are often further stoked by the clinical setting and medical professionals. Studies have shown that parents of intersex children typically prefer terminology that refers to disorders of sex development (DSDs) rather than to intersex because the latter negatively implies that their child is "between genders," trans, queer, lesbian, bisexual, or gay (Greenberg 2012, 93). Queerphobia fuels many parents' attempts to distance themselves and their child from LGBTQIA2 issues and identifiers. DSD discourse helps to pacify parents' queerphobic concerns because it opposes the idea that their intersex child is queer or "in between" male and female. DSD discourse emphasizes that the child has one, true, consistent (heterosexual) sex and gender. The true sex simply needs to be uncovered and inscribed into/onto the child's body-mind in order to fulfill the child's heterosexual destiny.[3] DSD nomenclature seemingly soothes parents' anxieties surrounding queerness, but the narrative does not always aid parents in forging positive bonds with their intersex child. Parents fear that others will treat their intersex child differently because of the social stigma surrounding intersex and queerness. However, parents themselves may be the ones who treat their child differently. For instance, some parents are hypervigilant about guarding against their intersex child's non/conforming gender performances and more lenient with their endosex siblings' performances (Karkazis 2008). Strict gender policing can result in strained familial ties (Orr and Watson 2021).

Ironically, in the attempt to straighten things out via curative violence, queer people are formed. By performing various procedures on intersex subjects, Roen (2005, 270) contends,

Clinicians (surgeons, endocrinologists, psychiatrists, and others) inevitably create newly queer beings. Surgical and psychotherapeutic processes carried out in childhood are not forgotten. Even when carried out on newborns, the body remembers. No matter how much the technological procedures are perfected, the experience of treatment is not erased. Furthermore, for adults who are able to articulate their own understandings of identity, the surgical reconstruction of queer bodies does not ultimately determine what, or how, those bodies become.

Queer or strange body-minds and memories are created; experiences of pathologization and curative violence haunt. Roen's argument echoes Morgan Holmes's (2000) claim that surgical interventions fashion queer sexes (see also Spurgas 2009). Ultimately, body-minds are not heteronormalized or rendered dyadic through medical intervention.

Martha Coventry's and Tiger Devore's testimonies supplement this argument. Coventry (1998) explains, "The truth is that the very thing surgery claims to save us [intersex people] from – a sense of differentness and abnormality – it quite unequivocally creates." Devore (1999, 80) similarly notes, "The doctors insist that you can't let a child go to school with ambiguous genitals, but the genitals they created were certainly strange looking."

The surgeries intended to normalize Devore's (in G. Harrison 2011) body-mind were "unnecessary failures" that did not produce dyadic genitals that "work." These interventions created queer, different beings and/or, as with Devore, "strange" genitals. Moreover, medical intervention does not prevent people from be(com)ing or identifying as queer. Although heterosexuality and dyadism are framed as compulsory, medical professionals, intersex people, and intersex folks' parents/proxies cannot anticipate the ways that heterosexuality and dyadism will not and cannot be internalized, embodied, or achieved.

Compulsory heterosexuality and dyadism underpin curative responses to the spectre of intersex. For this reason, it is imperative to acknowledge, as bioethicists Jason Behrmann and Vardit Ravitsky (2013) insist, that parents' decisions to use PGD in order to choose against intersex "may ... conceal biases against same-sex attractedness and gender nonconformity." I am disinclined to claim that queerphobia "may" only possibly influence choices and clinicians' recommendations. Although some people and (potential) parents resist queerphobia and are not invested in reproducing this form of discrimination, many do not actively resist the cultural imperative to be heterosexual and have internalized queerphobia. Or others may claim that they support LGBTQIA2 people but rationalize choosing against queerness for the "welfare" of the child. Researching women's complex relationships with amniocentesis, anthropologist Rayna Rapp (1999, 93) has learned that people "who choose to abort after a diagnosis of sex chromosome anomalies in their fetuses ... believed those anomalies would lead to homosexuality ... The fear of a homosexual orientation was so profound that sex chromosome problems and sexual 'problems' were irrevocably conflated." It is reasonable to suggest that people confronting the same diagnoses detected by PGD react in a similarly interphobic and queerphobic way, whether consciously or unconsciously. It is also reasonable to suggest that these discriminatory ideologies influence clinicians' recommendations.

To combat queerphobia, Behrmann and Ravitsky (2013) propose that (potential) parents who think about selecting against intersex via PGD should be provided with resources about interphobia, intersex anatomies, support groups, and intersex people living fulfilling lives. These resources may change (potential) parents' minds about intersex and, by extension, queerness. Getting this information into fertility clinics and into (potential) parents' possession will be difficult. Historically, medical professionals have largely failed to provide this type of information.[4] Medical professionals have stifled the spread of this information and support by telling intersex people and their family members that they are lone anomalies. Emily Quinn (2015, 109), an intersex activist with complete androgen insensitivity syndrome (CAIS), explains that her doctor "did not direct me to any actual support," even though there is plenty of information about CAIS and even though there are support groups for people with CAIS. Like Karen A. Walsh (2015), Kimberly Zieselman (2015), and Pidgeon Pagonis (2015a), among many others, Quinn (in Wall et al. 2015) was told, "There is nobody else like me." Accurate information and support have been historically withheld. I am therefore skeptical that this sort of information will be welcomed into fertility clinics and provided to (prospective) parents in the near future. Nevertheless, we ought to insist that such information be readily available. Another cumbersome barrier that would prevent this information from entering fertility clinics is the chasm between clinical terminology and the depathologizing nomenclature employed by intersex activists and intersex studies scholars. Medical professionals in fertility clinics, just like in other medical environments, do not use the word "intersex" or destigmatizing expressions like "intersex variations" or "intersex traits." Attempting to bridge this language gap via collaboration has been difficult and highly contested in medical, activist, and scholarly communities.

One may expect, given that DSD nomenclature has become standard in medical settings, that fertility clinics and governmental documents that regulate reproductive technologies employ the same terminology. Yet evaluating, for example, Canada's PGD regulations and various fertility clinics reveals that intersex is abstracted, misrepresented, and pathologized, but it is not explicitly pathologized through DSD terminology. More broad and elusive language is used, such as "sex-linked disorders or diseases" (S. O'Neill and Blackmer 2015, 10). Ottawa Fertility Centre (n.d.) uses similarly broad phrases on its "Fertility Treatments" webpage: "sex-linked genetic disorders," "gene defects," and "chromosomal disorders." And Best Start: Ontario's Maternal, Newborn and Early Childhood Development Resource Centre and the Halton Region Health Department's (2007, 61) guide for providers of fertility services in Ontario refers to "sex-chromosome disorders" and "major congenital anomalies." So many variations fall under these often unclear, wide-ranging categories, including, as noted in the guide, the intersex variation Klinefelter syndrome. Being born with this variation, so the Resource Centre and Health Department implies, does not offer one the "Best Start."

In addition to classifying Klinefelter syndrome as a "major congenital anomal[y]," the Resource Centre and Health Department (2007, 78) define

Klinefelter syndrome as "an abnormal condition in a male characterized by two X chromosomes and one Y chromosome, leading to infertility, smallness of the testes, sparse facial and body hair." These characteristics and descriptions are at odds with heterosexual hegemonic masculinity and, therefore, could stoke queerphobic concerns with potentially having an intersex child. Moreover, the words "major" and "anomaly" as well as the definition are misleading, if not false. Studies estimate that between 1 in 500 to 1,000 people have this variation (Bojesen, Juul, and Gravholt 2003; Fullerton, Hamilton, and Maheshwari 2010). Klinefelter is hardly anomalous. Hence, Gail Fullerton, Mark Hamilton, and Abha Maheshwari (2010, 588) refer to Klinefelter as "common." Further, people with Klinefelter syndrome are not necessarily infertile.[5] People with Klinefelter mosaic cell lines may have reproductive sperm and can fertilize an egg without reproductive technologies. Further, with the development of microsurgical techniques and reproductive technologies, many people with Klinefelter can and do have biological children. Given these findings and developments, "the label of infertile should be reevaluated" (Fullerton, Hamilton, and Maheshwari 2010, 595). At any rate, a person is not innately queerly disabled, disordered, or diseased if they cannot (or do not) reproduce or if they have small testes and sparse body hair.

Ultimately, the language used in these sorts of documents is at odds with the fact that intersex traits themselves cause few, if any, medical problems. The discourses are misleading, rooted in fear-mongering terminology (e.g., "disease," "major," "syndrome," and "defect"), incorrect, and esoteric, which enables medical professionals to maintain power over intersex "treatment." The nature of these descriptions and the foregrounding of disability also allow the queerphobia that underpins choosing against intersex to go largely undetected. The discourses cultivate the best conditions for queerphobic, interphobic eugenic choices. Ultimately, given the evident gap between activist, medical, and fertility discourses, it is tragically unlikely that positive and accurate information about intersex will be instituted in fertility clinics anytime soon. More difficult, and possibly painful, linguistic collaboration is needed for resources to be made readily available in fertility clinics.

In addition to queerphobia underpinning medical professionals' recommendations and (potential) parents' motivations to avoid intersex, queerphobia is evident in Sparrow's (2013) argument for intersex eugenics. Sparrow maintains that selecting against intersex is permissible because of potential harms caused by the social environment. Sparrow (2013, 33) writes, "If [intersex] children are at risk of psychological harms from being teased or persecuted for having 'different' genitals, this is clearly a social problem." However, his notion of social harms quickly becomes queer-phobic, interphobic, and medicalized when he begins sympathizing with a very narrow definition of "properly functioning genitals." Sparrow's (2013, 33–34) concern for intersex people's welfare also becomes questionable when he voices concern for intersex people's potential sex partners:

> While the empirical claim that children born with ambiguous genitalia suffer consequent social and psychological harms may be controversial, it is also plausible (Elliot 1998; Warne and Bhatia 2006) and – if true – might justify PGD out of concern for the welfare of the future child ... If we think of "healthy" genitalia as granting the capacity for intercourse leading to re-production, eliciting sexual attraction in mates, and providing pleasure, then relations with other people are essential to the first two of these and will often be central to the third. Genitals that don't "fit" with the genitals of other people, that fail to elicit desire in one's sexual partners, and/or that render pleasure difficult to achieve in the prevailing social circumstances (which include access – or lack of access – to vibrators and/or other sex toys) are arguably functionally deficient. Establishing that the difficulties associated with being born intersex are a function of social context would not therefore itself rule out their being the appropriate *objects* of medical intervention. (Emphasis added)

The claim that *people* – rather than, in Sparrow's words, *objects* – born with variant genitals and other intersex traits confront social and psychological harm should not be controversial.[6] However, the three key "biological func-tions" that indicate "health" are contentious. To unpack this quotation, I interrogate each noted biological function and the idea of genital "fit." I then close this section and lead into the next section on ableism by problematiz-ing Sparrow's use of the term "healthy."

The idea that healthy genitals lead to reproduction via, it is implied, penis-in-vagina sex – unless otherwise impeded by, for example, contracep-tion, abortion, or nonconsensual sterilizing violence – is often assumed to reflect the heterosexual natural order of things. Lee Edelman (2004, 11, 2) refers to this belief as rooted in the "absolute logic of reproduction" and the cultural investment in "reproductive futurism." The cultural investment in, or demand for, dyadic sex (i.e., compulsory dyadism) and therefore heterosexual sex (i.e., compulsory heterosexuality) and reproduction (i.e., compulsory reproduction) is not "natural" but rather an "unquestioned value" (Edelman 2004, 4). The undisputed logic of reproduction creates "a hierarchical system of sexual value" in which able-bodied, "marital, reproductive heterosexuals are alone at the top of the erotic pyramid" (Rubin 1998, 107). The pro-natal hierarchy is so naturalized that having children is, for example, represented as and reasoned to be "the natural destiny of all women and marriage the only legitimate means for its fulfillment" (Carroll 2012, 27). Rather than being the natural order of things, the logic of reproduction is a cultural construct that is institutionalized through and propagated by, for instance, the secular and religious institutions of marriage, medical professionals, and certain scholars like Sparrow (2013).

People who do not or cannot fulfill compulsory dyadism, able-bodiedness, heterosexuality, and reproduction are often pathologized and demonized. Edelman (2004, 11) writes, "Whatever refuses this [reproductive] mandate by which our political institutions compel the collective reproduction of the Child must appear as a threat not only to the organization of a given social order but also, and far more ominously, to social order as such." The "whatever," in this context, is the queer: "The queer comes to figure the bar to every realization of futurity" (Edelman 2004, 4). Also, people – primarily women – "whose desires or social roles escape this [reproductive] function [e.g., spinsters] confound the ideological construction" that women's biological destiny is to reproduce (Carroll 2012, 27). Or, as with Sparrow's (2013) claim, intersex people with variant genitals or intersex people who cannot reproduce are deemed unhealthy precisely because they confound the "absolute logic of reproduction" (Edelman 2004, 11); they are near or at the bottom of the "erotic pyramid" (Rubin 1998, 107) and threaten "social order as such" (Edelman 2004, 11). Variant genitals are not innately unhealthy or pathological if they cannot or do not lead to reproduction. (However, it is important to keep in mind that many intersex people's ability to biologically reproduce is taken away via sterilizing curative violence.) They are pathologized only because they do not conform to the apparent heteronatural, pro-natal order of things. Claiming that intersex eugenics is in the interest of potential intersex people because they may not be able to reproduce becomes difficult to defend when one questions the intersecting logics of compulsory reproduction, dyadism, able-bodiedness, and heterosexuality. The potential intersex child is not being protected. Pro-natal, discriminatory ideologies are being safeguarded.

Seemingly rooted in evolutionary theory or objectivist aesthetic theory, another supposed function of healthy genitals that Sparrow (2013) proposes is that they elicit attraction and desire in one's sexual partner/s. Variant genitals – queer, disordered, disabled, crip genitals – apparently do not elicit such desire; they are, Sparrow suggests, innately unattractive. The idea of an objective genital aesthetic standard, although untenable, reinforces culturally mandated ways of being and justifies intersex eugenics under the guise of protecting the potential intersex person from teasing, bullying, and rejection for ostensibly having innately ugly genital characteristics. There is no objective genital aesthetic standard, even though Western philosophers have attempted to provide objectivist aesthetic theories for centuries (see Aristotle 1984; Plato 1962; and Plotinus 1952). Attractiveness is also not merely subjective (i.e., "beauty is in the eye of the beholder"), as many aesthetic subjectivist philosophers suggest in opposition to objectivists (Hume 1894, 1988; Kant 1997). Which characteristics are deemed attractive or unattractive – beautiful or grotesque – is an ideological assessment and political value judgment.[7] Influenced by, for example, racism, sexism, and anti-Semitism, standards of genital beauty, attraction, and health have shifted through time and space. And these shifts demonstrate the political nature of which genital features are deemed un/healthy and un/attractive.

Historically, due to anti-Semitism, the circumcised penis was construed as a mark of pathological sexual difference, disease, impairment, and incompleteness (Gilman 1991). This understanding has shifted. Currently, due to inconclusive and highly contested medical and scientific studies and aesthetic claims, uncircumcised penises are often regarded as ugly, unhygienic vectors of disease in countries where circumcision is common practice (e.g., the United States and Canada) (Hellsten 2004). Or, consider the current increase in female genital cosmetic surgeries performed on endosex, cis women who want to attain the more "desirable," "normal," albeit prepubescent, "tucked-in look," as seen in mainstream pornography (participant quoted in Braun 2009, 242; see also F.J. Green 2005; and Liao and Creighton 2007). Racist cultural views also underpin assessments that Black women, and women of colour in general, have "ugly," "too dark," "unclean," "malconformed," or "ambiguous" genitals.[8] Discriminatory cultural assumptions and representations of genitals reproduce and inform our understandings of genital attraction. Genitals are not inherently un/desirable, ugly, or beautiful. Specific socio-political ideas and cultural contexts influence people's aesthetic evaluations.

Variant genitals are not inherently unattractive. They challenge the assumed normality of white heterosexuality and dyadic sex. They challenge people's (hetero)sexual imagination. Moreover, given that interphobia relies on racialized/racist understandings of proper or beautiful genitals, one cannot ignore the racist underpinnings of claiming that variant genitals will not illicit desire in others and, therefore, are innately ugly. Sparrow's (2013) concern with (potential) intersex people's (potential) sex partners reveals more about his limited sexual imaginary and about his ability to subtly reproduce racist, interphobic, and ableist ideologies than it does about any genuine concern for (potential) intersex individuals' well-being. In other words, even though Sparrow insists that he is concerned for (potential) intersex people's welfare and health, voicing a concern for potential lovers' aesthetic stance on variant genitals indicates otherwise. Beauty is not a marker of health; beauty is a political, ideological appraisal.

Another function of healthy genitals, Sparrow purports, is that they provide pleasure. I was initially confounded by the notion that variant genitals may not provide pleasure or may render pleasure, in Sparrow's (2013, 33) terms, "difficult to achieve." If an intersex person escapes surgical curative violence, genital sensation and orgasm are not hindered. Be that as it may, Sparrow (2013, 34) mentions "one's sexual partners" while discussing the functions of healthy genitals; he appears to be concerned with intersex people's partners' assumed lack of pleasure. An intersex person's partner will apparently struggle to be pleasured by variant genitals, and/or the partner will struggle to pleasure the intersex person with variant genitals because they are illegible. The former suggestion, receiving pleasure will be "difficult," is only logically consistent if one takes for granted the belief that endosex, heterosexual, penis-in-vagina sex is the most sexually satisfying or, in Sparrow's (2013, 34) words, if we assume that "the prevailing social circumstances" are endosex and heterosexual.

Assuming that such circumstances are optimal for sexual gratification reproduces compulsory dyadism and heterosexuality. This assumption also neglects the fact that heterosexual, penis-in-vagina sex is frequently not optimal for endosex, cis women with vaginas/vulvas because there is no, or not enough, clitoral stimulation (E.A. Armstrong, England, and Fogarty 2012; Koedt 2000; Mahar, Mintz, and Akers 2020). This type of sex is optimal for heterosexual, endosex, cis men with penises. Like the insistence of so many medical professionals that assigned girl intersex children need medical interventions so that a prospective "normal"-sized penis can fit inside, Sparrow's concern with potential men's easy sexual satisfaction smacks of phallogocentrism and heterosexual male entitlement to vaginal pleasure. Overall, despite Sparrow's claim that he is concerned for (potential) intersex people's welfare, his concern about potential lovers' (primarily or presumably men's) inability to be *easily* sexually pleased indicates otherwise. It is hard not to question Sparrow's (2013, 34) legitimate concern for intersex people when he refers to them as "functionally deficient ... appropriate objects of medical intervention" because their genitals may "render pleasure difficult."

The latter suggestion, that providing pleasure to people with variant genitals will be difficult, reminds me of sexist stereotypes about women with vulvas, vaginas, and clitorises: they are impossible to decode, women take longer than men to orgasm, and reaching orgasm is challenging for women (E.A. Armstrong, England, and Fogarty 2012; Koedt 2000; Mahar, Mintz, and Akers 2020). These false stereotypes have long histories of sexist pathologization and have material consequences today. In addition to women being shamed and pathologized, women's sexual needs are often ignored and silenced; in turn, there is remarkable orgasm inequity between endosex, cis, heterosexual men and women. Echoing the assumption that women are difficult to please because of a biological deficit, Sparrow (2013) suggests that intersex people are difficult to please because of an innate biological problem or hindrance. As the literature about these sexist stereotypes and the orgasm gap show, there is no inherent, pathological problem with vaginas, vulvas, and clitorises. There is a sexist, social, and education problem. Similarly, variant genitals are not intrinsically difficult to please; there is an interphobic, queerphobic, social, and education problem.

Crosscutting all of these claims about "healthy" genitals is the premise that variant genitals do not naturally "fit," I presume, with ostensibly endosex genitals or perhaps even with other variant genitals. This anxiety regarding fit is also evident in the preoccupation with normalizing or "straightening" out variant genitals. But genitals are not puzzle pieces. To the homophobic proposal that men with penises who have sex with men with penises is unnatural because "the parts don't fit," writer Duane Simolke (2005, 23) cheekily responds, "You obviously lack imagination." Simolke (2005, 23) also suggests that proponents of this claim should read some publications, "whether erotic or clinical," to broaden their sexual horizons. Borrowing from Simolke, I recommend thinking more creatively and queerly about the notion that variant genitals do not fit with supposed endosex people's genitals. Thinking queerly reminds one that people's genitals can and do fit in and/or are placed in, around, and on numerous places, subjects, and objects to experience pleasure. In fact, Sparrow (2013, 34) invites us to think about some obvious options when he refers to "social circumstances" that may "include access – or lack of access – to vibrators and/or other sex toys." Nevertheless, Sparrow (2013, 33, 34) still proposes that variant genitals do not naturally "fit" in "prevailing circumstances" and are "arguably functionally deficient." Thinking queerly challenges the queerphobic, interphobic, pro-natal notion that genitals have an essential purpose or a natural place to fit.

Historically framed by religious discourses, the accusation that certain genital formations do not fit together has long been used to pathologize LGBTQIA2 people, primarily gay men. Wayne R. Dynes (2014, 81) summarizes and historicizes this rationalization in *The Homophobic Mind*:

> Simple observation shows that the sexual organs of the male body protrude, while the female genitalia are concave. The organs fit together like an electrical plug in its socket. For this reason heterosexual couplings are simple, direct, and inviting, while homosexual ones are awkward, contrived, and unsatisfactory ... This claim represents a subset of the argument from design. Popular in the seventeenth and eighteenth century, the argument has been revived in recent years by Creationists, who hold that God's imprint is found everywhere in the world in the form of "intelligent design."

Based on the same sort of reasoning as the often-referenced human eyeball argument – the human eyeball is so complex that God must have designed it – the queerphobic idea that penises and vaginas were constructed by God to fit together is espoused. More recently the idea of "fit" has been transformed and taken up in medico-biological, evolutionary, and secular discourses to pathologize queer sex/uality and intersex people with variant genitals. In any case, Dynes (2014, 82) writes,

> Modern sex research has pointed to crucial biological discrepancies that have weakened the old notion of the perfect suitability of male and female sexual organs. For one thing, the "fit" of the penis to the vagina is not notably better than its fit to the anus ... In addition, the male and female biorhythms summoned by sexual excitation show notable difference, and much negotiation and adjustment is required to achieve mutual satisfaction ... If this argument were conclusive, everyone would experience more pleasure and satisfaction from opposite-sex couplings than same-sex ones. Yet many do not.

Echoing the research from which Dynes draws, post-structuralist, queer, trans, feminist, crip, disability, asexuality, and intersex studies scholars have discredited the essentialist claim that anatomical parts have natural purposes and ought to perform certain sex acts or gendered labour. Think-ing imaginatively and queerly about what to do with, how to touch, and where to put genitals and other erogenous zones – as queer, trans, intersex, asexual, disabled, and crip people do – is not simply about exploring sexual-ity and sexual stimulation. Doing so contributes to anti-queerphobic, anti-ableist, and anti-interphobic projects like the systemic disabling of intersex people and intersex eugenics. So, as Simolke (2005) suggests, let us stimu-late our imaginations, read some literature, and think queerly.

Interphobia and Ableism

Sparrow's (2013) suggestion that variant genitals are "unhealthy" is one of the many characterizations of intersex traits that leads me to consider intersex eugenics, like the treatment of intersex people in general, as a dis-ability issue. Additionally, queerness and race cannot be separated from disability when considering (the prospect of) an intersex embryo, fetus, or child. Disorder, health, disability, racialization, and queerness interlock and overlap. A disability lens is requisite when analyzing intersex eugenics and PGD technologies in order to fully understand why intersex eugenics is presumed benevolent, "perhaps even morally required" (Sparrow 2013, 29). A disability studies approach reveals that intersex anatomies are presumed to be and are represented as fundamentally disordered, disabled, diseased, and in Sparrow's (2013, 34) terms, "functionally deficient." The fact that intersex is being successfully assimilated into conventional notions of dis-ability and ill health is clear. Put simply, a disability approach reveals that intersex eugenics is justified by explicitly ableist discourses.

Although queerphobia and racism undeniably figure in arguments for intersex eugenics, queerphobic and racist sentiments are more implicit when compared to ableist discourses. In fact, queerphobic and racist ideol-ogies are justified via ableist discourses about, for example, what is deemed un/healthy, ab/normal, and species a/typical. Yet the bioethical literature concerning intersex eugenics overwhelmingly does not unpack the ableism present in arguments for intersex eugenics. Intersex is strategically discur-sively constructed as a disability precisely so that ableist narratives can prominently figure in conversations about PGD – and in intersex medical management in general – because doing so allows, in Georgiann Davis's (2015, 70) terms, "for medical professionals to reassert their authority and maintain their exclusive jurisdiction over intersex." That is, harnessing ableist logics is at present easier – more culturally admissible – than ex-plicitly employing queerphobic and racist rhetoric. Of course, queer people face myriad forms of discrimination and harassment. Homonormative expressions and representations of queerness, however, are increasingly common, celebrated, and accepted (see Dryden and Lenon 2015; McCaskell 2016; and Puar 2007, 2013). Indeed, many nations actively position themselves as accepting of queer people. Without a doubt, racialized people are still systemically brutalized and marginalized. Moreover, due to anti-racist scholars and activists, it is clear that anti-racist rhetoric, campaigns, and transnational movements, like the Black Lives Matter movement, are gaining considerable support on the global stage.[9] Hence, queerphobia and racism cannot be as readily or explicitly mobilized in policies or (scholarly) conversations concerning PGD, intersex eugenics, or intersex medical maltreatment. Doing so would immediately be interpreted as discriminatory. Unlike queerphobic and racist discrimination, ableism is rarely construed as discrimination. Ableism remains generally undetected because it is perceived to be natural and a matter of common sense. Ableist narratives, therefore, are liberally mobilized. Whichever form of oppression and discrimination is explicitly culturally admissible will be overtly mobilized to justify intersex eugenics and curative violence. Although one discriminatory narrative may dominate at a given time, these narratives remain braided together and must be understood as still working together. Nevertheless, the fact that ableism figures so prominently in conversations about intersex eugenics and PGD without receiving much attention reveals that, in order to combat intersex eugenics, we must combat ableism; we must crip our intersex analyses of PGD.

Drawing on disability studies scholars to complicate the seemingly straightforward and objective descriptors "healthy" and "unhealthy," I further unpack Sparrow's (2013) suggestion that variant genitals are unhealthy. I also critique how intersex is conflated with paradigmatic disabilities. And I identify and examine the ways that medical professionals and fertility clinics misrepresent intersex by conflating intersex traits with life-threatening diseases like cancer. Representing intersex as a disability or disease in these medical/izing contexts is a means to exploit ableist sentiments for intersex eugenic projects. Presenting intersex as a disability or disease in circumstances that devalue disability is a discursive manoeuvre to ensure that medical professionals retain authority over intersex and reify compulsory able-bodiedness, dyadism, and heterosexuality as well as whiteness.

It's a ... Baby: Unhealthy, Sexless Intersex Infants
The necessity of a disability approach is highlighted by reading Sparrow's

(2013) proposition that variant genitals are unhealthy alongside the disability studies analysis of "healthy" births offered by disability studies scholar Danielle Peers (2015, 339):

> Judith Butler (1988) argues that one of the first constituting acts of subjectivity is the sexing of newborns. The movement from *it* to *girl* in the declaration "It's a girl!" is the first of many sexing technologies that secure an essential part of our subjectivity. Yet, before the celebratory announcement of the sex of a newborn (or fetus), there is almost always an equally critical qualifier, namely, *healthy*. Indeed, my strong breath and normative number of digits marked my movement from thing to human just as much as my vagina did. Borrowing from Butler, I contend that discrete health and ability statuses – not unlike "discrete genders" – "are part of what 'humanizes' individuals within contemporary culture" (522). Objectified knowledges of gender and health, along with their corresponding technologies of division and normalization, have each fundamentally constituted me not only as a person, but also as a particular *sort* of person to be recognized, treated, and acted upon in corresponding ways.

Intersex and feminist studies scholars identify that a problem arises when the constituting act of sexing and gendering a newborn baby cannot instantly take place because of identifiable (queer) intersex traits (see Fausto-Sterling 2000; Kessler 1998; and Preves 1999, 2003). Considering Peers's apt observation that being legibly healthy constitutes one as human together with both the pathologization of intersex and Sparrow's suggestion that variant genitals are unhealthy complicates the idea that the "problem" with intersex is solely a sex or queer issue.

Upon an encounter with an intersex newborn with variant genitals, a gender qualifier is not immediately applied, and the equally critical, humanizing qualifier "healthy" is also not applied. Rather than the declaration "It's a healthy baby girl/boy," a parent may be met with the unnerving declaration "It's a ... baby." Or, as Vincent Guillot's (in Lohr 2016) mother was, a parent may be told that they "had given birth to a monster." Or, as Baseema (quoted in Gough et al. 2008, 500) was, a parent may be met with unnerving silence: "I said 'is it a girl or a boy?', and they didn't, they just didn't say anything. They did not have a word" (see also Zeiler and Wickström 2009). In other words, health is often defined in terms of normalcy. And, given this construction, intersex infants are subjected to literal curative sexing technologies.[10] The variant genital "problem" is an intersecting queer and disability issue – a crip intersex issue. Intersex newborns with variant genitals are not rendered fully human because they are assumed "sexless" and, therefore, "unhealthy." In order to prevent this situation from occurring, reproductive sexing technologies (e.g., PGD) are made available. Or, to ostensibly remedy the unhealthy situation, curative sexing technologies are deployed, including intersex genital mutilation (IGM), hormone replacement therapy (HRT), and genital examinations. The assumption that atypical characteristics are innately unhealthy and inferior remains intuitively correct to bioethicists concerned with people having the "healthiest" children, or in bioethicist Julian Savulescu's (2001, 413) terms, having the "best children" who will be able to lead "the best" lives. Yet, as disability studies demonstrate, health is not an objectively inherent or apolitical quality or state of being; it is an ideology. To quote disability studies scholar Dan Goodley (2011, 82), "Health and illness are aspects of larger systems and are not located entirely within the single person." Un/healthy states of being are not wholly rooted in the body-mind. They are political, relational, and discursively constructed and, in turn, create un/healthy or dis/abled subjects.

Intersex infants born with variant genitals are not fundamentally unhealthy; their visible sex traits queer and crip sex and gender systems. Drawing from feminist philosopher Julia Kristeva (1982, 4), I note that "it is ... not lack of cleanliness or health that causes abjection but what disturbs identity, system, order. What does not respect borders, positions, rules. The in-between, the ambiguous, the composite." Innate unhealthiness is not what renders intersex traits shocking, spectral, or abject – capable of literally silencing medical professionals and striking fear in parents. Intersex variations are abject because they disturb boundaries and compulsory ways of being. Locating the problem with intersex in the intersex trait itself opens up a space to restore identity, system, and order. And medical professionals fill that space with various technologies of gender and "health," such as IGM, HRT, and PGD. The taken-for-granted premise that intersex variations are unhealthy portrays these eugenic technologies – tools apparently capable of exorcising the spectre – as necessary, curative, and benevolent.

Intersex, Leglessness, and Deafness: Conflating Intersex with Paradigmatic Disabilities

According to Sparrow (2013, 34), like "deafness and leglessness," intersex variations are unhealthy, species-atypical, medical problems. Conflating intersex with these sorts of paradigmatic disabilities integrates intersex into conventional notions of disability, exploits ableist sentiments, and works to depoliticize intersex eugenics. Interestingly, Sparrow attempts to illustrate that intersex is primarily a medical problem by appealing to disability studies scholars. Sparrow (2013, 32) states that disability scholars maintain that "medical problems [e.g., deafness and leglessness] have a social component." This delineation of disability scholars is misrepresentative and not nuanced. In addition to critiquing the medical model of disability (i.e., disability is an innate defect and medical problem), disability studies scholars critique the social model of disability (i.e., all disabilities are purely a social problem) when they account for impairments like chronic pain and cancer, noting that some people seek medical intervention and cure.[11] Nuanced theories, like Alison Kafer's (2013, 4) "political/relational model" (P/R model), prove that disability or disabled body-mind classifications are much more complex than the medical-social binary and propose that disability is political and relational. Sparrow (2013), however, incorrectly implies that disability scholars support the idea that all disabilities are *principally* "medical problems" and have "a social component" – perhaps just one social component. In doing so, Sparrow wrongly insinuates that disability studies scholars understand medicine and society as distinct entities. Medicine is a social, political, relational, cultural practice; it is fundamentally a part of politics, culture, and society.

Working with this misrepresentative iteration of disability theories, Sparrow (2013, 32) proceeds to claim that there is "a rough consensus" that "a failure to develop legs,"[12] "leglessness," and "deafness" are medical issues because they "are deviations from species-typical functioning which will raise barriers and reduce opportunities." As a result, "selection against these traits looks to be justified by concern for the life prospects of the future child" (Sparrow 2013, 32). After naming and reviewing the key biological functions of healthy genitalia, Sparrow (2013, 34) concludes,

> It seems likely that some intersex conditions should properly be thought of as analogous to leglessness or deafness – that is, as medical conditions that significantly restrict an affected individual's welfare and opportunities in the range of environments that it is reasonable to expect them to encounter. In such cases, PGD to avoid the condition is morally permissible – and perhaps even morally required ([J.] Harris 2001).
>
> Some may be tempted to argue, as per the "disability critique" of prenatal testing (Asch 1988 and 2000; Wendell 1996; Saxton 1997; Kaplan 1993), that selection is morally problematic even in these cases. However, the environmental analogy foregrounds the implausible nature of the claim

that such intersex conditions should be thought of as "mere variations" rather than harmful deviations from species-typical functioning.

Sparrow argues that, like people who do not have legs and deaf individuals, people with intersex anatomies are fundamentally and harmfully species-atypical because their body-minds are not readily accommodated by current ableist infrastructures and gender, sex, and linguistic systems. Therefore, selecting against these (potential) body-minds is, for Sparrow, benevolent and not ableist. Sparrow's logic is backwards. These folks are not innate deviations because they do not reflect compulsory modes of being, do not fit neatly into dominant ideological systems, or do not move freely in ableist infrastructures. Rather, instituted culturally mandated ways of being create discursive and literal environments that exclude and fail to value the full diversity of human body-minds.

Sparrow's focus on individuals' assumed welfare masks the ableism that unpins his argument. This "individual discourse," Goodley (2011, 8) explains, "creates a number of 'fault lines': disability is cast as an essentialist condition (with organic aetiologies)," and "disabled people are treated as objects rather than as authors of their own lives." Recall Sparrow (2013, 34) referring to intersex people as "objects" appropriate for curative violence, not active subjects. Consequently, "'person fixing' rather than 'context changing' interventions are circulated" (Goodley 2011, 8). Or, where PGD is concerned, preventative technologies are promoted as benevolent. Medical professionals' power over intersex is maintained, and productively combatting discriminatory logics remains off the table. Presenting intersex traits and (other) disabilities as species-atypical defects – exploiting taken-for-granted ableist reasoning – enables one to more readily evade the charge that selecting against these variations is discriminatory and eugenic.

The assumption that intersex is like a disability or is a disability is also reflected in the language employed by fertility clinics. In 2016, for example, Rainbow Fertility's webpage "Additional Options with IVF" explained that this clinic provides PGD to "detect anomalies" and "abnormal chromosomes," like "Turner Syndrome," an intersex variation, in order to prevent the "adverse outcomes" of "the birth of a child with physical and/or mental disabilities." The webpage has since deleted most of these phrases and simply suggests talking to a specialist for more information (Rainbow Fertility 2020). Similarly, for years, City Fertility's "Genetic Testing" webpage stated that PGD is a tool used to screen out "genetic abnormalities" "that may prevent implantation to the uterine lining, lead to pregnancy loss, or result in the birth of a child with physical and/or mental disabilities. PGD may help prevent these adverse outcomes." Such abnormalities, this webpage stated, include "Down syndrome or Trisomy 21" and "Klinefelter syndrome (XXY)," an intersex variation, which may result in "physical differences and mental retardation." Like Rainbow Fertility, City Fertility (2020) has since changed much of its wording, but the message is clear: PGD can prevent "the birth of a child with physical and/or mental disability," and this outcome is presented as de facto good. The shift in language seemingly functions to mask the discriminatory and eugenic underpinnings of PGD deployment. But the fact that variations like intersex and Down syndrome are deemed innate body-mind deformities and failures that ought to be avoided at all costs via exorcising technologies is clear. Ultimately, explicitly or implicitly reproducing the rhetoric of tragedy – employing pathologizing, ableist, and culturally disconcerting terms like "adverse," "abnormal," and "disabilities" – frames intersex as an innate disability that ought to be avoided.

Sparrow's position and the discourses used by fertility clinics are not unique. Yet Sparrow's essentializing comparison/conflation of intersex with deaf people in his 2013 article is noteworthy because it thoroughly contradicts his 2005 article, "Defending Deaf Culture: The Case of Cochlear Implants." Like many disability studies scholars, Sparrow (2005, 137) argues that the disadvantages that deaf people confront are produced by ableist "social and institutional causes and could be rectified by changes in the way society is organized." Echoing Kafer's P/R model, he challenges the idea that disability is an innate defect and works to expand the confines of normal human variation or species-typical functioning. Indeed, Sparrow (2005, 138–39) implies that deafness is relational and political:

> Deafness is a disability because hearing is one of the six senses that humans characteristically possess ... But a moment's thought reveals ... the limits of normal human capacities will be the result of who we consider to be part of the range of normal human variation amongst persons. If we include the deaf, then hearing will not be something that all normal people have. It will instead become a less important mark of difference, like hair or eye color ...
>
> It is also timely here to emphasize how far the boundaries of the 'normal' have already shifted. For much of the history of Western culture the 'normal' person was white, male and propertied. Women, non-whites and working class people were thought to be inferior examples of the human form.

If one recognizes how ideologies concerning ab/normality and dis/ability shift, as Sparrow previously did, then it is clear that intersex variations are not innately deviant, abnormal, or species-atypical, contrary to what Sparrow (2013) more recently suggests. The oppression that intersex people experience, as Sparrow (2005, 137) says of the disadvantages that deaf people confront, "could be rectified by changes in the way society is organized." Reductive, objectifying, and derivative explanations of sex, gender, health, and disability do not resolve injustices but exacerbate them and cultivate the best conditions for new eugenics. In other words, "a moment's thought" (Sparrow 2005, 138) demonstrates that dispelling the myth of normality, innate disability, sex dyadism, and "the myth of a normal child" is vital to remedying social injustices (Baglieri et al. 2011, 2124).

Interphobia and Ableism: Conflating Intersex with Diseases

As discussed at length in Chapter 1, intersex traits are often falsely compared to and regarded as though they were life-threatening diseases. Regarding intersex variations as diseases/diseased and (potentially) cancerous or comparing intersex to diseases enables medical professionals to more readily justify exorcising and eugenic technologies like PGD. That is, this discourse enables state regulators to support access to PGD, and it enables fertility clinicians to rationalize promoting and employing PGD for intersex eugenics.

In addition to medical professionals problematically comparing "intersex traits to dangerous diseases, despite the fact that most intersex traits have minimal, if any, health risks" (G. Davis 2015, 69), intersex is also misrepresented as a disease in some national PGD regulations. For example, recall that although sex selection is prohibited in Canada, "sex selection for the purpose of preventing, diagnosing, or treating sex-linked disorders or *diseases* is permitted in Canada" (S. O'Neill and Blackmer 2015, 10, emphasis added). Without explicit definitions of and distinctions between disease and disorder, intersex variations are misrepresented as and can be misconstrued to be life-threatening diseases. Disease, then, as it relates to intersex in this context, is a strategic metaphor. And, as Phil Smith (2004) explains, "the disease metaphor" is a useful means to create body-mind differences and to justify eliminating what is culturally disruptive or perceived to be "repulsive and revolting." Hence, like medical professionals, Canada's policy exploits (potential) parents' anxieties about chronic ill health, disabilities, and death to justify eugenic screening technologies like PGD. (Potential) parents are likely understandably distressed by this rhetoric and believe that they are acting in the best interests of the (potential) fetus or child when they agree to interventions like PGD. Yet this fact does not mean that they are not colluding with discriminatory and eugenic logics or technologies.

Conclusion: "Choosing" PGD and Intersex Eugenics

Reflecting on the fact that reproductive technologies are deployed to prevent the implantation of embryos or the gestation and birth of fetuses with (perceived) disabilities, defects, and atypical traits, disability studies scholar Bill Hughes (2000, 564) states,

> The ghosts of imperfection and impairment haunt modern medicines' art of iatromechanics. Prenatal genetic diagnosis is the exorcist ... Disabled people have, in the past, been singled out by "genetic inquisitions" and identified as "suspect sires" ... The new genetics disavows this disreputable ancestry but disabled people have good reason not only, to remain unconvinced by such assurances, but also to affirm the import of Tom Shakespeare's (1995, p. 22) suggestion that the new genetics is a case of "back to the future" ... The new genetics establishes a framework for distinguishing people – not to mention cellular entities *in utero* and *in vitro* – on the basis of the amount of "genetic capital" that can be identified in a given sample of DNA. An embryonic system of biological and aesthetic stratification is inherent in the framework.

The spectre of racialization, queerness, and intersex and/is/as disability haunts contemporary reproductive technologies. Hence, eugenic practices and ideologies have not been eradicated; they have been transformed. The exorcist of old eugenics simply has access to new technologies and discourses; the exorcist just appears to wear a kinder mask and to wield gentler instruments. As a result, as this chapter underlines, disabled, intersex, crip, queer, and/or racialized individuals have good reason to remain unconvinced by medical assurances and legal narratives alleging that eugenics is over.

In addition to remaining unconvinced that eugenics is over, I argue that the active promotion of PGD, particularly the ironic promotion to LGBTQIA2 communities, provides us with the opportunity to question the liberal, homonational discourses of LGBTQIA2 acceptance and inclusion. Narratives of queer diversity or tolerance cannot be taken seriously, not simply because diversity does not equal equity and tolerance does not equal celebratory acceptance but also because PGD is used to prevent the implantation of queerly disabled, crip, racialized intersex embryos and their possible subsequent gestation and birth. Technologies employed to detect and prevent the gestation and birth of fetuses with intersex variations (as well as other pathologized characteristics) tell us that intersex, crip, disabled, queer, and/or racialized people are not and should not be wanted in the future. As a result, when PGD is promoted to LGBTQIA2 groups, we need to be self-reflexive and to interrogate the ways that we are called to be complicit in reinforcing intersecting forms of discrimination. In doing so, we recognize the relationship between intersex, queerness, race, and disability and the constitutive connection between racism and compulsory dyadism, heterosexuality, able-bodiedness, and reproduction. Given this relationship, there is good reason for intersex, queer, disability, crip, antiracist, and feminist pro-choice activists to actively align with each other.

Many disability activists and scholars note that pro-choice advocates must engage with disability activists because pro-choice advocates often appeal to ableist narratives in order to justify access to reproductive technologies.[13] For instance, some pro-choice activists argue that people should have access to later-term abortions if they discover that the fetus has a disability. According to queer and disability activist Lenzi Sheible (2014),

> This strategy attempts to justify later abortions to anti-choicers by trading on the rhetoric that some abortions – of fetuses with "abnormalities" – are inarguably necessary. Rather than reasoning that all abortions should be equally accessible no matter what, many pro-choice advocates lean on the argument that of *course* people, including anti-choicers, would opt out of having a disabled child if they had the means.

Likewise, pro-choice advocates need to be mindful of the ways that not only ableism but also interphobia, racism, and queerphobia underpin arguments that seek to justify or deny people's access to reproductive technologies. People's right to reproductive technologies need not implicitly or explicitly be made at the expense of any group of people. Ensuring that such discriminatory discourses are not employed resists dehumanizing and re/marginalizing several communities.

The idea and legislation of reproductive "choice" are complicated when taken alongside the discriminatory, new eugenics discourses used to justify access to reproductive technologies. Indeed, returning to the language of haunting, (potentially) pregnant people confront the narrative that they could, but ought not to, implant, house, and gestate an unviable, monstrous, "gender-disabled" (K.P. Morgan 2005, 301), "sideways"-growing (Stockton 2009, 1) phantasm. Furthermore, people who give birth to "spectral" babies with (perceived) disabilities, differences, or diseases are often blamed and shamed for doing so.[14] These blaming narratives and shaming practices create a cultural, moral imperative to "choose" the "viable" embryo or fetus – to "choose" to engage with the diagnostic exorcist.

Consider Sparrow's (2013, 29) ghostly language: "Confronted with the spectre of intersex, modern medicine makes choices available to parents and physicians." PGD is one of these choices. The ghostly rhetoric unequivocally communicates that the prospect of implanting an intersex embryo, gestating an intersex fetus, and giving birth to an intersex baby is a frightening possibility. Sparrow presents choosing for intersex, or not choosing against intersex, as a prima facie poor choice, perhaps even an immoral choice. Choosing for or not choosing against the phantasm, according to Sparrow's narrative, suggests that the parent does not have the future child's welfare in mind. He creates a moral imperative to select against intersex – to "choose" new eugenics. As Jeff Nisker (2013, 47) explains, "once a difference [e.g., intersex] becomes a medical disorder to which the medical profession is dedicating time and resources to prevent, procedures to this end become endowed with appropriateness and thus threaten a woman's ability to reject."

(Potentially) pregnant people's engagement, or lack thereof, with preventative, eliminative, and exorcising reproductive technologies is not simply about freely making a choice. Choice and coercion, like freedom and cultural imperatives, are coextensive. As disability studies and bioethics scholar Tom Shakespeare (1998, 666) writes, "The medical profession and the context in which reproductive decisions are made, undermines the capacity for free choice, and promotes eugenic outcomes." Eugenic sentiments are promoted, but they are masked as apolitical personal choices. Reflecting on the ways that parents of intersex children are coerced into agreeing to early surgical interventions, G. Davis (2015, 23) explains that "medical professionals ... place the responsibility for medical decisions entirely on parents, thereby avoiding responsibility for questionable interventions." Similarly, by placing responsibility on (potential) parents to avoid implanting certain "unviable" embryos and gestating "defective" fetuses while narrating this responsibility as a choice, medical professionals, reproductive technology researchers, and governments are able to avoid responsibility for eugenic interventions.

Considering who benefits from more reproductive "choices" is illuminating. As this chapter illustrates, these sorts of reproductive technologies do not benefit people with the culturally devalued characteristics that these technologies seek to eliminate. Rather, they further exacerbate stigma. Moreover, many (potentially) pregnant people do not necessarily feel liberated when more diagnostic technology choices are made available to them (Rapp 1999). Legalizing, under/unregulating, and making these technologies easily accessible are measures that benefit nation-states invested in reproducing a (hetero)normative, neoliberally "productive" workforce while avoiding explicitly endorsing discriminatory logics and eugenics (Kaposy 2018; Thompson 2005). These technologies also greatly benefit the capitalistic corporate bodies, clinics, and researchers that economically profit from developing, providing, and promoting reproductive technologies with eugenic implications. Considering the reproductive technologies used to test for Down syndrome, bioethicist Chris Kaposy (2015) explains, "The arms race to develop these tests is not being driven by the needs of people with Down syndrome or the needs of their families ... Devotion to create a test that helps parents to avoid the birth of people who tend to enjoy their lives seems somehow ... off the mark." Similarly, activist and researcher Morgan Carpenter (2016) acknowledges that "conflicts of interest ... arise when clinicians making decisions on what constitute 'serious genetic disorders' financially benefit from conducting those tests." The fact that people profit from coercive new eugenics discourses and from the eugenic deployment of reproductive technologies is extraordinarily disconcerting.

To be clear, I *do not* propose that anyone's access to reproductive technologies should be limited. In fact, I maintain that access to reproductive and sexual education, health care, and technologies – including, but not limited to, contraception, abortion, testing for sexually transmitted infections (STIs), and prenatal health care – desperately needs to be expanded so that all people can access them, not just the most privileged. As a result, Morgan Holmes's (2008b, 178) position resonates with me: "I insist on the right of women to terminate pregnancies, even in cases where I might prefer they decide otherwise."[15] I defend, insist on, and celebrate the rights of all people who can become pregnant or are pregnant to terminate pregnancies or choose one embryo over another embryo, even in cases where I am troubled by the ideological underpinnings of said decision. People who can become pregnant or who are pregnant are required to make unbelievably difficult decisions about their body-minds, well-being, health, future, relationships, economic stability, careers, housing, and so on. Rather than reducing these complex situations by implying that these people make entirely free decisions in a vacuum, we must critically question why eugenic choices are marketed as and seem ethical, benevolent, and even required. We need to evaluate what dominant political, social, health care, economic, and infrastructure systems make these eugenic decisions desirable.

In his book *Choosing Down Syndrome: Ethics and New Prenatal Technologies*, Kaposy argues that more people should have children with Down syndrome and resist the ableist forces that devalue individuals with Down syndrome. Drawing from studies and accounts of parents and children with Down syndrome, Kaposy proves that having a child with Down syndrome is fulfilling and that people with Down syndrome do not lead miserable lives. Indeed, Kaposy (2018, 1) opens his book with the following: people with Down syndrome "are beloved members of families. People with Down syndrome go to school, make friends, graduate, have jobs, get married, have sexual relationships, pursue hobbies and interests, start businesses, pursue higher education, and so on. It seems odd to create such a list since it is a list of common things that most people do." Likewise, I hope that I have demonstrated that intersex people do not lead insufferable lives. Indeed, there are families out there who celebrate their intersex children. Again, although I (like Kaposy) do not advocate restricting access to reproductive technologies, I think that more people should have children with intersex traits and resist the discriminatory forces that so thoroughly devalue intersex people.

Ultimately, we must be diligent in celebrating and supporting all people with diverse body-mind variations and culturally devalued modes of be(com)ing. Doing so means that scholars and activists need to continue to demand that medical professionals, traditional bioethicists, and the general population rethink the systemic pathologization and active eugenic erasure and elimination of intersex variations, disabilities, differences, and racialized, queer, and crip ways of being. As Holmes (2008b, 175, 179) states, it is imperative that we "recognise the inherent value in a life lived with and through difference" and ensure that all people can "exercise their own level of qualified autonomy within the networks of social support that enable the qualified autonomy of all persons."

Conclusion
Eradicating Exorcisms

Against all the forces that seek to shame and eradicate people with intersex characteristics, Pidgeon Pagonis (2015c) declares in their art, "The future is intersex." Having witnessed and experienced interphobic violence, Sean Saifa M. Wall (2015c) asserts, "We are here. We exist. And we are moving forward."[1] Intersex people are *here*. Intersex *is* in the future; intersex people are imagining vibrant futures. In spite of all the institutionalized powers that confront the spectre of intersex by attempting to surveil, defer, and destroy it, intersex will always haunt. Intersex is, after all, indiscriminate; it is "a perpetually shifting phantasm in the collective psyche of medicine and culture," and it is a relatively new, but growing, identity category (Holmes 2002, 175). The indefensibility of the sex dyad and the inevitable catastrophic failure of curative violence to exorcise intersex prove that intersex will always haunt. And this haunting should be welcomed and celebrated, not feared, hunted down, and exorcised.

I am hopeful that intersex will not always haunt through the nonlinear effects of pathologization, diagnosis, curative violence, imposed disabilities, sexual assault, lies and deceit, traumatizing stigmatization, and humiliating body-mind scrutiny. There are possible futures where the ever-shifting queer, crip, racialized intersex spectre is not demonized but instead politicized, celebrated, accepted, and anticipated. Intersex is an always-in-process discursive project and embodied phantasm and, therefore, probably can never be fully known, transparent, or taken "out of the shadows" (Caplan-Bricker 2017). Nevertheless, one can be contented and even excited by future intersex iterations, embodiments, and identities as long as they are not met with violence – as long as they are not regarded as sites of "no good future" (Kafer 2013, 3).

Through the diligent and brilliant labour performed by scholars, activists, and advocates, the Intersex Rights Movement has, for decades now, offered up exciting visions of intersex futures devoid of compulsory dyadism and all its harms. For these futures to manifest – in order to deinstitutionalize compulsory dyadism – intersex projects must be cripped. Given not only the pathologization of intersex but also the successful integration of intersex into traditional, ableist conceptions of disability, as well as the contemporary reliance on ableist discourses to justify myriad forms of compulsory dyadism, the most effective instruments to add to the anti-interphobic tool box right now are the tools offered by feminist disability and crip studies. Compulsory dyadism and able-bodiedness are too bound up and indistinguishable to treat as distinct issues, experiences, or embodiments. Crip intersex projects concentrate on the interconnection between interphobia and ableism and underscore the fact that compulsory dyadism and able-bodiedness sustain each other. When one crips intersex academic theorizations, activist initiatives, and imaginings of pro-intersex futures, they do not fall short.

As illustrated by the various testimonies and stories that we bear witness to throughout this book, dominant discriminatory logics that conceptualize pathologization and futurity as antithetical render intersecting intersex, disabled, queer, crip, and racialized embodiments as sites of no good futures. Recall, for example, all the queer, crip, racialized, intersex futures that were stolen – or, in Tiger Devore's (in Lahood 2012) terms, "taken away" – from intersex people via curative violence. Medicalizing logic insists that intersex futures are or will be inescapably bleak, hopeless, and tragic because they deviate from culturally mandated ways of being. Recall that athletes like Caster Semenya are presumed to have no rightful future in sport because of their racialized, suspect intersex, crip, queer embodiments and are denied claims to femininity and womanhood. Or, at the risk of misrepresenting myself as anti-choice, consider all the ostensibly disabled, racialized, queer, crip, intersex embryos or fetuses that are discarded in the name of benevolently saving them from lives of living with "species-atypical functioning" or with "genitals that don't fit" or "that fail to elicit desire in one's sexual partners" (Sparrow 2013, 32, 33–34). Given these complex inter-sections, I do not regard Wall's or Pagonis's assertions that intersex is here now and in the future as entirely distinct from other activist mantras and claims to rightfully being and belonging in the future.

Proclamations of intersex futurity remind me of the work of multidisci-plinary visual artist and educator Alisha B. Wormsley (n.d.), whose mantra "There are black people in the future" aligns with Afrofuturist philoso-phies that "[imagine] possible futures through a black cultural lens" (Ingrid LaFleur, quoted in Womack 2013, 9). Wormsley (quoted in Conley 2016) recounts,

> I was working in this neighborhood [i.e., Homewood, Pittsburgh] where young men are shot and killed and incarcerated. There was this idea of being able to see myself in the future, including my students ... I feel that it's a mantra, that if I say it, then it will happen...there are Black people in the future ...
>
> For me it became important to say it and phrase it. If I print this, it has some merit with people who are trying to kill us ...
>
> We will always exist because we exist right now ... Those things that are trying to attack us will never be successful.

In addition to developing the mantra "There are black people in the future," Wormsley has produced a remarkable art project of the same name to ex-plore and illustrate Black people's survival, brilliance, and (future) presence. All the forces that seek to enslave, incarcerate, brutalize, or pursue the ex-termination of Black people are resisted by Afrofuturists, critical race and anti-colonial theorists, activists, and artists who know that there are Black people in the future. There is a course of Black futurity that is magical and anti-racist.[2]

I am also reminded of Alison Kafer's (2013, 46) observation that "dis-abled people are continually being written out of the future, rendered as the sign of the future no one wants." "Disability is disavowed" in the future, Kafer (2013, 3) explains, in two main ways:

> First, the value of a future that included disabled people goes unrecognized, while the value of a disability-free future is seen as self-evident; and second, the political nature of disability, namely its position as a category to be con-tested and debated, goes unacknowledged. The second failure of recogni-tion makes possible the first; casting disability as a monolithic fact of the

body, as beyond the realm of the political and therefore beyond the realm of debate or dissent, makes it impossible to imagine disability and disability futures differently ... Rather than assume that a "good" future naturally and obviously depends upon the eradication of disability, we must recognize this perspective as colored by histories of ableism and disability oppression. Thus, in tracing these two failures of recognition – the disavowal of disability from "our" futures – I imagine futures otherwise, arguing for a cripped politics of access and engagement based on the work of disability activists and theorists ...

I am yearning for an elsewhere – and, perhaps, an "elsewhen" – in which disability is understood otherwise: as political, as valuable, as integral.

Numerous feminist disability and crip scholars and activists counter the taken-for-granted "truth" that Kafer describes – the ideological hatred for disabled futures – and claim that disability is in the future. We imagine, demand, and construct disability futures where the value, beauty, and political nature of disability are understood and appreciated. We imagine, demand, and construct crip futurities, anti-ableist futures, and utopias – "The Future We Want" (del Cura 2017).[3]

The queer rallying cry "We're here, we're queer, get used to it," which insists on the current presence and a future existence of queer people, also comes to mind. People need to "get used to it" because we are here and are not going anywhere. Queer Nation NY (2016), a New York City LGBTQIA2 organization founded in 1990 by the HIV/AIDS activists of ACT UP, popularized the now ubiquitous motto during demonstrations opposing the various forms of violence against LGBTQIA2 people. Often, representations of queer futures are depicted as diminished, violent, diseased, and nonexistent because they do not follow heteronormative scripts. They do not follow "straight time" – heteronormative, marital, reproductive futurity (Tom Boellstorff, in Latour et al. 2015). Combatting these representations, queer activists and scholars have long imagined and theorized "queer futures," "anti-futures," and even "no futures" where queer temporalities and lives are not invested in straight time.[4] Queer people ideate, insist on, and live on the boundaries or outside the constraints of straight temporality and develop alternative futures.

Lastly, reflect on the mantra "The future is female." Championing this phrase, many lesbians in the 1970s, especially those involved in lesbian separatist politics, popularized T-shirts emblazoned with this vision of the future, rejecting limited, violent futures fashioned by patriarchal control

(Burckhardt 2017). This feminist, pro-woman, pro-lesbian mantra has been contested for its seemingly biologically essentializing rhetoric and because it has been problematically co-opted for capitalist and neoliberalist gains. Nevertheless, this motto has resonated with many women, particularly lesbians, for decades.[5] Although many people take issue with the mantra and its uptake, some still claim that there is power in the sentiment. Liza Cowan, a lesbian separatist in the 1970s, maintains that the phrase is still an empowering incantation to conjure liberatory futures. Cowan (quoted in Gush 2015) conceives of the "female" as a kind of attitudinal or political lens:

> The beauty of the phrase is that there is no precise meaning ... It is a dynamic phrase, a lively phrase ... If we are to have a future, it must be female, because the rule of men – patriarchy – has just about devastated life on this beautiful planet. The essence and the spirit of the future must be female. So the phrase becomes not just a slogan, but a spell. For the good of all.

Some use the phrase to express anger with patriarchal violence: "The Future Is Female. And She's Furious" (C. Young 2019). According to others, a female future offers a safer space where women can grow beyond – or smash – patriarchal constraints and the demands of compulsory motherhood and heterosexuality (Krauzo 2018). Although the phrase (or spell) has been met with warranted critique, women demand and deserve nonviolent, equitable futures.

In rejecting discursive and literal subjugation, erasure, and eradication, these marginalized groups assert that they/we are in the future and that just futures are possible to conceive and create. And, as intersectional thinkers attest, all of these embodiments and subsequent forms of institutionalized oppression are not distinct but wrap around and support each other to form a complex labyrinth. Adding to Eli Clare's (2009, 143) observation that "gender reaches into disability; disability wraps around class; class strains against abuse; abuse snarls into sexuality; sexuality folds on top of race," I argue that race envelops intersex and that intersex extends out to disability, "everything finally piling into a single human body." And, given that the intersex spectre indiscriminately haunts this labyrinth, we require "intersextional" futures (Preciado 2005, 155).

By continually trying to spot the spectre of intersex in this maze and by venturing back to the largely untrodden thoroughfares where intersex and disability – as well as compulsory dyadism and able-bodiedness – meet in this complex maze, I have identified several sites where intersex and/as/is/

with disability manifest and interconnect. In untangling this intersextion, I have re/imagined and theorized possible futures without compulsory dyadism and the curative violence that so quickly follows. I have envisioned futures where the diverse, valuable, and political ways that intersex and/as/is/with disability become (visible) and haunt together in unobstructed and respected ways. And, as this future takes shape, everyone will encounter intersex with disability in more unexpected, multiple, phantasmal, and inter-sexy ways.

Future Crip Intersex Projects

Policies and ideologies need to be fundamentally restructured in order for intersex people to thrive, no matter their diverse body-minds and uniquely intersecting embodiments, experiences, and identities. As anti-interphobic scholars, activists, and advocates continue working toward this restructuring effort, disability must be centralized; compulsory dyadism cannot be undone without undoing compulsory able-bodiedness. Moreover, as we crip intersex to undermine other sites of compulsory dyadism, we need to think creatively. What forms of interphobic discrimination require a crip intersex lens? What modes of compulsory dyadism are rendered matters of common sense and, subsequently, undetectable? How do infrastructures, education, and accepted methods of cultural celebration uphold compulsory dyadism? And how do feminist disability and crip theories help to destabilize this culturally mandated way of be(com)ing? What future crip intersex theoretical and activist projects are needed? I offer four possible crip intersex projects.

In the introduction, I alluded to one such project: a crip intersex analysis of same-sex marriage. Typically, debates about same-sex marriage imply that this is a lesbian, gay, and possibly bisexual and trans issue. However, marriage – whether same-sex or different-sex – is a disability, crip, intersex issue. We need to recognize, as Robert McRuer (2006) and other queer and disability studies scholars note, that some arguments for institutionalizing same-sex marriage relied on ableist discourses. Same-sex marriage was justified on the grounds that instituting it would be an adequate remedy to the spread of HIV/AIDS, a highly stigmatized, disabling chronic illness. Conflating queerness with the supposed horrific spread of disability, disease, and degeneracy unnecessarily restigmatizes queer folks and (queer) people with HIV/AIDS.

A crip analysis of same-sex/different-sex marriage draws one's attention to the fact that people with disabilities are often denied the chance to get married or to express their sexual and romantic desires at all (McRuer and Mollow 2012; D. Richards et al. 2009; Wilkerson 2002). People with disabilities are presumably asexual, undesirable partners, outside of the romantic/sexual economy, and incapable of giving or receiving love and pleasure in romantic/sexual partnerships. A crip intersex analysis of same-sex/different-sex marriage further nuances these discussions. Contemporary iterations of same-sex/different-sex marriage institutionalize compulsory dyadism; only two sexes are recognized. "Disabled" intersex people are systematically subjected to curative violence so that they fit into all the systems of compulsory dyadism, including the same-sex/different-sex marriage model. Intersex is not recognized or accommodated; rather, intersex characteristics are exorcised so that they fit – so that intersex people become loveable or, in Kira Triea's (1999, 143) terms, "fuckable." However, these attempts to make intersex people fit within this system inevitably fail.

Although many intersex people cultivate fulfilling sexual, romantic, and loving relationships and get married, some intersex people report struggling with physical intimacy or finding a partner because of the trauma and disabilities caused both by curative violence and by the response to their anatomical traits in general. For example, as explained by Peter Trinkl (in Lahood 2012), an intersex person subjected to curative violence,

> People get labelled and dumped into the so-called "faggot bag." That's where a guy who doesn't sort of, you know, conform to traditional notions of masculinity must be gay because of their nonconformity. And I got put into that bag. That was a very painful place to be in. My orientation is heterosexual ... When I was nineteen [or] twenty, I tried dating a few times, and it usually went nowhere because ... they see my difference, and I freeze up or stare at the ceiling, and it was like a disaster. I basically sort of became asexual in the face of all of this. I'm an elderly guy, unmarried, sort of outside the mainstream, and I'm still read as gay ... That's what's going to happen in my lifetime.

Not only do many intersex people feel shame regarding their physical characteristics and/or anger about the abilities that were removed, such as the ability to orgasm and the ability to biologically reproduce, but the violent interventions also result in limiting their positions in the economy of sexual pleasure and romantic partnership. Curative violence does not even inevitably result in intersex people fitting into the same-sex/different-sex model.

Some intersex people, for example, identify as nonbinary or genderqueer. And curative violence creates queer, crip, and/or – as with Devore (1999, 80) – "strange" genitals. Overall, analyzing the institution of marriage through a crip intersex lens will offer fruitful insights into how sex, gender, and dis/ability are discursively and literally created. A crip intersex approach to marriage signals that we need to look beyond access to the altar or marriage licences – that we must look into doctors' offices and medical theatres.

Another needed project involves bathrooms. Bathrooms are a site of compulsory dyadism given that they are overwhelmingly literally structured around the male-female sex dyad. In analyses of bathrooms both as a litmus test for biological sex and as volatile cites of gender policing, the discrimination that trans, genderqueer, nonbinary, queer, and gender non-conforming people face is central. Bathrooms are also disability and accessibility issues. Too few bathrooms are structured for people with varying disabilities, such as people who use wheelchairs or walkers, individuals who are blind or have vision impairments, or people with arthritis: bathroom doors and stalls are too small, toilets are hard to find, guide dogs cannot fit or manoeuvre, there are no handle bars, the lighting is too low, the toilets are too low or too high, the faucets and paper towel dispensers are too high or difficult to use, and so on. However, this "bathroom problem" (Halberstam 2005, 20) extends beyond bathroom walls and is not simply a trans, queer, or disability issue; it is an intersecting disability, intersex, trans, queer problem that requires a crip intersex approach (Orr 2019). Given that intersex people are subjected to curative violence in order to fit into the male-female sex binary and are typically left with disabilities, we need to look beyond the bathroom walls – into medical theatres – in order to fully comprehend how violent and far-reaching the bathroom problem is.

In addition to the anxiety and violence that gender non-conforming, genderqueer, queer, nonbinary, and trans folks experience in bathrooms, for intersex people, bathrooms become sites of trauma because of the curative violence that they have endured. For instance, as recounted in Chapter 2, for Daniela Truffer (2015, 111), going to the bathroom consistently causes pain because, she explains, "when I was two, our family doctor stuck his finger into my urethral opening; I was screaming very loud, my father says. My mother had to put me into warm water because every time I had to pee I screamed in pain. Later I was hurried to the hospital with a bad infection. Still today my urethra often hurts after going to the toilet." Moreover, medical management does not always make fitting into sexed and gendered bathrooms easy, especially for children recovering from surgery and dealing with disabilities. As discussed in Chapter 2, Devore (in G. Harrison 2011) recalls,

> I would go back to school [after undergoing surgery during summer holiday], and I would have a tube running into my body with a sack on my leg underneath my pants that would collect my urine. So I didn't use boys' bathrooms. I didn't use girls' bathrooms. I had to go to the nurse's office ... to empty out this sack. So I didn't really have a sense of belonging to a sex on the basis of bathroom choice.

Bathrooms, for a variety of reasons, are sites of unease, fear, and trauma for people with intersex traits, particularly for those who have been subjected to curative violence and for those who are trans, genderqueer, nonbinary, queer, and/or gender non-conforming. Crip intersex projects theorizing about sex-segregated bathrooms will nuance conversations about urinary violence as well as dis/ability and sex/gender policing.

An additional project that demands attention involves inter/sex education. Sex education needs to be radically revamped at all levels to include destigmatizing information about inter/sex, gender, sexuality, and dis/ability. However, I will focus on one specific example here: what future medical professionals are taught about inter/sex. Prospective medical practitioners are taught that there are only two real, legitimate sexes: male and female. As a result, they are taught very little about intersex. When intersex is mentioned in textbooks used to teach these students (e.g., Dudek 2014; and Standring 2016), the text may include decades-old photographs of naked intersex people (emphasizing their genitals), typically children, always white. Echoing arguments made by disability studies scholars,[6] intersex studies scholars argue that these photographs should not be used as teaching aids because they are objectifying, have been unethically acquired, and in no uncertain terms communicate that intersex traits are disordered and must be "fixed" via curative violence (Creighton et al. 2002; Topps 2015). These analyses are apt, but they can be nuanced if we ask why all the photographs are of white people. It seems to me that the photographs constitute an unlikely archive of the racism and ableism that are so bound up with interphobia.

When contemporary surgery on intersex people became common practice in the Global North in the mid-twentieth century (largely due to John Money's theories), the idea that Black people were more likely to be sexually "ambiguous" was still being circulated, and these issues persist today. Zine

Magubane (2014, 771) writes of the rise of intersex medical management in America that surgery on white patients was "imperative to establish the normality of whiteness. An ambiguously gendered white body needed to be corrected to retain its whiteness, whereas an ambiguously gendered black body was seen as confirming the essential biological difference between whites and blacks." These operations were needed to retain not only these people's whiteness and rights as white people but also, and in turn, their heterosexual able-bodiedness. Black intersex people were construed as fundamentally pathologically ambiguous – unsalvageable. Given that "corrective" surgery was presumed crucial for white intersex children, they were the ones in medical theatres. They were the ones "available" to be photographed. Their images were and still are found in textbooks that prospective medical practitioners view.

In addition, white people were more likely than people of colour – particularly socio-economically disadvantaged or rural people of colour – to give birth in hospitals and to regularly engage with the medical institution; people of colour who were invested in culturally traditional home births (or had no other option), who had different cultural relationships with the sex dyad, or who were/are rightly skeptical of the racist medical industry would avoid hospitals (see A. Davis 2003; Dawley 2003; and J. Nelson 2003). As a result, it stands to reason that some racialized intersex infants were not subjected to the surgical knife. They were not there to be photographed and are, therefore, not found in contemporary teaching tools.

Recounting conversations that they had with other intersex people of colour, Pagonis (2017a) explains that, although the medical industry "has no space for" Black, Indigenous, and other people of colour,

> on the flip side of that coin, there's also some positives that happen ... So say you can't afford to go to a hospital or [going to the hospital] just wasn't in your culture ... and you had home birth and you had a doula that's from your community and this doula, because I've met some people like this, this doula saw the baby who had intersex genitalia at birth and the doula was like, their ancestral knowledge was like, it's ok, this baby should be loved and reared ... and seen as like a blessing, instead of rushed off to the hospital.

So the photographs are undeniably ethically reprehensible and should not be used as teaching tools. Additionally, the photographs of exclusively white intersex people that prospective medical practitioners view reproduce a complex, discriminatory story that must be attended to. This line of thinking will not only nuance intersex studies scholarship but also lend to and extend research in disability, anti-racist, queer, and education studies.

Overall, looking closely at what tools are used to teach prospective medical doctors suggests that the serious lack of intersex-competency education will negatively impact the patient-practitioner relationship, clinical assessments, and treatment, as well as the relationship between intersex children and their parents/proxies (see Karkazis 2008; and Orr and Watson 2021). Educators and textbook authors, rather than reaffirming and reinstitutionalizing the male-female sex dyad to the detriment of intersex patients, must actively oppose compulsory dyadism, a cultural mandate that is rooted in racism, queerphobia, and ableism. One pragmatic way to remedy these issues is by actively centralizing intersex people's knowledges – especially racialized intersex people's knowledges – in the education process or, more aptly put, the re-education process. This process must include teachers, students, *and* textbook authors.

The last needed project that I propose here involves the proliferation and popularization of gender-reveal parties. Critiquing these parties demands a crip intersex approach. A gender-reveal party, as described by Florence Pasche Guignard (2015, 479), "is an example of the new forms of ritualization that take place during pregnancy in 21st-century North America. Typically, the focal point of the party is when the future parents cut a cake whose inside color (blue or pink) reveals the sex of the fetus." These events reproduce compulsory dyadism, cisgenderism, and heteronomativity. They effectively reduce a fetus's gender and, by extension, (hetero)sexuality to their expected genitals. But, as intersex activist Jim Costich (in Lahood 2012) notes, "People have genitals. People are not genitals." In a variety of ways, these parties erase and punish intersex, trans, genderqueer, non-binary, and gender non-conforming people because these groups of people defy the sex and gender binaries.

A crip intersex analysis of gender-reveal parties also allows us to keep in mind that events like gender-reveal parties are also a crip, disability issue. If reproductive technologies reveal that the fetus is intersex, said fetus cannot be readily sexed or gendered and is therefore deemed unhealthy, pathological, and disabled. So what are prospective parents to do? They may be called to pathologize or abort said fetus or coerced into doing so. Or, after the party, what are parents to do if the newborn exhibits intersex traits and the sex is unclear? Explaining to one's family and community that the revealed sex/gender at the party was incorrect because the baby is intersex is typically not even considered to be an option; indeed, parents would likely not have the support from medical professionals to pursue this route. Parents are called to view their child as disordered or diseased and at a pathological risk of being queer; they are systematically called to agree to curative violence. The popularization of these parties puts even more, already profound pressure on parents to reinforce the sex dyad and the pathologization of intersex-as/is-disability. And, if these increasingly popular, yet seemingly innocuous, events are not subjected to crip intersex critiques, people remain complicit in upholding intersecting forms of oppression.

Continuing to crip intersex projects will result in more robust, nuanced, and effective theories, methods, and initiatives. By engaging intersex studies' theories of inter/sex and by bridging this field with feminist disability and crip theories of pathologization, a crip intersex approach demands that an intersex politics and studies be rooted in a disability and crip politics and studies. Drawing attention to the intersextion of intersex and disability refines our theoretical understanding of the relationship between inter/sex, sexuality, gender, disability, race, and colonialism, expands our comprehension of how compulsory dyadism and able-bodiedness circulate and are maintained, and helps intersex studies scholars and activists to combat interphobia in new, successful ways. Ultimately, I call other scholars and activists invested in intersex human rights to crip intersex.

Building Alliances

I recognize that this work is and will continue to be difficult given that I have identified some stigmaphobic distancing from disability and given that I am encouraging intersex studies scholars to integrate an entire, complex field of research into their projects. However, intersex studies scholars can round out their already extensive tool collection by adding the invaluable theoretical and methodological instruments that feminist disability and crip scholars have developed. They will not have to reinvent the wheel. Intersex activist groups can learn from disability activist groups' nuanced critiques of the medical-social and P/R models of disability and can bolster intersex human rights claims by appealing to legislations and policies that pertain to people with disabilities. And intersex folks may find solace in forging alliances with disability groups because they can offer spaces for intersex people to share their experiences of pathologization and living with body-mind disabilities caused by curative violence.

I remain cognizant, however, that a material activist alignment or alliance between intersex and disability groups may not always be constructive.

There are possible drawbacks and limitations to proposing this alliance, particularly when topics of identity, awareness, education, and activist funding are broached. The (contested) alliance between intersex and LGBTQIA2 communities serves as an example.[7] Some intersex people align and/or identify with queer identities, communities, and activist organizations. For some intersex people, queerness reflects their identities, subjectivities, and experiences in the world as lesbian, gay, bi, trans, queer, asexual, and/or intersex subjects. Queer organizations, groups, and gatherings provide these folks with spaces to reflect on and share their experiences and to take part in instrumental activist labour, love, and community-building projects. Intersex individuals' engagement in LGBTQIA2 spaces have enriched these spaces and the conversations and initiatives that occur. However, other intersex people reject this association because it may lead many people to believe that all intersex people are, or identify as, queer in one way or another. Other individuals rightly note that adding the "I" to the LGBTQA2 acronym is often an empty gesture. Interphobia and compulsory dyadism are frequently afterthoughts or not actively integrated into or taught to LGBTQIA2 activist groups. This lack of education has resulted in many people (in and outside of queer communities) conflating intersex with trans embodiments, identities, and subjectivities. Or, when specific LGBTQA2 organizations add the "I," intersex issues are often not given ample space, funding, or education opportunities.

Similar to how LGBTQIA2 environments function for certain intersex people, as noted above, forging an alliance with disability groups may provide locations and forums for intersex people who do not identify as queer to share their experiences of pathologization and medical violence (Cornwall 2009). Even though I am not at all comfortable policing how people identify, many intersex people could, I believe, claim disability and crip as identities and enter these spaces to build bonds, take part in activist work, and provide unique perspectives. Yet it seems that most intersex people do not identify with disability or crip. Although some intersex individuals may distance from disability for a variety of reasons, some intersex people, and I hypothesize here, may feel like they cannot claim disability or crip. They may believe that they are infringing on disability and crip boundaries and spaces.

Despite the fact that "what is interpretable as disability" or a disability issue "need not be tethered to a disability identity" and the fact that what is interpretable as intersex or an intersex issue need not be tethered to an intersex identity, when intersex and disability groups align and work together, difficult (yet familiar) conversations about identity – who is "in" and who is "out" – will occur in activist and academic circles (Mollow and McRuer 2012, 13). Challenging discussions about the re/distribution of organizational funding and about educational logistics will also take place. To be clear, I say "*when* intersex and disability groups align" because I am optimistic about a crip intersex future and because I want to emphasize that intersex, crip, queer, racialized, and disabled embodiments are not going anywhere; they are in the future.

I began this book with a lofty request, asking possible understandably discontented readers to forbear in order to see what benefits emerge from theorizing intersex and compulsory dyadism through a feminist disability and crip lens. I am profoundly grateful for my readers' attention and engagement as I have explored and demonstrated that such theorizing accrues many benefits and is, in fact, necessary. Compulsory dyadism cannot successfully be dismantled without undermining compulsory able-bodiedness. These ghosts haunt together, so we must welcome and celebrate them together. If the vibrant, beautiful future is indeed intersex, it is also dangerously and gorgeously crip.

Notes

ACKNOWLEDGMENTS

1 I must note that some of the ideas in Part 3 of this book, "New Eugenics: Pre-implantation Genetic Diagnosis and Compulsory Dyadism," were initially developed in a chapter titled "(Liberatory) Reproductive Technologies and (Eugenic) Interphobic Selection," first published by Inter-Disciplinary Press and later re-released by Brill. Additionally, a few of the ideas found in Chapter 2, "Medical Interventions and Acquired Body-Mind Disabilities," as well as in the concluding chapter, "Eradicating Exorcisms," were originally developed in an article titled "Resisting the Demand to Stand: Boys, Bathrooms, Hypospadias, and Interphobic Violence," featured in *Boyhood Studies: An Interdisciplinary Journal*.

INTRODUCTION: INTERSEX AND/AS/IS/WITH DISABILITY

1 Curative violence (Kim 2017, 27) "describe[s] the exercise of force to erase differences for the putative betterment of the Other. Curative violence occurs when cure is what actually frames the presence of disability as a problem and ends up destroying the subject in the curative process." In Eunjung Kim's (2017, 2, 14, 9) terms, the "curative process" that many intersex people are subjected to involves "physical and material violence" and can "[destroy] the subject"; hence, "cure and disability coexist as a process" (see also Clare 2017; and Erevelles and Minear 2010).

2 The notion that "sitings" or "locations" of intersex need not be bound to identity is a rather commonplace idea in intersex studies literature and activist work. Intersex as an identity (not merely anatomical traits or diagnosis) is relatively new, but it is becoming increasingly common, particularly in intersex activist circles. However, physical characteristics deemed intersex, sexually "ambiguous," variant, or disordered (i.e., DSD) are not always tied to intersex identity. Some people with intersex traits

do not claim intersex as an identity or diagnosis, other folks welcome DSD nomenclature or identify with disorder, and other individuals reject intersex and DSD labels as colonial impositions and celebrate their own culturally specific identities, social categories, languages, and traditions. Intersex is not always tethered to an identity. Challenging compulsory dyadism and fighting for people's body-mind autonomy are not dependent on identification.

3 See Colligan 2004; Cornwall 2013; Koyama 2006; Y. Menon 2011; Spurgas 2009; and Wilkerson 2012.

4 Ethan Levine (2014, 186) also cites and analyzes this quotation.

5 Likewise, speaking of nation-states' inability to grant full citizenship status to people with disabilities, Sharon L. Snyder and David T. Mitchell (2010, 119) claim that because intersex people have a disability that is "less easy to accommodate" to citizenship proper, they have disability citizenship. Different language and theoretical tools are used by scholars who theorize intersex people's citizenship status but do not integrate disability theory. For example, Georgiann Davis (2015) employs the notion of "biological citizenship" to analyze the fact that intersex individuals are not rendered full citizens, as evidenced by, for instance, the fact that intersex people's body-mind integrity and self-determination are not legally protected. Emily Grabham (2007) refers to intersex people's limited access to citizenship proper as "intersex citizenship." These discourses of intersex, disability, and biological citizenship are not necessarily mutually exclusive. In fact, braiding all of these theorizations together would provide a very nuanced picture of how intersex people's citizenship, autonomy, and self-determination are denied and re/negotiated.

6 Despite the seemingly apparent nature of biological sex dyadism, this belief was not always maintained. Thomas Laqueur (1992, 5) outlines that before the late eighteenth century, when sex dimorphism came to dominate Western popular consciousness and medical theory, men and women were not understood to be "different in every conceivable aspect of body and soul, in every physical and moral aspect" (see also Daston and Galison 2007; Fausto-Sterling 2000; Herdt 1994; Oudshoorn 1994; and Warnke 2011). Rather, sex differences and observable differences in morphologies were thought of as variations of one type of possible body: male. Women and men were not wholly different; women were understood to be underdeveloped men turned inside out. Claiming that the one-sex-two-gender model gave way to the "correct" two-sex-two-gender model because of scientific advancements and "discoveries" may seem reasonable. Yet this claim is misguided. There is no scientific evidence that proves body-minds are (or ought to be) dimorphous. In Laqueur's terms (1992, 169), "sexual difference was created despite, not because of, new discoveries." Science does not reveal objective truths about the body-mind; rather, science and scientific discourses constitute the body-mind as sexed and gendered.

7 See, for example, Clare 2017; Oliver 2004; Shakespeare 2013; C. Thomas 2004; and Tremain 2002.

8 See, for example, Chase 1998; Guillot, Bauer, and Truffer 2016; Jordan-Young 2010; Karkazis 2008; Méndez 2016; and Roen 2009.

9 *Pamela Crawford and John Mark Crawford v. Medical University of South Carolina and South Carolina Dept. of Social Services, 2013CP4002877 (2017).* See also Albritton 2015; and Baumgartner 2017.

10 For more information about the law and intersex, refer to Julie A. Greenberg's (2012) book *Intersexuality and the Law.*

11 See also Clare 2017; Erevelles and Minear 2010; and Kafer 2013.

12 For texts concerning restorative justice, see Daly 2000; Daly and Stubbs 2006; Strang and Braithwaite 2002; and van Wormer 2009.

13 See also Costello 2012b, 2013; Inter/Act n.d.; and Plattner 2011.

14 Texts concerning these culturally mandated ways of being include Butler 2006; Deifelt 2005; Edelman 2004; Kafer 2003, 2013; Kelly and Orsini 2016; McRuer 2006, 2011, 2013; Mitchell and Snyder 2000; Puar 2009; Rich 1980; and Snyder and Mitchell 2010.

15 Furthermore, an "isomer" refers to one of two or more compounds, radicals, or ions that contain the same number of atoms of the same elements but differ in structure.

16 Or, as similarly described by the Australia Human Rights Commission (2018), endo-sex "refers to people whose sex characteristics meet medical and social norms for typical 'male' or 'female' bodies."

17 See, for example, Bödeker 2000; Carpenter 2019; Costello 2019a, 2019b; Grinspan and Carpenter 2018; Holzer 2019; Kids Helpline 2020; Marquez 2019a; Schulter 2017; and Sumerau 2020.

18 For additional haunting imagery, see Gurney 2007; and Spurgas 2009.

19 Trevor L. Hoag (2014, 10) writes, "Everyone is haunted by someone or something; everyone senses the peculiar 'presence/absence' of that which they have lost, whether it is a loved one, a material object, a shattered ideal."

CHAPTER 1: THE QUESTION OF HEALTH RISKS AND INTERSEX VARIATIONS

1 Other texts that also note these beliefs include Ahmed et al. 2016; Carpenter 2018; G. Davis 2015; Dreger 1999b; Lee et al. 2016; Sparrow 2013; and Trafimow 2013.

2 I do not construe Walsh's assertion that HRT is a poor substitute for the real thing as commentary about or commentary that can be applied to trans, intersex, gender-queer, and nonbinary individuals who need, consent to, and are fully informed of the possible risks and benefits of HRT. On this topic, David Cameron (2007, 164) claims that it is terribly ironic that trans people who can give legal consent struggle to access HRT (as well as other gender-affirming procedures and forms of care), whereas HRT is often forced upon intersex youths even though they cannot give legal consent.

3 Given that intersex is represented as being akin to cancer, it is unsurprising that a tool was developed to assess the psychological states of parents of intersex children. The tool is essentially the same one used to assess the psychological states of parents whose children were recently diagnosed with cancer. David E. Sandberg and Tom Mazur (2014, 109) write, "The Psychosocial Assessment Tool ..., a tool originally designed for families of newly diagnosed children with cancer, is among the earliest instruments to be administered in the DSD-TRN [Disorders of Sex Development Translational Research Network] to screen for psychosocial risk [i.e., stress and coping mechanisms] in families." They explain that "the Psychosocial Assessment Tool (PAT), developed out of the Pediatric Psychosocial Preventative Health Model framework (Pai et al., 2008), was designed to screen for psychosocial risk in families of children newly diagnosed with cancer (Nielsen-Bohlman, [Panzer, and Kindig,

eds.] 2004). With *minor* modifications, it has been modified for use in DSD" (Sandberg and Mazur 2014, 100–1, emphasis added). Rather than supplying parents with accurate resources about sex variations, intersex people, and support groups, parents are encouraged to understand their child as diseased – cancerous. As Vickie Pasterski and colleagues (2014, 373) note, it is unsurprising that parents of intersex children "reported overall levels of PTSS [post-traumatic stress symptoms] that were comparable to those reported by parents of children diagnosed with other disorders, in this case cancer."

4 See Iuvone et al. 2011; Reimers 2009; M.A. Smith et al. 2010; and Woodgate et al. 2016. I present statistics about children with brain cancer rather than adults because when discussing the medical management of intersex variations, the focus is typically "fixing" intersex infants and children.

5 As explained by M. Joycelyn Elders, David Satcher, and Richard Carmona (2017, 2), former surgeons general of the United States, "a gonadectomy can create a need for hormone replacement therapy, and may also preclude fertility ... In short, surgeries whose purpose is to ensure physical and psychological health too often lead to the opposite result."

6 See, for example, Byers et al. 2017; Inacio et al. 2011; Jung et al. 2017; and Mendonca et al. 2009.

7 See Dolmage 2014; Mitchell and Snyder 2000; Hesford and Brueggemann 2007; Titchkosky 2005; Schor 1999; and Vidali 2010.

8 There are a variety of blind metaphors, such as "one is blind to reality," as well as several stereotypes about and representations of blind people, who are said to have superhuman hearing abilities, to be musically inclined, to be helpless, to be spiritual, and so on (see Ben-Moshe 2005; Hesford and Brueggemann 2007; Schor 1999; and Vidali 2010).

9 Literature concerning this matter includes Arana and Human Rights Commission Staff 2005; Koyama 2003; Orr and Watson 2021; and G. Wilson 2012.

10 See, for example, Brouwers et al. 2007; S. Kumar et al. 2016; Nordenvall et al. 2020; and Örtqvist et al. 2017.

11 See, for example, Damani, Mittal, and Oates 2001; Fullerton, Hamilton, and Maheshwari 2010; Gianpiero et al. 1998; Paduch et al. 2008; Schiff et al. 2005; and Wikström et al. 2006.

12 See also Butler 2006; Rich 1980; and Rubin 1998.

13 Holmes (2008a, 148) reports that Gearhart "deeply regrets" making such a statement.

CHAPTER 2: MEDICAL INTERVENTIONS AND ACQUIRED BODY-MIND DISABILITIES

1 See Chase 1998, 2006; G. Davis 2015; Holmes 2009a; Karkazis 2008; Kessler 1998; Monro, Crocetti, and Yeadon-Lee 2019; Morland 2009; Pidgeon Pagonis, quoted in Schoenberg 2018; Preves 1999, 2003; Roen 2005; and Viloria 2017.

2 For more such analyses, see Spurgas 2009.

3 See Eckert 2009; Fausto-Sterling 2000; Jordan-Young 2010; Klöppel 2009; Laqueur 1992; and Oudshoorn 1994.

4 Additionally, Ulrike Klöppel (2009, 173) explains that the discovery of "sex chromosomes" in the 1950s also undermined the sex dyad. People learned that there are more than two chromosome formations. In addition to XX and XY, Myra J. Hird

(2000, 354) explains, "there are many variations of 'sex' [chromosomes]: XXY, XXXY, XXXXY, XXYY, XXXYY to name only a few ... The only thing that does not exist is a pure (Y or YY) male."

5 See Bao and Swaab 2010; Brizendine 2006; Dörner 2010; Jordan-Young 2010, 2012; Swaab 2004; Valla and Ceci 2011; and Velazquez, Mateos, and Erra 2019.

6 I do not construe Walsh's assertion that HRT is a poor substitute for the real thing as commentary about or commentary that can be applied to trans, intersex, gender-queer, and nonbinary individuals who need, consent to, and are fully informed of the possible risks and benefits of HRT. On this topic, Cameron (2007, 164) claims that it is terribly ironic that trans people who can give legal consent struggle to access HRT (as well as other gender-affirming procedures and forms of care), whereas HRT is often forced upon intersex youths even though they cannot give legal consent.

7 Dreger (1999a) also outlines other historical "ages" of intersex management. Klöppel (2009) complicates Dreger's historical accounts and descriptions.

8 As explained by M. Joycelyn Elders, David Satcher, and Richard Carmona (2017, 2), former surgeons general of the United States, "surgeries whose purpose is to ensure physical and psychological health too often lead to the opposite result."

9 For similar observations, see Bauer and Truffer 2016; and Klöppel 2016.

10 For commentary regarding the sanism that underpins pairing surgery with psycho-logical evaluations or, perhaps, replacing surgery with psychiatric interventions, see Orr and Peters, n.d.

11 Genital examinations are medically necessary sometimes. However, I am speaking of the frequent genital examinations, exposures, and manipulations that are medic-ally unnecessary but nevertheless take place.

12 This perception is explicitly reflected in Vincent Guillot's story. When Guillot (in Lohr 2016) was born with intersex traits, his mother was told that "she had given birth to a monster."

13 See Clare 2009; Couser 2009; Garland-Thomson 1996a; Hevey 2013; and Jarmakani 2008.

14 In contrast to the examples that Kessler (1998) highlights, there are numerous note-worthy humanizing self-/representations of intersex people. Such examples are typ-ically created and produced by intersex people or in collaboration with intersex people, or they centralize intersex people's knowledges and experiences.

15 See Abbott 2011; Chase 2006; Creighton et al. 2002; Garland-Thomson 2000, 2005, 2009; Hevey 2013; Longmore 2005; Snyder, Brueggemann, and Garland-Thomson 2002; Topps 2015; and J. Wilson 2000.

16 Sometimes, unnecessary surgery occurs in tandem with medical displays. Hida Viloria (2017, 82) recounts hearing Robin's story at a conference: "Robin is next to speak, and she also remembers growing up before her surgery. She was initially raised as a boy, but then her parents and doctors decided she wasn't developing enough as a male. So they performed a surgery on her in what she calls a 'teaching theatre,' where hordes of doctors and med students shuffled through the OR [oper-ating room] to study her unusual genitals."

17 The various ways that intersex people testify to the myriad disabling traumas – in film, at conferences and conventions, in print, on online forums, and through art –

teach/force viewers, to meet the intersex gaze so that they can see and conceptualize intersex people *as people.*

18 Some medical examinations, after initial inspection, also include dilating socio-medically assigned girl children and adolescents whose vaginas are deemed too small or shallow. As noted in the previous chapter, dilators – hard dildo-like instruments – are used to nonsurgically deepen vaginas that are deemed too short for a penis to fit inside. Medical professionals employ the ableist metaphor "blind pouch vagina" to justify dilating these people's vaginas. Dilation is painful and humiliating and can cause chronic pain, dryness, urinary problems, burning, friable tissue, bleeding, and discomfort during penetrative sex.

19 See Ashley 1962; Cornwall 2014; G. Davis 2015; Dreger 1998; Fausto-Sterling 2000; Money 1968; Money and Ehrhardt 1972; Natarajan 1996; and Preves 2003.

20 See Arana and Human Rights Commission Staff 2005; Coventry 1998; Harper 2007; and Hester 2006.

21 For more on intersex people, self-destructive behaviour, and mental health, see Mazur et al. 2004; Rosenwohl-Mack et al. 2020; Schützmann et al. 2009; and Warne et al. 2005.

22 See Chapter 1 for comments about inflated and contested cancer claims.

CHAPTER 3: IS THERE MEDICAL RECOGNITION OF THE DISABILITIES CREATED?

1 For more on medicine and mistakes, see Claridge and Fabian 2005; and Porter 1998.

2 Exceptions include, for example, Bougnères 2017; Diamond and Sigmundson 1997; Elders, Satcher, and Carmona 2017; and Gregorio 2017.

3 See Bauer and Truffer 2015; Bracka 1995; Devine and Horton 2002; McNamara et al. 2015; Orr 2019; and Snodgrass et al. 1998. In addition, for historical accounts of how hypospadias was regarded and treated starting in the fourth century BCE, see Hadidi and Azmy 2004; Laios et al. 2014; Laios, Karamanou, and Androutsos 2012; and D.E. Smith 1997. In brief, in the fourth century BCE, Aristotle described hypospadias, noticing that affected boys had to sit to urinate due to the formation of their genitals. In the second century CE, Galen introduced the term "hypospadias." "Treatment," according to Galen, involved amputating the part of the penis that went beyond the urethral meatus.

4 For more information about complications and the disabling impacts of these surgeries, see McNamara et al. 2015; Safwat, Elderwy, and Hammouda 2013; Salle et al. 2016; and Stanasel et al. 2015.

5 See Cinman et al. 2012; Craig et al. 2014; Kampantais et al. 2012; C.J. Long et al. 2017; and Safwat, Elderwy, and Hammouda 2013.

6 See, for example, Adayener and Akyol 2006; Amukele, Stock, and Hanna 2005; Coskun and Seyhan 2003; Gill and Hameed 2011; Hrabovszky and Huston 2002; C.J. Long et al. 2017; and van der Werff and van der Meulen 2000.

7 James R. Craig and colleagues (2014, 196) similarly note that the term describes "individuals with remaining functional complications after multiple attempts at hypospadias repair."

8 In other words, "this 'crippling' isn't caused by the hypospadias; it's caused by the complications of surgeries to 'fix' hypospadias" (Dreger 2017).

9 Moreover, the fact that some of the articles concerning hypospadias repairs and hypospadias cripples are published in academic journals concerning plastic surgery reveals that medical professionals must understand that these procedures take place for cosmetic, not medical, reasons: *Annals of Plastic Surgery* (Coskun and Seyhan 2003); *Journal of Plastic, Reconstructive and Aesthetic Surgery* (Gill and Hameed 2011); *Plastic and Reconstructive Surgery* (van der Werff and van der Meulen 2000).

10 For more commentary about "failed" masculinity, see Barnes 2014; Carmeli and Birenbaum-Carmeli 1994; and Inhorn et al. 2009.

11 See Gorey and Leslie 1997; Kvam 2008; Putnam 2003; Scherer and Reyns 2019; and Sobsey and Doe 1991.

12 For an analysis of these sorts of representations that is rooted in "mad intersex studies," see Orr and Peters, n.d.

13 For literature concerning how medicine is never and never could be objective, see Daston and Galison 2007; Ehrenreich and Barr 2005; Paget 2004; and van Dijck 2005.

CHAPTER 4: TEMPORARILY ENDOSEX

1 Although many scholars and journalists impose assumed intersex and disorders of sex development (DSDs) on these women, none of the athletes listed above have publicly claimed DSD or intersex as an identity. Respecting these women's narratives and identities is important, while acknowledging the interphobic, racist, and sexist violence that they experience. Imposing identity or diagnostic categories on these athletes is a colonial act, as I discuss at greater length in Chapter 5.

2 See Magubane 2001, 2014; McClintock 1995; Orr and Watson 2018; Reis 2005, 2009; Somerville 2000; and Willis 2010.

3 The purported "Hottentot Venus," Saartjie Baartman, is the most widely known woman to have endured such violence and been reduced to her biological characteristics, namely her buttocks and genitals. Baartman was a South African woman who was captured, enslaved, examined, and enfreaked for European audiences. Even after her death, Baartman's body was subjected to dehumanizing examination and treatment by Georges Cuvier, surgeon general to Napoleon Bonaparte. Baartman's body was cut apart, and many pieces, including her genitals, were pickled in laboratory jars. These bottles, along with a plaster cast of her body, were displayed in the Musée de l'Homme in Paris. European audiences continued to enfreak and gawk at her body until 1974. After years of petitioning, Baartman's remains were finally returned to her homeland in 2002. For a comprehensive text about Baartman's life, as well as the racist symbolic construction of Black women, see Deborah Willis's (2010) edited collection *Black Venus 2010: They Called Her "Hottentot."*

4 See, for example, Ball 2004; Garfinkel and Stoller 1967; Preves and Eyler 1999; and Warren, Sutherland, and Lenz 1994.

5 See, for example, Lightman et al. 2009; Peers 2012; Samuels 2003; and Valle and Connor 2019.

6 See, for example, Catalano 2015; Garrison 2018; and Soucek 2014.

7 For texts that address transexclusionary radical feminists and/or the pathologization of trans people, see Baril 2015a; Baril and Trevenen 2014; G. Davis, Dewey, and Murphy 2016; Koyama 2016; Serano 2007, 2012; and Tosh 2016.

8 See also Baril 2015b; J.L. Davis 2012; and Stevens 2011.

9   One may be compelled to label these people "transintersex," but that expression is reserved for intersex people whose gender identity differs from the socio-medically assigned gender. In addition, the term "transintersex" detracts from the centrality of disability in conversations about intersex variations.

10 For texts concerning mad studies, see LeFrançois, Menzies, and Reaume 2013; McWade, Milton, and Beresford 2015; and Reaume 2002.

11 Furthermore, when intersex people are referred to psychologists for support, they are often sent there because they have resisted medical intervention. As I and Meg Peters (Orr and Peters) explain, "in the attempt to impose and justify curative violence, medical practitioners may send disobedient intersex patients to psychologists." "Difficult" patients who challenge doctors' orders have been sent "to psychologists for psychiatric 'treatment'" that supports doctors' desires and discriminatory ideologies (G. Wilson 2012). Despite the presumed "natural" desire to not change one's anatomical traits, when intersex people voice their desire not to do so, they are pathologized in a new way.

CHAPTER 5: CRIPPING SPORT SEX TESTING

1   For texts that address these women's experiences, see Abdul 2019; Blatchford 2016; Gugala 2014; Jordan-Young and Karkazis 2019; and Mitra 2014a, 2014b.

2   For discussions of this period, see Pieper 2014, 2016; and Wackwitz 1996, 2003.

3   See also Donnellan 2008; and Pieper 2014, 2016.

4   See also Cahn 2015; Cohen 2009; Dworkin and Cooky 2012; and Kane 1995.

5   For texts that address this literal and symbolic violence, see Adams and Leavitt 2018; Billings and Young 2015; Chadwick, Chanavat, and Desbordes 2016; Cunningham 2003; Daddario 1998; Jordan-Young and Karkazis 2019; and Travers 2008.

6   It is not unheard of for women who compete in other sports to be rendered suspect intersex and subjected to sex testing (Cohen 2009). For example, during the "1990 Asian Games held in Beijing, an Indian female hockey player was reportedly expelled after failing the requisite gender verification test" (Pieper 2014, 1566). Overwhelmingly, however, women athletes who compete in track and field events have historically and currently been the focus.

7   See, for example, Buzuvis 2010; Camporesi and Maugeri 2016; McDonagh and Pappano 2008; Messner 2002; Milner and Braddock 2016; Zaccone 2010.

8   Phelps retired from competitive swimming in 2012 but came back in 2014. He did not compete in the 2020 Olympic Games, but as of 2021, there were murmurs that he would return to competition.

9   See, for example, Dalbey 2019; Dunbar 2019; Jordan-Young and Karkazis 2019; Lindahl 2019; and Vikander 2019.

10 As demonstrated in Chapter 3, current dominant medical standards for intersex patients constitute discriminatory medical malpractice; the "treatments" are gratuitously disabling, mutilating, violent, and tortuous.

11 See Cavanagh and Sykes 2006; Jordan-Young and Karkazis 2012; Kane 1995; Krane 2001; Magubane 2014; Orr and Watson 2018; and Pieper 2014, 2016.

12 See Cooky, Dycus, and Dworkin 2013; G. Davis 2015; Jordan-Young and Karkazis 2019; Karkazis 2016a; Magubane 2014; Mitra 2014a, 2014b; Munro 2010; Nyong'o 2010; and Orr and Watson 2018.

13 Kłobukowska was forced to retire and was publicly defamed. Consequently, she experienced severe depression, broke off contact with the sports world, and underwent surgery and HRT "to reassess her sex as woman" (Martínez-Patiño et al. 2010, 315; see also Carlson 2005). Even decades later, Kłobukowska's sex characteristics are discussed and shamed in the media. In an infantilizingly titled news article penned for the *Times*, "Girls Will Be Girls at the Beijing Olympics – Sex Tests Will Prove It," published in 2008 before the Beijing Olympics, Jane Maccartney and Hattie Garlick (2008) discuss "suspicious-looking female athletes" and note that "Kłobukowska ... was the first athlete to be unmasked as a man when she failed an early form of chromosome test in 1967."

14 See Collins 2004; Deliovsky 2008; Ferguson and Satterfield 2017; Hamilton et al. 2019; Kane 1995; Orr and Watson 2018; Pieper 2014, 2016; and Somerville 2000.

15 Chand became India's first "out" gay athlete. She notes that she decided to speak publicly about her sexuality after the Indian Supreme Court decriminalized gay sex in 2018 (Ives 2019).

16 For texts that take colonialism into account while analyzing sport, see Gems 2006; Magubane 2014; Orr and Watson 2018; Sykes 2017; and Sykes and Hamzeh 2018.

17 To be clear, when I speak of race and African and Black people here, I am not conflating Blackness with African identity or citizenship, and I am not merely retrospectively applying contemporary understandings of Black, white, race, or racism to historical contexts. Race, whiteness, and Blackness have been constructed very differently through time and space (see McClintock 1995; McClintock, Mufti, and Shohat 1997; Goldberg 1990; Schiebinger 1993; and Willis 2010). Race categories were and, in many respects, remain unsteady. Indeed, Magubane (2001, 823) writes, "Skin color and hair textures were not stabilized as markers of racial difference until fairly late in the nineteenth century." When I speak of the historical construction or understanding of many African women's physical attributes and genitals, I do not suggest that they understood themselves to be or thought of themselves as Black or that they were necessarily understood to be Black by others. Nevertheless, the shift in racial and racist discourses and beliefs that rooted Blackness in, for example, darker skin and hair texture occurred alongside the maintenance of the belief in sexually ambiguous African women, and African women were constructed as Black. That is, my aim here is to trace the ideological construction and imposition of sexual ambiguity in order to contextualize how this construction and imposition are articulated through current sex-testing practices.

18 See Cooky, Dycus, and Dworkin 2013; Klein 2016; Magubane 2014; Munro 2010; and Orr and Watson 2018.

19 I must note that some scholars and historians are not certain that Truth said those exact words because the question did not appear in the first transcription of the event. Nevertheless, this question became a motto and cultural touchstone – and remains so to this day – in the fight against the intersecting logics of racism and sexism.

20 See, for example, Florida 2005; Fox 2014; Ghemawat 2009; and Stiglitz 2006.

21 See Atluri 2012; Lugones 2007; N. Menon 2011; Mitra 2014a; Mposo 2017; and Reddy 2005.

22 For information about these identities, see Hossain 2018; Johari 2014; Khan et al. 2009; and Mposo 2017.

23 See Cooper 2010; Dreger 2010; Kalra, Kulshreshtha, and Unnikrishnan 2012; and Mitra 2014a.

24 For literature concerning the presumed athletic hyperabilities of Black people, see K.C. Harrison and Lawrence 2004; and Miller 2015.

25 In response to all the slandering remarks and articles coming from the West after the 800-metre race, particularly about Semenya, hashtags like #BlackExcellence, #HandsOffCaster, and #BlackGirlMagic began trending. Alyssa Klein (2016) recounts some of the tweets that appeared in defence of Semenya. @Thabo_Shinange tweeted, "The threat of black excellence creates stupidity from the white world #HandsOffCasterSemenya #HandsOffCaster"; @Kmoeti tweeted, "#HandsOffCaster because Black women shouldn't have to hold back their greatness to coddle your insecurities & bigotry"; and @KaZihlandlo tweeted, "Whiteness so fragile, questioning whether Caster Semenya should run with women. GTFOH [get the fuck out of here]! #HandsOffCaster #WeLoveCaster."

26 See, for example, Critchley 2016; Flanagan 2016; Kanayama 2016; T. Morgan 2016; and Parker 2016.

CHAPTER 6: SPORT SEX AND DIS/ABILITY DE/SEGREGATION

1 See Brittain and Beacom 2018; Goggin and Newell 2000; Martin 2017; Misener et al. 2019; Peers 2009, 2012, 2015; and N. Thomas and Smith 2008.

2 See, for example, Berger 2008; Goggin and Newell 2000; Grue 2016; Howe 2011; and Maika and Danylchuk 2016.

3 For work concerning "origin stories" and sport, see Peers 2012, 2015.

4 Such interpersonal circumstances and labour are often emphasized in sexist coverage about and interviews with able-bodied women athletes. Women athletes' coaches and/or husbands are often credited for the athletes' achievements, effectively discrediting the women's achievements. It is implied that these women would never have been able to reach such elite levels without men. For example, when Hungarian swimmer Katinka Hosszú beat the world record in the 400-metre medley at the Rio Olympics in 2016, an NBC commentator said that her husband and coach, Shane Tusup, was "the person responsible for her performance" (see Bogart 2016; Mei 2016; and Park 2016).

5 For these notable exceptions, see Gilbert and Schantz 2008; Heilpern 2016; Howe 2008; D. Rose 2012; and Springer 2016.

6 See, for example, Berger 2013; Clare 2009; Gordon and Rosenblum 2001; Linton 1998; N. Watson and Vehmas 2019; and Wendell 1996.

7 For a critique of "the myth of Olympic unity," see Devitt 2011.

8 For more information about decolonizing sports, see Appadurai 2015; Bale 2002; Darby 2002; Darnell and Hayhurst 2011; Hayhurst 2014; Hern 2013; MacLean 2019; Orr and Watson 2018; and Sykes 2017.

9 For information about various Indigenous communities' and nations' alternative sex, gender, and sexuality models and how these models have been decimated by colonial forces, see Bear 2016; Cannon 1998; Driskill 2004; N. Menon 2011; Mitra

2014b; O'Sullivan 2021; Picq 2020; Reddy 2005; Ristock et al. 2019; Roscoe 1992, 1998; TallBear 2018; Tuck and Yang 2012; Vigneault 2011; Warnke 2011; and W.L. Williams 1992.

10 I especially cherish my first marathon participation medal because I was trained and encouraged by a supportive stepsister, Bronwen Douglas, and I trained alongside and celebrated our achievements with my dear friend and fellow runner Lisa Nazarenko.

11 See also Chu et al. 2009; Golden 2009; Kokozos and Gross 2015; Real 1998; Reichert et al. 2012; Vogel et al. 2011; Ward 2019; and Way et al. 2014.

CHAPTER 7: INTERSEX, PGD, AND THE EUGENICS AGENDA

1 I must note that the ethical implications of using reproductive technologies to select against Tay-Sachs are not straightforward but instead hotly debated and contested (see Holland 2002; Saxton 2017; and Shakespeare 1998).

2 See, for example, Astorino 2015; Carpenter 2014; Costello 2014c; Holmes 2008b; and Preves 2003.

3 In addition to voiced concerns about PGD and interphobic selection, scholars and activists are also troubled by the experimental drug dexamethasone (DEX) (see Dreger, Feder, and Tamar-Mattis 2012; Reis and Kessler 2010; and Sytsma 2006). DEX, a drug prescribed to people who are pregnant with a fetus with congenital adrenal hyperplasia, is intended to avert genital and behavioural "masculinization" or "virilization" of the fetus. Even at the risk of the pregnant person's and fetuses' safety, DEX is prescribed to prevent the development of nonfatal variant genitals and to reduce the chance of the infant looking or acting "unfeminine" and developing "lesbianism" or "bisexuality."

4 See Crotty, Rodwell, and Germov 2000; L.J. Davis 2013; Hansen and King 2001; Magnet 2013; McLaren 2014; and Shakespeare 1998.

5 MaterniT21 is a relatively new screening test on the market. Intended to replace amniocentesis and CVS, MaterniT21 is noninvasive, does not carry the risk of miscarriage, and can accurately diagnose Down syndrome sooner. Jaime L. Natoli and colleagues (2012) report that, between 1995 and 2011, people terminated their pregnancies 60 to 90 percent of the time when their fetus was diagnosed with Down syndrome. Chris Kaposy (2013) notes that people typically refuse invasive screening tests because of the possibility of miscarriage, not because they are morally against testing for or aborting a fetus with Down syndrome. Because MaterniT21 is noninvasive and does not pose the risk of miscarriage, Kaposy (2013, 300) anticipates that termination rates will increase: "The introduction of MaterniT21 will likely increase the overall incidence of abortion after prenatal diagnosis of Down syndrome."

6 See L.J. Davis 1995; Green and Statham 1996; Hubbard 2013; Hull 2009; Kaposy 2013, 2018; and Waldschmidt 2015.

7 For examples of these bioethicists, medical professionals, and genetic counsellors, see CooperSurgical n.d.; Goh et al. 2019; Savulescu 2001, 2007; Sparrow 2013; Speechley and Nisker 2010; and Trafimow 2013.

8 Statistics concerning how commonly PGD is used to detect and select against intersex variations are not available. However, there are some statistics concerning how

frequently people choose to abort a fetus diagnosed with an intersex trait. Caroline Mansfield, Suellen Hopfer, and Theresa M. Matrau (1999) conducted a meta-analysis of fetal termination rates after prenatal diagnosis of Down syndrome, spina bifida, anencephaly, Turner syndrome (an intersex variation), and Klinefelter syndrome (an intersex variation) and concluded that, on average, 58 percent of fetuses diagnosed with Klinefelter syndrome were terminated and 72 percent of fetuses with Turner syndrome were terminated. Céline M. Girardin and Guy Van Vliet (2011) compiled the rates of pregnancy termination following prenatal diagnosis of Klinefelter syndrome from various places, including British Columbia from 1971 to 1997, at 88 percent; Switzerland from 1980 to 2001, at 74 percent; California from 1983 to 2003, at 70 percent; Germany from 1989 to 1998, at 17 percent; and Denmark from 1970 to 2000, at 70 percent. The second edition of the *World Atlas of Birth Defects* (World Health Organization 2003, 123), which compiles data from 1993 to 1998, indicates that the pregnancy termination rate for fetuses prenatally diagnosed as "indeterminately sexed" was, for example, 20 percent in Alberta, 47 percent in Switzerland, and 16.68 percent in Australia. For more information on this matter, see Bauer, Truffer, and Plattner (2014)

9 Behrmann and Ravitsky (2013, 39) add that "as this [integration of PGD] happens, many more conditions may 'creep' into the screening process." In addition to intersex, which is already "creeping" into screening processes, other culturally devalued characteristics and disabilities are likely to creep into PGD screening, such as autism and cleft lip or palate. The genetic factors for clefting and autism have not been entirely determined. However, speaking of autism, Sher Fertility Institute (n.d.), an American institution with numerous fertility clinics, claims that the situation "could all change in the next few years with the rapid advancement in genetic research." Likewise, Marie M. Tolarova (2015) reports, "With rapidly advancing knowledge in medical genetics and with new DNA diagnostic technologies, more cleft lip and palate anomalies are diagnosed." Sebastiaan Mastenbroek and colleagues (2007) report a couple of cases where PGD detected cleft lip and palate (see also Paterson et al. 2011). Disability scholars and activists critique the idea that autism is "a crippling disability" (Orsini 2009, 115) and they critique the focus on cure and eliminating both autism and clefting. They are understandably and justifiably concerned about the ableism that fuels employing reproductive technologies to eliminate these variations, as well as about medical professionals "steering" (Bingham 2013) parents to abort fetuses with these characteristics (see Chew 2013; Cox 2014; Paterson et al. 2011; P. Walsh et al. 2011; C. Williams, Alderson, and Farsides 2002).

10 That being said, many people who apparently do not have fertility issues still have to pay for IVF. Some folks include gay men who hire a surrogate and egg donor and use their own sperm, trans men who can become pregnant only through IVF, and lesbian couples who hope to have one woman carry the child and the other woman contribute her egg. Hence, "fertility issues" are quite narrowly defined and, as a result, the OHIP coverage excludes many queer folks who desire to be biologically related to their (potential) child. Even though the rhetoric used to promote the IVF coverage seems inclusive, a number of LGBTQIA2 individuals cannot access this coverage. Some queer family formations are, therefore, prevented.

11 See G. Allen 1989; Campbell 2000; Crotty, Rodwell, and Germov 2000; L.J. Davis 2013; Grekul, Krahn, and Odynak 2004; and McLaren 2014.

12 Sparrow (2013) does not use the phrase "intersex eugenics." He primarily refers to the practice as "selecting against intersex traits." However, as I demonstrate above, using PGD for this type of selection is eugenic. Hence, I refer to it as such.

13 For analyses concerning activist stereotypes, see Bashir et al. 2013; G. Brown 2007; and Lindblom and Jacobsson 2014.

14 For a discussion of the urban-rural binary, spatiality, and the assumptions that urban places are more tolerant of diversity, that diversity is always more visible in urban places, and that visibility is always desirable, see Gray, Gilley, and Johnson 2016; Kazyak 2011, 2012; Prest 2016; and Thomsen 2016.

15 For texts that concern consequentialism, see Korsgaard 2013; Mulgan 2001; O. O'Neill 2013; and Railton 1984.

16 The specific philosophical traditions that I am thinking of include utilitarian ethics (i.e., happiness must be maximized) (Quinton 1973; Shaw 1999) and Kantian ethics (i.e., the categorical imperative, which insists that morality must be based on a rational, objective foundation) (Kant 1997).

17 See, for example, Bourne, Douglas, and Savulescu 2012; Sandel 2007; and Savulescu 2001, 2007, 2012.

18 See, for example, Collins 1986, 1989, 2000; Gilligan 1982; Haraway 1988, 1990, 1991; Harding 1986, 1991; Hartsock 1981, 1983, 1987, 1990; Noddings 1984; Potter 2006; Shildrick and Mykitiuk 2005; D. Smith 1979, 1987, 1990; and Tuana 1992.

19 That includes this book. *Cripping Intersex* would not have been possible without intersex people sharing their knowledges in the mediums noted above.

20 For texts that effectively undermine the idea of objective truths about body-mind morphologies, see Daston and Galison 2007; G. Davis 2015; L.J. Davis 1995; Erevelles 2011; Fausto-Sterling 2000; Garland-Thomson 2009; Jordan-Young 2010; McRuer 2006; and van Dijck 2005.

21 As Rosemarie Garland-Thomson (1997, 279) writes, "normal" traits are "assumed to possess natural corporeal superiority."

22 See Alexander 2010; Bucerius and Tonry 2014; Connor, Ferrir, and Annamma 2016; Edney 2004; Evans et al. 2020; Puar 2007, 2013; V. Smith 2013; Solomos 2020; and Sudbury 2013.

CHAPTER 8: A CRIP INTERSEX APPROACH TO PGD

1 Chinyere Ezie (2011) similarly argues that the violence that intersex people face is, or at least can be legally framed as, sex discrimination.

2 See, for example, Amato 2016; Orr and Watson 2021; Pagonis 2015b; Preves 2003; and Triea 1999.

3 Perhaps parents prefer DSD discourse to intersex terminology because a medical condition, disorder, or disability may be easier to cope with than coming to terms with a queerly embodied child. Be that as it may, disability and queerness are not distinct issues here; disorder, disability, and queerness intersect.

4 See Arana and Human Rights Commission Staff 2005; G. Davis 2015; Garcia 2015; L.S. Long 2015; Preves 2003; Truffer 2015; and Wall 2015b.

5 See Damani, Mittal, and Oates 2001; Fullerton, Hamilton, and Maheshwari 2010; Gianpiero et al. 1998; Paduch et al. 2008; Ramasamy et al. 2009; Schiff et al. 2005; and Wikström et al. 2006.

6 I add "other intersex traits" because Sparrow (2013) problematically conflates variant genitals with intersex. Not all people with intersex anatomy have variant genitals.

7 See Collins 2004; Garland-Thomson 1997, 2000, 2009, 2011; Hobson 2003; Kessler 1998; and Tate 2007.

8 See Fahs 2014; Magubane 2014; McClintock 1995; and Somerville 2000.

9 See Ostertag 2020; Sawyer and Gampa 2018; Sobo, Lambert, and Heath 2020; and Walcott and Abdillahi 2019.

10 Put differently, "medical claims are couched in terms that attempt to conceptualize deviance," abnormality," or atypicality "as a medical problem" that requires treatment, cure, and/or alteration rather than an ideological shift (Conrad and Schneider 1992, 266).

11 See, for example, Clare 2017; Kafer 2013; Oliver 2004; Shakespeare 2013; C. Thomas 2004; and Tremain 2002.

12 Disability scholars would never claim that one had "failed" to develop legs, as Sparrow (2013) posits, because doing so reinforces pathologizing practices and compulsory able-bodiedness.

13 See, for example, Clare 2017; Henry 2013; Knight 2017; Sharp and Earle 2002; and Stapleford 2014.

14 See Clare 2009; Fentiman 2019; Rapp 1999; and Waggoner 2015.

15 For similar stances, see Kaposy 2018; and Thomsen 2013.

CONCLUSION: ERADICATING EXORCISMS

1 Likewise, reflecting on Morgan Holmes's (2009a) edited collection *Critical Intersex,* Robert McRuer (2009, 245, 250) thinks about "The Future of Critical Intersex," noting that the authors in *Critical Intersex* "dare to imagine" "unforeseeable freedoms beyond binary assurances that they envision, and for the intersex futures that they welcome."

2 Works that address Black futurity and Afrofuturism include R. Anderson 2016; Dean and Andrews 2016; Eshun 2003; Fisher 2013; Holbert, Dando, and Correa 2020; Yaszek 2006; and Zamalin 2019.

3 More texts concerning crip and disabled futures include Fritsch 2016; Heisinger-Nixon 2017; Jerreat-Poole 2020; Kelly 2018; Mackey 2009; Rice et al. 2017; and Schlauderaff 2020.

4 Literature about queer futures includes Boellstorff 2007; Edelman 2004; Fritsch 2016; Goltz 2009; Halberstam 2005, 2011; Keeling 2019; and Valentine 2015.

5 Works that address this adage and the debates surrounding it include A. Harris 2004; Kingston 2018; Krauzo 2018; Segal 1987; and C. Young 2019.

6 See Abbott 2011; Garland-Thomson 2005; Hevey 2013; Longmore 2005; and Snyder, Brueggemann, and Garland-Thomson 2002.

7 Works that address this (contested) alliance include Astorino 2013; Cornwall 2009; and Viloria 2017.

Works Cited

Abbott, Natalie. 2011. "'Nothing Is Uglier Than Ignorance': Art, Disability Studies, and the Disability Community in the Positive Exposure Photography Project." *Journal of Literary and Cultural Disability Studies* 5 (1): 71–90. https://doi.org/10.3828/jlcds.2011.5.

Abdul, Geneva. 2019. "This Intersex Runner Had Surgery to Compete. It Has Not Gone Well." *New York Times,* December 16. https://www.nytimes.com/2019/12/16/sports/intersex-runner-surgery-track-and-field.html.

Adams, Carly, and Stacey Leavitt. 2018. "'It's just girls' hockey': Troubling Progress Narratives in Girls' and Women's Sport." *International Review for the Sociology of Sport* 53 (2): 152–72. https://doi.org/10.1177/1012690216649207.

Adayener, Cüneyt, and Ilker Akyol. 2006. "Distal Hypospadias Repair in Adults: The Results of 97 Cases." *Urologia Internationalis* 76 (3): 247–51. https://doi.org/10.1159/000091628.

Affleck, John. 2016. "Why Do the Paralympics Get So Little Media Attention in the Unites States?" *The Conversation,* September 15. https://theconversation.com/why-do-the-paralympics-get-so-little-media-attention-in-the-united-states-65205.

Agamben, Giorigo. 2005. *State of Exception.* Trans. Kevin Attell. Chicago: University of Chicago Press.

Ahmed, Faisal S., et al. 2016. "Society for Endocrinology UK Guidance on the Initial Evaluation of an Infant or an Adolescent with a Suspected Disorder of Sex Development (Revised 2015)." *Clinical Endocrinology* 84 (5): 771–88. https://doi.org/10.1111/cen.12857.

Albritton, Joshua C. 2015. "Intersexed and Injured: How *M.C. v. Aaronson* Breaks Federal Ground in Protecting Intersex Children from Unnecessary Genital-

Normalization Surgeries." *Tulane Journal of Law and Sexuality* 24: 163–87. https://journals.tulane.edu/tjls/article/view/2879.

Alexander, Michelle. 2010. *The New Jim Crow: Mass Incarceration.* New York: New Press.

Allen, Garland E. 1989. "Eugenics and American Social History, 1880–1950." *Genome* 31 (2): 885–89. https://doi.org/10.1139/g89-156.

Amato, Viola. 2016. *Intersex Narratives: Shifts in the Representation of Intersex Lives in North American Literature and Popular Culture.* Bielefeld, Germany: transcript Verlag.

Amukele, Samuel A., Jeffery A. Stock, and Moneer K. Hanna. 2005. "Management and Outcome of Complex Hypospadias Repairs." *Journal of Urology* 174 (4): 1540–43. https://doi.org/10.1097/01.ju.0000176420.83110.19.

Anderson, Len. 2009. "On What Basis Was Caster Tested?" *Sowetan Live,* August 24. http://www.sowetanlive.co.za/sowetan/archive/2009/08/24/on-what-basis-was-caster-tested.

Anderson, Reynaldo. 2016. "Afrofuturism 2.0 & the Black Speculative Arts Movement: Notes on a Manifesto." *Obsidian: Literature in the African Diaspora* 42 (1–2): 228–37. https://www.jstor.org/stable/44489514.

Anderson-Minshall, Diane. 2016. "Are We Witnessing the Birth of TV's Intersex Liberation?" *Advocate,* July 6. https://www.advocate.com/current-issue/2016/7/06/are-we-witnessing-birth-tvs-intersex-liberation.

Andrews, Charlotte Richardson. 2017. "Why Intersexuality Will Be the Next Civil Rights Frontier." *Huck Magazine,* April 14. https://www.huckmag.com/perspectives/intersexuality-will-next-civil-rights-frontier/.

Andropoulos, Dean B., and Michael F. Greene. 2018. "Anesthesia and Developing Brains – Implications of the FDA Warning." *New England Journal of Medicine* 376 (10): 905–7. doi:10.1056/NEJMp1700196.

Appadurai, Arjun. 2015. "Playing with Modernity: The Decolonization of Indian Cricket." *Altre Modernità* 14 (11): 1–24. doi:10.13130/2035-7680/6526.

Arana, Marcus de María, and Human Rights Commission Staff. 2005. *A Human Rights Investigation into the Medical 'Normalization' of Intersex People: A Report of a Public Hearing by the Human Rights Commission of the City and County of San Francisco.* San Francisco, CA: Human Rights Commission of the City and County of San Francisco. https://isna.org/files/SFHRC_Intersex_Report.pdf.

Aristotle. 1984. *The Complete Works of Aristotle.* Ed. Jonathan Barnes. Original 4th century BCE. Princeton, NJ: Princeton University Press.

Armstrong, Elizabeth A., Paula England, and Alison C.K. Fogarty. 2012. "Accounting for Women's Orgasm and Sexual Enjoyment in College Hookups and Relationships." *American Sociological Review* 77 (3): 435–62. https://doi.org/10.1177/0003122412445802.

Armstrong, James. 2015. "B.C. Group Wants Gender Removed from Birth Certificates in Canada." *Global News,* May 27. https://globalnews.ca/news/2020374/b-c-group-wants-gender-removed-from-birth-certificates-in-canada/.

Asch, Adrienne. 1988. "Reproductive Technology and Disability." In *Reproductive Laws for the 1990s,* ed. Sherrill Cohen and Nadine Taub, 69–124. Clifton, NJ: Humana.

–. 2000. "Why I Haven't Changed My Mind about Prenatal Diagnosis: Reflections and Refinements." In *Prenatal Testing and Disability Rights,* ed. Erik Parens and Adrienne Asch, 234–58. Washington, DC: Georgetown University Press.

Ashley, David James Burrows. 1962. *Human Intersex.* Philadelphia: Williams and Wilkins.

Asklund, Camilla, et al. 2010. "Semen Quality, Reproductive Hormones and Fertility of Men Operated for Hypospadias." *International Journal of Andrology* 33 (1): 80–87. https://doi.org/10.1111/j.1365-2605.2009.00957.x.

Associated Press. 2018. "IAAF Delays Testosterone Rules until Caster Semenya Case Verdict." *CBC,* October 22. https://www.cbc.ca/sports/olympics/trackandfield/ iaaf-delays-testosterone-rules-until-caster-semenya-case-verdict-1.4864869.

Astorino, Claudia. 2012. "'Dyadic'?" *Full-Frontal Activism: Intersex and Awesome,* September 10. http://fullfrontalactivism.blogspot.ca/2012/09/dyadic.html.

–. 2013. "Brought to You by the Letter I: Why Intersex Politics Matters to LGBT Activism." *Autostraddle,* September 23. https://www.autostraddle.com/brought -to-you-by-the-letter-i-why-intersex-politics-matters-to-lgbt-activism -192760/.

–. 2015. "Why I'm Disturbed by Screening for Intersex Traits in Utero." *Rewire,* March 11. https://rewire.news/article/2015/03/11/im-disturbed-screening -intersex-traits-utero/.

Atluri, Tara. 2012. "The Prerogative of the Brave: Hijras and Sexual Citizenship after Orientalism." *Citizenship Studies* 16 (5–6): 721–36. https://doi.org/10.1080/136 21025.2012.698496.

Aurenque, Diana, and Hans-Jörg Ehni. 2013. "For the Sake of 'Normality'? Medical Indication, Social Justification, and the Welfare of Children." *American Journal of Bioethics* 13 (10): 55–57. https://doi.org/10.1080/15265161.2013.828117.

Australia Human Rights Commission. 2018. "Terminology." https://www.humanrights. gov.au/our-work/lgbti/terminology.

Baglieri, Susan, et al. 2011. "[Re]claiming 'Inclusive Education' toward Cohesion in Educational Reform: Disability Studies Unravels the Myth of the Normal Child." *Teachers College Record* 113 (10): 2122–54. doi:10.1177/016146811111 301001.

Bailey, Steve. 2008. *Athlete First: A History of the Paralympic Movement.* Chichester, UK: John Wiley and Sons.

Baker, Bernadette. 2002. "The Hunt for Disability: The New Eugenics and the Nor- malization of School Children." *Teachers College Record* 104 (4): 663–703. doi: 10.1111/1467-9620.00175.

Bale, John. 2002. *Imagined Olympians: Body Culture and Colonial Representations in Rwanda.* Minneapolis: University of Minnesota Press.

Ball, Edward. 2004. *Peninsula of Lies: A True Story of Mysterious Birth and Taboo Love.* New York: Simon and Schuster.

Bao, Ai-Min, and Dick F. Swaab. 2010. "Sex Differences in the Brain, Behavior, and Neuropsychiatric Disorders." *Neuroscientist* 16 (5): 550–65. https://doi.org/ 10.1177/1073858410377005.

Baratz, Arlene B. 2017. "Risk of Anesthesia on Developing Brains: Another Alarm Signaling Danger of Early Cosmetic Genital Surgery." interACT: Advocates for

Intersex Youth, April 13. http://interactadvocates.org/anesthesia-dangerous -cosmetic-intersex-surgeries/.

Baril, Alexandre. 2015a. "'How dare you pretend to be disabled?' The Discounting of Transabled People and Their Claims in Disability Movements and Studies." *Disability and Society* 30 (5): 689–703. https://doi.org/10.1080/09687599.2015. 1050088.

–. 2015b. "Needing to Acquire a Physical Impairment/Disability: (Re)thinking the Connections between Trans and Disability Studies through Transability." *Hypatia* 30 (1): 30–48. https://doi.org/10.1111/hypa.12113.

Baril, Alexandre, and Kathryn Trevenen. 2014. "Exploring Ableism and Cisnormativity in the Conceptualization of Identity and Sexuality 'Disorders.'" *Annual Review of Critical Psychology* 11 (1): 389–416.

Barnes, Liberty Walther. 2014. *Conceiving Masculinity: Male Infertility, Medicine, and Identity.* Philadelphia: Temple University Press.

Bashir, Nadia, et al. 2013. "The Ironic Impact of Activists: Negative Stereotypes Reduce Social Change Influence." *European Journal of Social Psychology* 43 (7): 614–26. https://doi.org/10.1002/ejsp.1983.

Bastien-Charlebois, Janik. 2015. "Sanctioned Sex/ualities: The Medical Treatment of Intersex Bodies and Voices." https://www.academia.edu/17353174/Bastien_ Charlebois_2015_Sanctioned_sex_ualiti_es_The_medical_treatment_of_intersex _bodies_and_voices.

Bauer, Markus, and Daniela Truffer. 2015. *Intersex Genital Mutilations: Human Rights Violations of Children with Variations of Sex Anatomy.* NGO Report on the Answers to the List of Issues (LoI) in Relation to the Initial Periodic Report of Germany on the Convention on the Rights of Persons with Disabilities (CRPD). https://intersex.shadowreport.org/public/2015-CRPD-LoI-Germany_ NGO-Report_Zwischengeschlecht_Intersex-IGM.pdf.

–. 2016. *Intersex Genital Mutilations: Human Rights Violations of Children with Variations of Sex Anatomy.* NGO Report to the 5th Periodic Report of the United Kingdom on the Convention on the Rights of the Child (CRC). https://intersex. shadowreport.org/public/2016-CRC-UK-NGO-Zwischengeschlecht-Intersex -IGM_v2.pdf.

Bauer, Markus, Daniela Truffer, and Karin Plattner. 2014. *Intersex Genital Mutilations: Human Rights Violations of Children with Variations of Sex Anatomy.* NGO Report to the 2nd, 3rd, and 4th Periodic Report of Switzerland on the Convention on the Rights of the Child (CRC). https://intersex.shadowreport. org/public/2014-CRC-Swiss-NGO-Zwischengeschlecht-Intersex-IGM_v2.pdf.

Baumgartner, Nina. 2017. "Intersex Parenting: Ethical and Legal Implications of the Treatment of Intersex Infants and the Ramifications for Their Families." *Women Leading Change* 1 (3): 46–56. https://journals.tulane.edu/ncs/article/view/1121.

BBC. 2016. "Disabled Models and Athletes Outraged by Brazilian Vogue Paralympic Campaign Photo." *BBC*, August 26. http://www.bbc.co.uk/newsbeat/ article/37194585/disabled-models-and-athletes-outraged-by-brazilian-vogue -paralympic-campaign-photo.

Beamish, Rob, and Ian Ritchie. 2007. "Totalitarian Regimes and Cold War Sport: Steroid 'Übermenschen' and 'Ball-Bearing Females.'" In *East Plays West: Sport and the Cold War,* ed. Stephen Wagg and David L. Andrews, 11–26. New York: Routledge.

Bear, Tracy L. 2016. "Power in My Blood: Corporeal Sovereignty through the Praxis of an Indigenous Eroticanalysis." PhD diss., University of Alberta.

Beck, Theodric Romeyn, and John B. Beck. 1860. *Elements of Medical Jurisprudence.* Vol. 1. Philadelphia: Lippincott.

–. 1863. *Evidence of Medical Jurisprudence.* Vol. 2. Philadelphia: Lippincott.

Behrmann, Jason, and Vardit Ravitsky. 2013. "Queer Liberation, Not Elimination: Why Selecting against Intersex Is Not 'Straight' Forward." *American Journal of Bioethics* 13 (10): 39–41. https://doi.org/10.1080/15265161.2013.828131.

Belser, Julia Watts, and Sharon V. Betcher. 2013. "Call for Papers: Special Issue on Religion, Disability and the Environment, Fall 2014 – Worldviews: Global Religions, Culture, and Ecology." *Journal of Religion, Disability and Health* 17 (3): 344–45. https://doi.org/10.1080/15228967.2013.809890.

Ben-Moshe, Liat. 2005. "'Lame Idea': Disability Language in the Classroom." In *Building Pedagogical Curb Cuts: Incorporating Disability in the University Classroom and Curriculum,* ed. Lait Ben-Moshe et al., 107–15. Syracuse, NY: Syracuse University Press.

Bennett, Catherine. 2016. "Cheating in Sport Is Becoming Even Harder to Judge." *Guardian,* June 12. https://www.theguardian.com/commentisfree/2016/jun/11/sport-olympics-drugs-maria-sharapova-transgender.

Berger, Ronald J. 2008. "Disability and the Dedicated Wheelchair Athlete: Beyond the 'Supercrip' Critique." *Journal of Contemporary Ethnography* 37 (6): 647–78. https://doi.org/10.1177/0891241607309892.

–. 2013. *Introducing Disability Studies.* Boulder, CO: Lynne Rienner.

Bergman, Helena, and Barbara Hobson. 2002. "Compulsory Fatherhood: The Coding of Fatherhood in the Swedish Welfare State." In *Making Men into Fathers: Men, Masculinities and the Social Politics of Fatherhood,* ed. Barbara Hobson, 92–124. Cambridge, UK: Cambridge University Press. https://doi.org/10.1017/CBO9780511489440.

Bermon, Stéphane, and Pierre-Yves Garnier. 2017. "Serum Androgen Levels and Their Relation to Performance in Track and Field: Mass Spectrometry Results from 2127 Observations in Male and Female Elite Athletes." *British Journal of Sports Medicine* 51 (17): 1309–14. doi:10.1136/bjsports-2017-097792.

Best Start: Ontario's Maternal, Newborn and Early Child Development Resource Centre and the Halton Region Health Department. 2007. *Reflecting on the Trend: Pregnancy after Age 35: A Guide to Advanced Maternal Age for Ontario Service Providers, Including a Summary of Statistical Trends, Influencing Factors, Health Benefits, Health Risks and Recommendations for Care.* Toronto: Best Start: Ontario's Maternal, Newborn and Early Child Development Resource Centre. https://www.beststart.org/resources/rep_health/pdf/bs_pregnancy_age35.pdf.

Billings, Andrew, and Brittany D. Young. 2015. "Comparing Flagship News Programs: Women's Sport Coverage in ESPN's *SportsCenter* and FOX Sports 1's *FOX Sports Live.*" *Electronic News* 9 (1): 3–16. https://doi.org/10.1177/1931243115572824.

Bingham, John. 2013. "MPs: Abortions Being Carried out for Cleft Palates." *Telegraph* (London), July 17. http://www.telegraph.co.uk/news/politics/10183668/MPs-Abortions-being-carried-out-for-cleft-palates.html.

Binswanger-Mkhize, Hans P. 2013. "The Stunted Structural Transformation of the Indian Economy." *Economic and Political Weekly* 48 (26–27): 5–13.

Blackless, Melanie, et al. 2000. "How Sexually Dimorphic Are We? Review and Synthesis." *American Journal of Human Biology* 12 (2): 151–66. https://doi.org/10.1002/(SICI)1520-6300(200003/04)12:2<151::AID-AJHB1>3.0.CO;2-F.

Blackwell, Tom. 2016. "'Huge' Demand for IVF Treatment in Ontario – Where It's Fully Funded – Has Waitlists Stretching to 2018." *National Post,* May 20. https://nationalpost.com/health/huge-demand-for-ivf-treatment-in-ontario-where-its-fully-funded-has-wait-lists-stretching-to-2018.

Blair, Konrad. 2015. "When Doctors Get It Wrong." *Narrative Inquiry in Bioethics* 5 (2): 89–92. doi:10.1353/nib.2015.0029.

Blatchford, Christie. 2016. "Female Athletes Competing against 'Intersex' Women a Difficult, Complex Issue." *National Post,* August 21. https://nationalpost.com/sports/olympics/christie-blatchford-female-athletes-competing-against-intersex-women-a-difficult-complex-issue.

Bloom, Ben. 2016. "Caster Semenya Destroys Rest of the Field to Claim Easy Gold in Women's 800m Final – Can Anyone Beat Her?" *Telegraph* (London), August 21. http://www.telegraph.co.uk/olympics/2016/08/20/caster-semenya-womens-800m-final-rio-olympics-lynsey-sharp-team/.

Bödeker, Heike. 2000. "Symposium on Intersexuality." European Federation of Sexology Congress, Berlin.

Boellstorff, Tom. 2007. "When Marriage Falls: Queer Coincidences in Straight Time." *GLQ* 13 (2–3): 227–48. https://doi.org/10.1215/10642684-2006-032.

Bogart, Nicole. 2016. "Rio 2016: Sexist Coverage Highlights Challenges Facing Women in Sport." *Global News,* August 10. https://globalnews.ca/news/2875239/rio-2016-sexist-coverage-highlights-challenges-facing-women-in-sport/.

Bojesen, Anders, Svend Juul, and Claus Højbjerg Gravholt. 2003. "Prenatal and Postnatal Prevalence of Klinefelter Syndrome: A National Registry Study." *Journal of Clinical Endocrinology and Metabolism* 88 (2): 622–66. https://doi.org/10.1210/jc.2002-021491.

Bougnères, Bouvattier, et al. 2017. "Deferring Surgical Treatment of Ambiguous Genitalia into Adolescence in Girls with 21-Hydroxylase Deficiency: A Feasibility Study." *International Journal of Pediatric Endocrinology* 2017 (3): 1–5. https://doi.org/10.1186/s13633-016-0040-8.

Bourne, Hannah, Thomas Douglas, and Julian Savulescu. 2012. "Procreative Beneficence and *In Vitro* Gametogenesis." *Monash Bioethics Review* 30 (2): 29–48. doi:10.1007/BF03351338.

Bowcott, Owen. 2011. "Caster Semenya Has One of the 46 Types of 'Intersex' Conditions." *Guardian* (London), September 11. https://www.theguardian.com/sport/2009/sep/11/caster-semenya-runner-intersex.

Bracka, Aivar. 1995. "Hypospadias Repair: The Two-Stage Alternative." *British Journal of Urology* 76 (6): 31–41. https://doi.org/10.1111/j.1464-410X.1995.tb07815.x.

Braga, Luis H., et al. 2017. "Canadian Urological Association-Pediatric Urologists of Canada (CUA-PUC) Guideline for the Diagnosis, Management, and Followup of Cryptorchidism." *Canadian Urological Association* 11 (7): E251–60. doi:10.5489/cuaj.4585.

Braun, Virginia. 2009. "'The Women Are Doing It for Themselves': The Rhetoric of Choice and Agency around Female Genital 'Cosmetic Surgery.'" *Australia Feminist Studies* 24 (60): 233–49. https://doi.org/10.1080/08164640902852449.

Brittain, Ian, and Aaron Beacom, eds. 2018. *The Palgrave Handbook of Paralympic Studies*. London: Palgrave Macmillan. doi:10.1057/978-1-137-47901-3.

Brizendine, Louann. 2006. *The Female Brain*. London: Bantam.

Brouwers, Marijn M., et al. 2007. "Risk Factors for Hypospadias." *European Journal of Pediatrics* 166 (7): 671–78. https://doi.org/10.1007/s00431-006-0304-z.

Brown, Chris, and Chris Corday. 2016. "Classification System Can Be a Hurdle for Paralympic Athletes." *CBC*, September 9. http://www.cbc.ca/sports/paralympics/paralympics-classification-amy-burk-1.3755689.

Brown, Gavin. 2007. "Mutinous Eruptions: Autonomous Spaces of Radical Queer Activism." *Environmental and Planning* 38 (11): 2685–98. https://doi.org/10.1068/a38385.

Brunner, Franziska, et al. 2015. "Gender Role, Gender Identity and Sexual Orientation in CAIS ('XY-Women') Compared with Subfertile and Infertile 46,XX Women." *Journal of Sex Research* 53 (1): 109–24. https://doi.org/10.1080/00224499.2014.1002124.

Bucerius, Sandra M., and Michael Tonry, eds. 2014. *The Oxford Handbook of Ethnicity, Crime, and Immigration*. Oxford: Oxford University Press.

Burckhardt, Anna. 2017. "Research Spotlight: The Radical Story behind the Famous 'The Future Is Female' Graphic T-Shirt." *Medium*, December 7. https://medium.com/items/research-spotlight-the-radical-story-behind-the-famous-the-future-is-female-graphic-t-shirt-accdbbe37b65.

Burfoot, Amby. 2019. "After Latest Swiss Court Ruling, the Odds Are against Caster Semenya." *LetsRun.com*, August 2. https://www.letsrun.com/news/2019/08/after-latest-swiss-court-ruling-the-odds-are-against-caster-semenya/.

Butler, Judith. 1988. "Performative Acts and Gender Constitution: An Essay in Phenomenology and Feminist Theory." *Theatre Journal* 40 (4): 519–31. doi:10.2307/3207893.

–. 1993. *Bodies That Matter: On the Discursive Limits of Sex*. New York: Routledge. https://doi.org/10.4324/9780203828274.

–. 2004. *Undoing Gender*. New York: Routledge.

–. 2006. *Gender Trouble*. 1990. Reprint, New York: Routledge. https://doi.org/10.4324/9780203824979.

Buzuvis, Erin E. 2010. "Caster Semenya and the Myth of the Level Playing Field." *Modern American* 6 (2): 36–42. https://digitalcommons.wcl.american.edu/tma/vol6/iss2/.

Byers, Heather M., et al. 2017. "Unexpected Ethical Dilemmas in Sex Assignment in 46,XY DSD Due to 5-Alpha Reductase Type 2 Deficiency." *American Journal of Medical Genetics* 175 (2): 260–67. https://doi.org/10.1002/ajmg.c.31560.

Cadet, Peggy, and Marc D. Feldman. 2012. "Pretense of a Paradox: Factitious Intersex Conditions on the Internet." *International Journal of Sexual Health* 24 (2): 91–96. https://doi.org/10.1080/19317611.2011.629287.

Cahn, Susan K. 2015. *Coming on Strong: Gender and Sexuality in Twentieth-Century Women's Sport.* 2nd ed. Urbana: University of Illinois Press.

Cairns, James. 2017. *The Myth of the Age of Entitlement: Millennials, Austerity, and Hope.* Toronto: University of Toronto Press.

Cameron, David. 1999. "Caught Between: An Essay on Intersexuality." In *Intersex in the Age of Ethics,* ed. Alice Domurat Dreger, 91–96. Hagerstown, MD: University Publishing Group.

–. 2007. "My Intersex Journey: From Awkward Teenager to Human Rights Activist." In *21st Century Sexualities: Contemporary Issues in Health, Education, and Rights,* ed. Gilbert H. Herdt and Cymene Howe, 163–65. New York: Routledge.

Campbell, Fiona Kumari. 2000. "Eugenics in a Different Key? New Technologies and the 'Conundrum' of 'Disability.'" In *"A Race for a Place": Eugenics, Darwinism, and Social Thought and Practice in Australia,* ed. Martin Crotty, Grant W. Rodwell, and John Germov, 307–18. Newcastle, Australia: University of Newcastle Press.

Camporesi, Silvia, and Paolo Maugeri. 2016. "Unfair Advantage and the Myth of the Level Playing Field in IAAF and IOC Policies on Hyperandrogenism: When Is It Fair to Be a Woman?" In *Gender Testing in Sport: Ethics, Cases and Controversies,* ed. Sandy Montañoia and Aurélie Olivesi, 46–59. New York: Routledge.

Cannon, Martin. 1998. "The Regulation of First Nations Sexuality." *Canadian Journal of Native Studies* 18 (1): 1–18. http://www3.brandonu.ca/cjns/18.1/cjnsv18no1_pg1-18.pdf.

Caplan-Bricker, Nora. 2017. "Their Time." *Washington Post,* October 5. http://www.washingtonpost.com/sf/style/2017/10/05/the-intersex-rights-movement-is-ready-for-its-moment/?utm_term=.bb06603cccd0.

Carlson, Alison. 2005. "Suspect Sex." *Lancet* 366: S39–40. https://doi.org/10.1016/S0140-6736(05)67842-7.

Carmack, Adrienne. 2014. *Reclaiming My Birth Rights: A Mother's Wisdom Triumphs Over the Harmful Practices of Her Medical Profession.* Distributed via Smashwords.

Carmeli, Yoram S., and Daphna Birenbaum-Carmeli. 1994. "The Predicament of Masculinity: Towards Understanding the Male's Experience of Infertility Treatment." *Sex Roles* 30 (9–10): 663–777. https://doi.org/10.1007/BF01544669.

Carneiro, Fernando. 2016. "Paralympic Athletes Replaced with Able-Bodied Models in Vogue Rio Campaign." *Ottawa Metro,* August 24. Accessed June 10, 2019. http://www.metronews.ca/news/world/2016/08/24/paralympic-athletes-replaced-withmodels-in-vogue-campaign.html.

Carpenter, Morgan. 2012. "Intersex Intersectionalities." Intersex Human Rights Australia, October 29. https://ihra.org.au/21214/intersex-and-disability/.

–. 2013. "Intersex Health – Morgan Carpenter's Presentation to Health in Difference Conference." Intersex Human Rights Australia, April 22. https://ihra.org.au/22160/intersex-health-hid2013-plenary/.

–. 2014. "Submission on the Ethics of Genetic Selection against Intersex Traits." Intersex Human Rights Australia, April 29. https://ihra.org.au/25621/submission-ethics-genetic-selection-intersex-traits/.

–. 2016. "LGBTI Sponsorship and the Elimination of Intersex Traits." Intersex Human Rights Australia, July 10. https://ihra.org.au/30555/sponsorship-elimination-intersex-traits/.

–. 2018. "The 'Normalization' of Intersex Bodies and 'Othering' of Intersex Identities in Australia." *Journal of Bioethical Inquiry* 15 (4): 487–95. https://doi.org/10.1007/s11673-018-9855-8.

–. 2019. "Identification Documents." Intersex Human Rights Australia, January 4. https://ihra.org.au/identities/.

Carr, Grace. 2017. "Here's What the 2018 Olympic Gender Regulations Look Like." *Daily Caller,* July 3. http://dailycaller.com/2017/07/03/heres-what-the-2018-olympic-gender-regulations-look-like/.

Carroll, Rachel. 2012. *Rereading Heterosexuality: Feminism, Queer Theory and Contemporary Fiction.* Edinburgh: Edinburgh University Press.

Casey, Bill. 2019. *The Health of LGBTQIA2 Communities in Canada: Report of the Standing Committee on Health.* Ottawa: House of Commons. https://www.cbrc.net/the_health_of_lgbtqia2_communities_in_canada_report_of_the_standing_committee_on_health.

Catalano, D. Chase J. 2015. "'Trans Enough?': The Pressures Trans Men Negotiate in Higher Education." *TSQ* 2 (3): 411–30. https://doi.org/10.1215/23289252-2926399.

Cavanagh, Sheila L., and Heather Sykes. 2006. "Transsexual Bodies at the Olympics: The International Olympic Committee's Policy on Transsexual Athletes at the 2004 Athens Summer Games." *Body and Society* 12 (3): 75–102. https://doi.org/10.1177/1357034X06067157.

Chadwick, Simon, Nicolas Chanavat, and Michel Desbordes, eds. 2016. *Routledge Handbook of Sports Marketing.* New York: Routledge.

Chang, Sydney. 2020. "Hypospadias: A Congenital Abnormality That Causes Male Factor Infertility." *Progyny,* February 3. https://progyny.com/education/male-infertility/hypospadias-male-factor-infertility.

Channel 4. 2016. "We're the Superhumans | Rio Paralympics 2016 Trailer." *YouTube,* July 14. https://www.youtube.com/watch?v=IocLkk3aYlk.

Chapman, Chris. 2016. "My Life with Hypospadias." *Mosaic,* October 3. https://mosaicscience.com/story/my-life-hypospadias/.

Charlewood, Godfrey. 1956. *Bantu Gynaecology.* Johannesburg: University of Witwatersrand Press.

Charlton, James I. 1998. *Nothing About Us Without Us: Disability Oppression and Empowerment.* Berkeley: University of California Press.

Chase, Cheryl. 1998. "Affronting Reason." In *Looking Queer: Body Image and Identity in Lesbian, Bisexual, Gay, and Transgender Communities,* ed. Dawn Atkins, 201–20. New York: Routledge. https://doi.org/10.4324/9780203047477.

–. 1999. "Surgical Progress Is Not the Answer." In *Intersex in the Age of Ethics,* ed. Alice Domurat Dreger, 147–60. Farnham, UK: University Publishing Group.

–. 2002. "'Cultural Practice' or 'Reconstructive Surgery'? U.S. Genital Cutting, the Intersex Movement, and Medical Double Standards." In *Genital Cutting and Transnational Sisterhood: Disputing U.S. Polemics,* ed. Stanlie M. James and Claire C. Robertson, 126–52. Robertson: University of Illinois Press.

–. 2006. "Hermaphrodites with Attitude: Mapping the Emergence of Intersex Political Activism." In *The Transgender Studies Reader,* ed. Susan Stryker and Stephan Whittle, 300–14. New York: Routledge. https://doi.org/10.4324/9780203955055.

Chemers, Michael M. 2008. *Staging Stigma: A Critical Examination of the American Freak Show.* New York: Palgrave Macmillan. doi:10.1057/9780230616813.

Chen, Mel Y. 2011. "Toxic Animacies, Inanimate Affections." *GLQ* 17 (2–3): 265–86. https://doi.org/10.1215/10642684-1163400.

Cherry, Gene. 2018. "Canada Group Has Serious Concerns of IAAF Hyperandrogenism Rule." *Reuters,* April 30. https://www.reuters.com/article/us-athletics-iaaf-hyperandrogenism-canad/canada-group-has-serious-concerns-of-iaaf-hyperandrogenism-rule-idUSKBN1I12CE.

Chew, Kristina. 2013. "Would You Abort a Disabled Child?" *Guardian* (London), April 22. https://www.theguardian.com/commentisfree/2013/apr/22/abort-down-syndrome-child-society-shares-blame.

Christensen, Ben. 2011. "Interfiling Intersex: How Dewey Classifies Intersex in Theory and in Practice." In *Serving LGBTIQ Library and Archives Users: Essays on Outreach, Service, Collections and Access,* ed. Ellen Greenblatt, 201–11. Jefferson, NC: McFarland and Company.

Chu, Judy Y., et al. 2009. "The Status of Boyhood Studies." *Boyhood Studies: An Interdisciplinary Journal* 3 (2): 111–54. https://doi.org/10.3149/thy.0301.111.

Church, Elizabeth. 2015. "Ontario Government Sets Age Limit at 43 for IVF Coverage." *Globe and Mail,* October 1. http://www.theglobeandmail.com/news/national/ontarios-liberal-government-to-fund-a-cycle-of-ivf-for-women/article26616360/.

Cinman, Nadya M., et al. 2012. "Acquired Male Urethral Diverticula: Presentation, Diagnosis and Management." *Journal of Urology* 188 (4): 1204–8. https://doi.org/10.1016/j.juro.2012.06.036.

City Fertility. 2020. "Genetic Testing." https://www.cityfertility.com.au/fertility-services/ivf-treatment/genetic-testing-pgd/.

Clare, Eli. 2009. *Exile and Pride: Disability, Queerness, and Liberation.* 1999. Reprint, Durham, NC: Duke University Press. https://doi.org/10.1215/9780822374879.

–. 2010. "Disability Pride." August 9. http://eliclare.com/disability/disability-pride.

–. 2017. *Brilliant Imperfection: Grappling with Cure.* Durham, NC: Duke University Press. https://doi.org/10.1215/9780822373520.

Claridge, Jeffery A., and Timothy C. Fabian. 2005. "History and Development of Evidence-Based Medicine." *World Journal of Surgery* 29 (5): 547–53. https://doi.org/10.1007/s00268-005-7910-1.

Clearway, Ajae, dir. 2007. *One in 2000.* Polyvinyl Pictures.

Cohen, Marilyn. 2009. *No Girls in the Clubhouse: The Exclusion of Women from Baseball.* London: McFarland.

Cole, C.L. 2000. "Testing for Sex or Drugs." *Journal of Sport and Social Issues* 24 (4): 331–33. https://doi.org/10.1177/0193723500244001.

Colligan, Simi. 2004. "Why the Intersexed Shouldn't Be Fixed: Insights from Queer Theory and Disability Studies." In *Gendering Disability*, ed. Bonnie G. Smith and Beth Huthison, 45–60. New Brunswick, NJ: Rutgers University Press.

Collins, Patricia Hill. 1986. "Learning from the Outsider Within: The Sociological Significance of Black Feminist Thought." *Social Problems* 33 (6): 14–32. https://doi.org/10.2307/800672.

—. 1989. "The Social Construction of Black Feminist Thought." *Signs: Journal of Women in Culture and Society* 14 (4): 745–73. https://doi.org/10.1086/494543.

—. 2000. *Black Feminist Thought: Knowledge, Consciousness, and the Politics of Empowerment.* 2nd ed. New York: Routledge.

—. 2004. *Black Sexual Politics: African Americans, Gender and the New Racism.* New York: Routledge.

Conley, Tameka Cage. 2016. "The Future Is Present and All Around: How Alisha B. Wormsley Remakes the World." *Offing*, February 16. https://theoffingmag.com/enumerate/the-future-is-present-and-all-around/.

Connell, Raewyn W., and James W. Messerschmidt. 2005. "Hegemonic Masculinity: Rethinking the Concept." *Gender and Society* 19 (6): 829–59. https://doi.org/10.1177/0891243205278639.

Connelly, Tony. 2016. "Media Cautioned over Use of 'Superhuman,' 'Brave' and 'Heroes' in Paralympic Reporting." *Drum*, September 5. http://www.thedrum.com/news/2016/09/05/media-cautioned-over-use-superhuman-brave-and-heroes-paralympics-reporting.

Connor, David J., Beth A. Ferrir, and Subini A. Annamma, eds. 2016. *DisCrit: Disability Studies and Critical Race Theory in Education.* New York: Teachers College Press.

Conrad, Peter, and Joseph W. Schneider. 1992. *Deviance and Medicalization: From Badness to Sickness.* 1980. Reprint, Philadelphia: Temple University Press.

Cooky, Cheryl, and Shari L. Dworkin. 2013. "Policing the Boundaries of Sex: A Critical Examination of Gender Verification and the Caster Semenya Controversy." *Journal of Sex Research* 50 (2): 103–11. https://doi.org/10.1080/00224499.2012.725488.

Cooky, Cheryl, Ranissa Dycus, and Shari L. Dworkin. 2013. "'What Makes a Woman a Woman?' versus 'Our First Lady of Sport': A Comparative Analysis of the Unites States and the South African Media Coverage of Caster Semenya." *Journal of Sport and Social Issues* 37 (1): 31–56. https://doi.org/10.1177/0193723512447940.

Cools, Martine, et al. 2006. "Germ Cell Tumors in the Intersex Gonad: Old Paths, New Directions, Moving Frontiers." *Endocrine Reviews* 27 (5): 468–84. https://doi.org/10.1210/er.2006-0005.

—. 2018. "Caring for Individuals with a Difference of Sex Development (DSD): A Consensus Statement." *Nature Reviews: Endocrinology* 14 (7): 415–29. https://doi.org/10.1038/s41574-018-0010-8.

Cooper, Emily J. 2010. "Gender Testing in Athletic Competitions – Human Rights Violations: Why Michael Phelps Is Praised and Caster Semenya Is Chastised." *Journal of Gender, Race, and Justice* 14 (1): 233–64.

CooperSurgical. n.d. "PGT-A." https://www.coopergenomics.com/pgta/.

Cornwall, Susannah. 2009. "Theologies of Resistance: Intersex/DSD, Disability and Queering the 'Real World.'" In *Critical Intersex*, ed. Morgan Holmes, 215–44. Farnham, UK: Ashgate. https://doi.org/10.4324/9781315575018.

–. 2013. "Asking About What Is Better: Intersex, Disability, and Inaugurated Eschatology." *Journal of Religion, Disability, and Health* 17 (4): 369–92. https://doi.org/10.1080/15228967.2013.840972.

–. 2014. *Sex and Uncertainty in the Body of Christ: Intersex Conditions and Christian Theology.* New York: Routledge.

Coskun, Sahin, and Tamer Seyhan. 2003. "Use of Buccal Mucsal Grafts in Hypospadia-Crippled Adult Patients." *Annals of Plastic Surgery* 50 (4): 382–86. doi:10.1097/01.SAP.0000037274.65665.FF.

Costa, Elaine Maria Frade, et al. 1997. "Management of Ambiguous Genitalia in Pseudohermaphrodites: New Perspectives on Vaginal Dilation." *Fertility and Sterility* 67 (2): 229–32. https://doi.org/10.1016/S0015-0282(97)81902-4.

Costello, Cary Gabriel. 2009. "Caster Semenya – An Intersex Perspective." *The Intersex Roadshow*, August 22. http://intersexroadshow.blogspot.ca/2009/08/caster-semenya-intersex-perspective.html.

–. 2012a. "How Common Is Intersex Status?" *The Intersex Roadshow*, March 13. https://intersexroadshow.blogspot.com/2012/03/how-common-is-intersex-status.html.

–. 2012b. "On Trans Gender Identity and the 'Intersex Brain.'" *Trans Fusion*, August 3. http://trans-fusion.blogspot.ca/2012/08/on-trans-gender-identity-and-intersex.html.

–. 2013. "Just-So Stories about Hermaphrodite Fish." *The Intersex Roadshow*, January 2. http://intersexroadshow.blogspot.ca/2013/01/.

–. 2014a. "Are Trans Communities Losing Intersex Allies in the TERF Wars?" *Trans Fusion*, September 14. http://trans-fusion.blogspot.ca/2014/09/are-trans-communities-losing-intersex.html.

–. 2014b. "Cis Gender, Trans Gender, and Intersex." *The Intersex Roadshow*, August 5. http://intersexroadshow.blogspot.ca/2014/08/cis-gender-trans-gender-and-intersex.html.

–. 2014c. "On Eugenic Abortion of the Intersex." *The Intersex Roadshow*, April 29. http://intersexroadshow.blogspot.ca/2014/04/on-eugenic-abortion-of-intersex.html.

–. 2015. "Cis Gender, Ipso Gender." *Trans Fusion*, June 30. http://trans-fusion.blogspot.ca/2015/06/cis-gender-ipso-gender.html.

–. 2016. "Intersex and Trans* Communities: Commonalities and Tensions." In *Transgender and Intersex: Theoretical, Practical, and Artistic Perspectives*, ed. Stephan Horlacher, 83–113. New York: Palgrave Macmillan. https://doi.org/10.1057/978-1-349-71325-7_4.

–. 2019a. "Intersex Experience and Fears about 'Gay Genetics.'" *The Intersex Road-show,* September 2. https://intersexroadshow.blogspot.com/2019/09/intersex
-experience-and-fears-about-gay.html.

–. 2019b. "Understanding Intersex Relationship Issues." In *Expanding the Rainbow: Exploring the Relationships of Bi+, Polyamorous, Kinky, Ace, Intersex and Trans People,* ed. Brandy L. Simula, J.E. Sumerau, and Andrea Miller, 231–45. Leiden: Brill Sense. https://doi.org/10.1163/9789004414105.

Côté, Anne. 2000. "Telling the Truth? Disclosure, Therapeutic Privilege and Inter-sexuality in Children." *Health Law Journal* 8: 199–216.

Court of Arbitration for Sport. 2017. "Media Release: Athletics: CAS Suspends the IAAF Hyperandrogenism Regulations until End of September 2017." July 28. https://www.tas-cas.org/fileadmin/user_upload/Media_Release_3759_July_2017.pdf.

Couser, Thomas. 2000. "The Empire of the 'Normal': A Forum on Disability and Self-Representation: Introduction." *American Quarterly* 52 (2): 305–10. doi:10.1353/aq.2000.0017.

–. 2009. *Signifying Bodies: Disability in Contemporary Life Writing.* Ann Arbor: Uni-versity of Michigan Press. doi:10.3998/mpub.915367.

Couture, Vincent, et al. 2013. "Gender Eugenics between Medicine, Culture, and Society." *American Journal of Bioethics* 13 (10): 57–59. https://doi.org/10.1080/15265161.2013.828129.

Coventry, Martha. 1998. "The Tyranny of the Esthetic Surgery's Most Intimate Violation." *On the Issues Magazine,* Summer. https://www.ontheissuesmaga-zine.com/1998summer/su98coventry.php.

–. 1999. "Finding the Words." In *Intersex in the Age of Ethics,* ed. Alice Domurat Dreger, 71–78. Hagerstown, MD: University Publishing Group.

Covington, Carter, dir. 2014–16. *Faking It.* Viacom Media Networks.

Cox, David. 2014. "Are We Ready for a Prenatal Screening Test for Autism?" *Guardian* (London), May 1. https://www.theguardian.com/science/blog/2014/may/01/prenatal-scrrening-test-autism-ethical-implications.

Craig, James R., et al. 2014. "Management of Adults with Prior Failed Hypospadias Surgery." *Transnational Andrology and Urology* 3 (2): 196–204. doi:10.3978/j.issn.2223-4683.2014.04.03.

Crawford, Catherine Leigh. 2019. "Handle with Care: Assessing Canadian Med-ical Policy for Children with Intersex Variations." MA thesis, Simon Fraser University.

Creighton, Sarah, et al. 2002. "Medical Photography: Ethics, Consent and the Intersex Patient." *BJU International* 89 (1): 67–72. https://doi.org/10.1046/j.1464-410X.2002.02558.x.

crippledscholar. 2016. "Can We Talk about That Paralympics Ad?" July 18. https://crippledscholar.com/2016/07/18/can-we-talk-about-that-paralympics-ad/.

Critchley, Mark. 2016. "Rio 2016: Fifth-Placed Joanna Jozwik 'Feels Like Silver Medalist' after 800m Defeat to Caster Semenya." *Independent* (London), August 22. http://www.independent.co.uk/sport/olympics/rio-2016-joanna-jozwik-caster-semenya-800m-hyperandrogenism-a7203731.html.

Crotty, Martin, Grant W. Rodwell, and John Germov, eds. 2000. *"A Race for a Place":* *Eugenics, Darwinism, and Social Thought and Practice in Australia.* Newcastle, Australia: University of Newcastle Press.

Crowe, Christine. 2000. "Inheriting Eugenics? Genetics, Reproduction and Eugenic Legacies." In *'A Race for a Place': Eugenics, Darwinism, and Social Thought and Practice in Australi,* ed. Martin Crotty, Grant W. Rodwell, and John Germov, 173–80. Newcastle, Australia: University of Newcastle Press.

Cunningham, George B. 2003. "Media Coverage of Women's Sport: A New Look at an Old Problem." *Physical Educator* 60 (2): 43–47.

Cuordileone, K.A. 2000. "'Politics in an Age of Anxiety': Cold War Political Culture and the Crisis in American Masculinity, 1949–1960." *Journal of American History* 87 (2): 515–45. doi:10.2307/2568762.

Cuvier, Georges. 1817. "Extrait d'observations faite sur le cadavre d'une femme connue à Paris et à Londres sous le nom de Vénus Hottentotte." In *Memoires du Musée d'histoire naturelle,* ed. Tome Troisième, 259–74. Paris: Chez A. Belin, Imprimeur-Libraire.

Daddario, Gina. 1998. *Women's Sport and Spectacle: Gendered Television Coverage and the Olympic Games.* Westport, CT: Praeger.

Dalbey, Alex. 2019. "The Scrutiny over Caster Semenya's Body Is a Study in Racism, Sexism, and Transphobia." *Daily Dot,* May 1. https://www.dailydot.com/irl/caster-semenya-cas-ruling/?fbclid=IwAR0_5JW3fLTX-nt6hoYCk8o224-zfTgxKLfBc5A-exANzwxZ3hH8Wwg434I.

Daly, Kathleen. 2000. "Restorative Justice in Diverse and Unequal Societies." *Law Context: A Socio-Legal Journal* 17 (1): 167–90.

Daly, Kathleen, and Julie Stubbs. 2006. "Feminist Engagement with Restorative Justice." *Theoretical Criminology* 10 (1): 9–28. https://doi.org/10.1177/1362480606059980.

Damani, Manish, Rajesh Mittal, and Robert D. Oates. 2001. "Testicular Tissue Extraction in a Young Male with 47,XXY Klinefelter's Syndrome: Potential Strategy for Preservation of Fertility." *Fertility and Sterility* 76 (5): 1054–56. https://doi.org/10.1016/S0015-0282(01)02837-0.

Darby, Paul. 2002. *Africa, Football, and FIFA: Politics, Colonialism, and Resistance.* London: Frank Cass. https://doi.org/10.4324/9781315039527.

Darnell, Simon C., and Lyndsay M.C. Hayhurst. 2011. "Sport for Decolonization: Exploring a New Praxis of Sport for Development." *Progress in Development Studies* 11 (3): 183–96. https://doi.org/10.1177/146499341001100301.

Darsey, James. 1991. "From 'Gay Is Good' to the Scourge of AIDS: The Evolution of Gay Liberation Rhetoric, 1977–1990." *Communication Studies* 42 (1): 43–66. https://doi.org/10.1080/10510979109368320.

Daston, Lorraine, and Peter Galison. 2007. *Objectivity.* New York: Zone Books.

Davis, Angela. 2003. "Racism, Birth Control, and Reproductive Rights." In *Feminist Postcolonial Theory: A Reader,* ed. Reina Lewis and Sara Mills, 353–67. New York: Routledge.

Davis, Colin. 2005. "Hauntology, Spectres and Phantoms." *French Studies* 59 (3): 373–79. https://doi.org/10.1093/fs/kni143.

Davis, Georgiann. 2013. "The Social Costs of Preempting Intersex Traits." *American Journal of Bioethics* 13 (10): 51–53. https://doi.org/10.1080/15265161.2013.828119.

–. 2014. "The Power in a Name: Diagnostic Terminology and Diverse Experiences." *Psychology and Sexuality* 5 (1): 15–27. https://doi.org/10.1080/19419899.2013.831212.

–. 2015. *Contesting Intersex: The Dubious Diagnosis.* New York: New York University Press.

–. 2016. "Intersexy Fat." *Intersex Day,* October 19. http://intersexday.org/en/intersexy-fat/.

–. 2017. "UNVL Professor Explores the 'Dubious Diagnosis' in Book about Intersex People." Interview with Casey Morell. *Nevada Public Radio,* March 3. https://knpr.org/knpr/2017-03/unlv-professor-explores-dubious-diagnosis-book-about-intersex-people.

Davis, Georgiann, Jodie M. Dewey, and Erin L. Murphy. 2016. "Giving Sex: Deconstructing Intersex and Trans Medicalization Practices." *Gender and Society* 30 (3): 490–515. https://doi.org/10.1177/0891243215602102.

Davis, Jenny L. 2012. "Narrative Construction of a Ruptured Self: Stories of Transability on Transabled.org." *Sociological Perspectives* 55 (2): 319–40. https://doi.org/10.1525/sop.2012.55.2.319.

Davis, Lennard J. 1995. *Enforcing Normalcy: Disability, Deafness, and the Body.* Brooklyn, NY: Verso.

–. 2013. "Introduction: Disability, Normality, and Power." In *The Disability Studies Reader,* 4th ed., ed. Lennard J. Davis, 1–16. New York: Routledge.

Dawley, Katy. 2003. "Origins of Nurse-Midwifery in the United States and Its Expansion in the 1940s." *Journal of Midwifery and Women's Health* 48 (2): 86–95. https://doi.org/10.1016/S1526-9523(03)00002-3.

Dean, Terrance, and Dale P. Andrews. 2016. "Introduction: Afrofuturism in Black Theology – Race, Gender, Sexuality, and the State of Black Religion in the Black Metropolis." *Black Theology: An International Journal* 14 (1): 2–5. https://doi.org/10.1080/14769948.2015.1131499.

De Bellefonds, Colleen. 2019. "Why Michael Phelps Has the Perfect Body for Swimming." *Biography,* June 26. https://www.biography.com/news/michael-phelp-perfect-body-swimming.

Deifelt, Wanda. 2005. "Beyond Compulsory Motherhood." In *Good Sex: Feminist Perspectives from the World's Religions,* ed. Patricia Beattie Jung, Mary E. Hunt, and Radhika Balakrisnan, 96–112. New Brunswick, NJ: Rutgers University Press.

del Cura, Mercedes. 2017. "The Future We Want: Demanding Rights for People with Disabilities during the Spanish Democratic Transition." *Public Disability History,* January 30. http://www.public-disabilityhistory.org/2017/01/the-future-we-want-demanding-rights-for.html.

Deliovsky, Kathy. 2008. "Normative White Femininity: Race, Gender and the Politics of Beauty." *Atlantis: Critical Studies in Gender, Culture and Social Justice* 33 (1): 49–59. https://journals.msvu.ca/index.php/atlantis/article/view/429.

Dembe, Joel. 2018. "Struggle with Paralympic Exposure in Canada Nothing New." *CBC,* March 8. https://www.cbc.ca/sports/paralympics/struggle-with-paralympic -exposure-in-canada-nothing-new-1.4565864.

Derrida, Jacques. 1994. *Specters of Marx: The State of the Debt, the Work of Mourning, and the New International.* Trans. Peggy Kamuf. Original 1993. New York: Routledge.

Devine, Charles J., and Charles E. Horton. 2002. "A One Stage Hypospadias Repair." *Journal of Urology* 167 (2, Part 2): 1169–74. https://doi.org/10.1016/S0022 -5347(02)80372-X.

Devitt, Mark Arthur. 2011. "The Myth of Olympic Unity: The Dilemma of Diversity, Olympic Oppression, and the Politics of Difference." MA thesis, University of Toronto.

Devore, Tiger. 1999. "Growing up in the Surgical Maelstrom." In *Intersex in the Age of Ethics,* ed. Alice Domurat Dreger, 79–82. Hagerstown, MD: University Publishing Group.

Diamond, Milton, and H. Keith Sigmundson. 1997. "Sex Reassignment at Birth: Long-Term Review and Clinical Implications." *Archives of Pediatrics and Adolescent Medicine Journal* 151 (3): 298–304. doi:10.1001/archpedi.1997.02170400084015.

Döhnert, Ulla, Lutz Wünsch, and Olaf Hiort. 2017. "Gonadectomy in Complete Androgen Insensitivity Syndrome: Why and When." *Sexual Development* 11 (4): 171–74. https://doi.org/10.1159/000478082.

Dolmage, Jay Timothy. 2014. *Disability Rhetoric.* New York: Syracuse University Press. doi:10.2307/j.ctt1j2n73m.

Donnellan, Laura. 2008. "Gender Testing at the Beijing Olympics." *Sport and the Law Journal* 16 (1): 20–28. http://www.britishsportslaw.com/wp-content/ uploads/2017/10/BASL-Vol-16-Issue-1-1.pdf.

Dörner, Günter. 2010. "Perinatal Brain Programming and Functional Teratology." *Journal of Perinatal Medicine* 38 (1): 1–2. doi:10.1515/jpm.2010.178.

Dreger, Alice Domurat. 1998. *Hermaphrodites and the Medical Invention of Sex.* Cambridge, MA: Harvard University Press.

–. 1999a. "A History of Intersex: From the Age of Gonads to the Age of Consent." In *Intersex in the Age of Ethics,* ed. Alice Domurat Dreger, 5–22. Hagerstown, MD: University Publishing Group.

–, ed. 1999b. *Intersex in the Age of Ethics.* Hagerstown, MD: University Publishing Group.

–. 2010. "Sex Typing for Sport." *Hastings Centre Report* 40 (2): 22–24. https://doi. org/10.1353/hcr.0.0250.

–. 2017. "Do You Have to Pee Standing Up to Be a Real Man?" *Pacific Standard,* June 14. https://psmag.com/social-justice/pee-standing-real-man-73133#.yfx7tme1k.

Dreger, Alice Domurat, Ellen K. Feder, and Anne Tamar-Mattis. 2012. "Prenatal Dexamethasone for Congenital Adrenal Hyperplasia." *Journal of Bioethical Inquiry* 9 (3): 277–94. https://doi.org/10.1007/s11673-012-9384-9.

Driskill, Qwo-Li. 2004. "Stolen from Our Bodies: First Nations Two-Spirits/Queers and the Journey to a Sovereign Erotic." *Studies in American Indian Literatures* 16 (2): 50–64. doi:10.1353/ail.2004.0020.

Dryden, OmiSoore H., and Suzanne Lenon, eds. 2015. *Disrupting Inclusion: Canadian Homonationalism and the Politics of Belonging.* Vancouver: UBC Press.

Dudek, Ronald W. 2014. *High-Yield Embryology.* 15th ed. Philadelphia: Lippincott Williams and Wilkins.

Duggan, Lisa. 2002. "The New Homonormativity: The Sexual Politics of Neoliberalism." In *Materializing Democracy: Toward a Revitalized Cultural Politics,* ed. Russ Castronova and Dana D. Nelson, 175–94. Durham, NC: Duke University Press. https://doi.org/10.1215/9780822383901.

Dunbar, Graham. 2019. "Caster Semenya Loses Appeal against IAAF Testosterone Rules." *CBC,* May 1. https://www.cbc.ca/sports/olympics/trackandfield/caster-semenya-appeal-1.5117936.

Dunn, Thomas R. 2016. *Queerly Remembered: Rhetorics for Representing the GLBTQ Past.* Columbia: University of South Carolina Press.

Dworkin, Shari L., and Cheryl Cooky. 2012. "Sport, Sex Segregation, and Sex Testing: Critical Reflections on This Unjust Marriage." *American Journal of Bioethics* 12 (7): 21–23. https://doi.org/10.1080/15265161.2012.680545.

Dynes, Wayne R. 2014. *The Homophobic Mind.* New York: Wayne R. Dynes.

Eckert, Lena. 2009. "'Diagnosticism': Three Cases of Medical Anthropological Research into Intersexuality." In *Critical Intersex,* ed. Morgan Holmes, 41–72. Farnham, UK: Ashgate. https://doi.org/10.4324/9781315575018.

Edelman, Lee. 2004. *No Future: Queer Theory and the Death Drive.* Durham, NC: Duke University Press. https://doi.org/10.1215/9780822385981.

Edney, Richard. 2004. "To Keep Me Safe from Harm? Transgender Prisoners and the Experience of Imprisonment." *Deakin Law Review* 9 (4): 327–38. https://doi.org/10.21153/dlr2004vol9no2art247.

Edwin, Ama Kyerewaa. 2008. "Don't Lie but Don't Tell The Whole Truth: The Therapeutic Privilege – Is It Ever Justified?" *Ghana Medical Journal* 42 (4): 156–61. https://www.ncbi.nlm.nih.gov/pmc/articles/PMC2673833/.

Egale Canada Human Rights Trust. 2019. *Supporting Your Intersex Child.* Toronto: Egale Canada Human Rights Trust. https://egale.ca/awareness/supporting-your-intersex-child/.

Ehrenreich, Nancy, and Mark Barr. 2005. "Intersex Surgery, Female Genital Cutting, and the Selective Condemnation of 'Cultural Practices.'" *Harvard Civil Rights-Civil Liberties Law Review* 40: 71–140. https://ssrn.com/abstract=2926589.

Elders, M. Joycelyn, David Satcher, and Richard Carmona. 2017. "Re-thinking Genital Surgeries on Intersex Infants." Palm Center, Blueprints for Sound Public Policy, June. https://www.palmcenter.org/wp-content/uploads/2017/06/Re-Thinking-Genital-Surgeries-1.pdf.

Elliot, Carl. 1998. "Why Can't We Go On as Three?" *Hastings Venter Report* 28 (30): 36–39. doi:10.2307/3528649.

English, Colleen. 2018. "Rewarding Participation in Youth Sport: Beyond Trophies for Winning (Premiando la participación en el deporte para jóvenes: más allá de los trofeos por ganar)." *Cultura, Ciencia y Deporte* 13 (38): 109–18. http://dx.doi.org/10.12800/ccd.v13i38.1066.

Erevelles, Nirmala. 2011. *Disability and Difference in Global Contexts: Enabling a Transformative Body Politics.* New York: Palgrave Macmillan. doi:10.1057/9781137001184.

Erevelles, Nirmala, and Andrea Minear. 2010. "Unspeakable Offenses: Untangling Race and Disability in Discourses of Intersectionality." *Journal of Literary and Cultural Disability Studies* 4 (2): 127–45. https://doi.org/10.3828/jlcds.2010.11.

Eshun, Kodwo. 2003. "Further Considerations of Afrofuturism." *CR: The New Centennial Review* 3 (2): 287–302. doi:10.1353/ncr.2003.0021.

Essack, Faatimah. 2016. "Caster Semenya Soars to Greatness: Intersex Gold Medalist." *Affinity*, August 22. http://affinitymagazine.us/2016/08/22/caster-semenya-soars-to-greatness-intersex-gold-medalist/.

Evans, Michele K., et al. 2020. "Diagnosing and Treating Systemic Racism." *New England Journal of Medicine* 383 (3): 274–76. doi:10.1056/NEJMe2021693.

Eveleth, Rose. 2012. "Does Double-Amputee Oscar Pistorius Have an Unfair Advantage at the 2012 Olympic Games?" *Smithsonian Magazine*, July 22. http://www.smithsonianmag.com/summerolympics/does-double-amputee-oscar-pistorius-have-an-unfair-advantage-at-the-2012-olympic-games-2655123/.

Ezie, Chinyere. 2011. "Deconstructing the Body: Transgender and Intersex Identities and Sex Discrimination – The Need for Strict Scrutiny." *Columbia Journal of Gender and Law* 20: 141–59. https://ssrn.com/abstract=1589519.

Fagerholm, Riitta, Risto Rintala, and Seppo Taskinen. 2013. "Lower Urinary Tract Symptoms after Feminizing Genitoplasy." *Pediatric Urology* 9 (1): 23–26. https://doi.org/10.1016/j.jpurol.2011.10.023.

Fahs, Breanne. 2014. "Genital Panics: Constructing the Vagina in Women's Qualitative Narratives about Pubic Hair, Menstrual Sex, and Vaginal Self-Image." *Body Image* 11 (3): 210–18. https://doi.org/10.1016/j.bodyim.2014.03.002.

Fallowfield, Lesley J., Victoria A. Jenkins, and Hazel A. Beveridge. 2002. "Truth May Hurt but Deceit Hurts More: Communication in Palliative Care." *Palliative Medicine* 16 (4): 297–303. https://doi.org/10.1191/0269216302pm575oa.

Fausto-Sterling, Anne. 1992. *Myths of Gender: Biological Theories about Women and Men.* New York: Basic Books.

–. 2000. *Sexing the Body: Gender Politics and the Construction of Sexuality.* New York: Basic Books.

Feldman, Marc D. 2000. "Munchausen by Internet: Detecting Factitious Illness and Crisis on the Internet." *Southern Medical Journal* 93 (7): 669–72.

Fentiman, Linda C. 2019. *Blaming Mothers: American Law and the Risks to Children's Health.* New York: New York University Press. doi:10.18574/nyu/9780814724828.001.0001.

Ferguson, Tomika, and James W. Satterfield. 2017. "Black Women Athletes and the Performance of Hyperfemininity." In *Critical Perspectives on Black Women and College Success*, ed. Lori D. Patton and Natasha N. Croom, 115–26. New York: Routledge.

Fichtner, Jan, et al. 1995. "Analysis of Meatal Location in 500 Men: Wide Variation Questions Need for More Meatal Advancement in All Pediatric Anterior

Hypospadias Cases." *Journal of Urology* 154 (2): 833–34. https://doi.org/10.1016/S0022-5347(01)67177-5.

Fiedler, Leslie. 1996. *Tyranny of the Normal: Essays on Bioethics, Theology and Myth.* Boston: David R. Godine.

Fisher, Mark. 2013. "The Metaphysics of Crackle: Afrofuturism and Hauntology." *Dancecult: Journal of Electronic Dance Music Culture* 5 (2): 42–55. https://doi.org/10.12801/1947-5403.2013.05.02.03.

Flanagan, Jane. 2016. "Is This the Most Bitter Rematch in Athletics? Controversial Gold Medalist Caster Semenya BEATS Her White Rivals Who Criticised Her 'Unfair' Advantage." *Daily Mail* (London), September 1. http://www.dailymail.co.uk/news/article-3769082/Is-bitter-rematch-athletics-Controversial-gold-medallist-Caster-Semenya-run-against-white-rivals-criticised-unfair-advantage-dedicates-sporting-award-haters.html.

Florida, Richard. 2005. "The World in Numbers: The World Is Spiky." *Atlantic Monthly,* October, 49–51.

Flower, William Henry, and James Murie. 1867. "Account of the Dissection of a Bushwoman." *Journal of Anatomy and Physiology* 1 (2): 189–208.

Ford, Kishka-Kamari. 2001. "'First, Do No Harm' – The Fiction of Legal Parental Consent to Genital Normalizing Surgery on Intersexed Infants." *Yale Law and Policy* 19 (2): 469–88.

Fox, Justin. 2014. "The World Is Still Not Flat." *Harvard Business Review,* November 3. https://hbr.org/2014/11/the-world-is-still-not-flat.

French, Liam, and Jill M. Le Clair. 2018. "Game Changer? Social Media, Representations of Disability and the Paralympic Games." In *The Palgrave Handbook of Paralympic Studies,* ed. Ian Brittain and Aaron Beacom, 99–121. London: Palgrave Macmillan. doi:10.1057/978-1-137-47901-3.

Friedman, Thomas L. 2005. *The World Is Flat: A Brief History of the Twenty-First Century.* New York: Farrar, Straus and Giroux.

Fritsch, Kelly. 2016. "Cripping Neoliberal Futurity: Marking the Elsewhere and Elsewhen of Desiring Otherwise." *Feral Feminisms* (5): 11–26. https://feralfeminisms.com/cripping-neoliberal-futurity/.

Fullerton, Gail, Mark Hamilton, and Abha Maheshwari. 2010. "Should Non-Mosaic Klinefelter Syndrome Men Be Labelled as Infertile in 2009?" *Human Reproduction* 25 (3): 588–97. https://doi.org/10.1093/humrep/dep431.

Galton, Francis. 2015. *Memories of My Life.* 1908. Reprint, New York: Routledge.

Gannon, Kenneth, Lesley Glover, and Paul Abel. 2004. "Masculinity, Infertility, Stigma and Media Reports." *Social Science and Medicine* 59 (6): 1169–75. https://doi.org/10.1016/j.socscimed.2004.01.015.

Garcia, Diana. 2015. "The Secret Inside Me." *Narrative Inquiry in Bioethics* 5 (2): 92–95. doi:10.1353/nib.2015.0034.

Garfinkel, Harold, and Robert J. Stoller. 1967. "Passing and the Managed Achievement of Sex Status in an 'Intersexed' Person." In *Studies in Ethnomethodology,* ed. Harold Garfinkel, 117–85. Englewood Cliffs, NJ: Prentice Hall.

Garland-Thomson, Rosemarie, ed. 1996a. *Freakery: Cultural Spectacles of the Extraordinary Body.* New York: New York University Press.

–. 1996b. "Introduction: From Wonder to Error – A Genealogy of Freak Discourse in Modernity." In *Freakery: Cultural Spectacles of the Extraordinary Body*, ed. Rosemarie Garland-Thomson, 1–19. New York: New York University Press.

–. 1997. *Extraordinary Bodies: Figuring Physical Disability in American Culture and Literature.* New York: Columbia University Press.

–. 2000. "Staring Back: Self-Representations of Disabled Performance Artists." *American Quarterly* 52 (2): 334–38. doi:10.1353/aq.2000.0024.

–. 2005. "Feminist Disability Studies." *Signs: Journal of Women's History* 30 (2): 1557–87. https://doi.org/10.1086/423352.

–. 2009. *Staring: How We Look.* Oxford: Oxford University Press.

–. 2011. "Integrating Disability, Transforming Feminist Theory." In *Feminist Disability Studies*, ed. Kim Q. Hall, 13–47. Bloomington: Indiana University Press.

Garrison, Spencer. 2018. "On the Limits of 'Trans Enough': Authenticating Trans Identity Narratives." *Gender and Society* 32 (5): 613–37. https://doi.org/10.1177/0891243218780299.

Gelman, Andrew. 2017. "Publish Your Raw Data and Your Speculations, Then Let Other People Do the Analysis: Track and Field Edition." *Statistical Modeling, Causal Inference, and Social Science*, August 21. http://andrewgelman.com/2017/08/21/publish-raw-data-speculations-let-people-analysis-track-field-edition/.

Gems, Gerald R. 2006. "Sport, Colonialism, and United States Imperialism." *Journal of Sport History* 33 (1): 3–25.

Gentile, Katie. 2016. *The Business of Being Made: The Temporalities of Reproductive Technologies, in Psychoanalysis and Culture.* New York: Routledge.

Geraedts, Joep P.M., et al. 2001. "Preimplantation Genetic Diagnosis (PGD), a Collaborative Activity of Clinical Genetic Departments and IVF Centres." *Prenatal Diagnosis* 21 (12): 1086–92. doi:10.1002/pd.249.

Ghemawat, Pankaj. 2009. "Why the World Isn't Flat." *Foreign Policy*, October 14. https://foreignpolicy.com/2009/10/14/why-the-world-isnt-flat/.

Gianpiero, Palermo D., et al. 1998. "Birth after Intracytoplasmic Injection of Sperm Obtained by Testicular Extraction from Men with Nonmosaic Klinefelter's Syndrome." *New England Journal of Medicine* 338 (9): 588–90. doi:10.1056/NEJM199802263380905.

Gilbert, Keith, and Otto J. Schantz, eds. 2008. *The Paralympic Games: Empowerment or Side Show?* Maidenhead, UK: Meyer & Meyer (UK).

Giles, Gillian. 2020. "PCOS and Intersex: A Case for Solidarity against the Binary." *Black Youth Project*, April 29. https://blackyouthproject.com/pcos-and-intersex-a-case-for-solidarity-against-the-binary/.

Gill, Nauman Ahmad, and Abdul Hameed. 2011. "Management of Hypospadias Cripples with Two-Staged Bracka's Technique." *Journal of Plastic, Reconstructive and Aesthetic Surgery* 64 (1): 91–96. https://doi.org/10.1016/j.bjps.2010.02.033.

Gilligan, Carol. 1982. *In a Different Voice.* Cambridge, MA: Harvard University Press.

Gilman, Sander. 1985. *Difference and Pathology: Stereotypes of Sexuality, Race, and Madness.* Ithaca, NY: Cornell University Press.

–. 1991. *The Jew's Body.* New York: Routledge.

Ginnane, Max, dir. 2011. *Too Fast to Be a Woman? The Story of Caster Semenya.* Rise Films and BBC.

Girardin, Céline M., and Guy Van Vliet. 2011. "Counselling of a Couple Faced with Prenatal Diagnosis of Klinefelter Syndrome." *Acta Pædiatrica* 100 (6): 917–22. https://doi.org/10.1111/j.1651-2227.2011.02156.x.

Givetash, Linda. 2017. "Effort to Remove Baby's Gender from Health Card Advances Equality: Experts." *Globe and Mail,* July 9. https://www.theglobeandmail.com/news/british-columbia/effort-to-remove-babys-gender-from-health-card-advances-equality-experts/article35624367/?ref=http://www.theglobeandmail.com&.

Goggin, Gerard, and Christopher Newell. 2000. "Crippling Paralympics? Media, Disability and Olympism." *Media International Australia* 97 (1): 71–83. https://doi.org/10.1177/1329878X0009700110.

Goh, Elaine Suk-Ying, et al. 2019. "Genetic Counselors' Preferences for Coverage of Preimplantation Genetic Diagnosis: A Discrete Choice Experiment." *Clinical Genetics* 95 (6): 684–92. https://doi.org/10.1111/cge.13531.

Goldberg, David Theo. 1990. *Anatomy of Racism.* Minneapolis: University of Minnesota Press.

Golden, Tom. 2009. "Boys and the Boy Crisis." *Boyhood Studies: An Interdisciplinary Journal* 3 (2): 194–200. https://doi.org/10.3149/thy.0301.194.

Goltz, Dustin Bradley. 2009. *Queer Temporalities in Gay Male Representation: Tragedy, Normativity, and Futurity.* New York: Routledge.

Goodley, Dan. 2011. *Disability Studies: An Interdisciplinary Introduction.* Los Angeles, CA: Sage.

Gordon, Avery. 2008. *Ghostly Matters: Haunting and the Sociological Imagination.* Minneapolis: University of Minnesota Press.

–. 2011. "Some Thoughts on Haunting and Futurity." *Borderlands* 10 (2): 1–21.

Gordon, Beth Omansky, and Karen E. Rosenblum. 2001. "Bringing Disability into the Sociological Frame: A Comparison of Disability with Race, Sex, and Sexual Orientation Statuses." *Disability and Society* 16 (1): 5–19. https://doi.org/10.1080/713662032.

Gorey, Kevin M., and Donald R. Leslie. 1997. "The Prevalence of Child Sexual Abuse: Integrative Review Adjustment for Potential Response and Measurement Bias." *Child Abuse and Neglect* 21 (4): 391–98. https://doi.org/10.1016/S0145-2134(96)00180-9.

Gough, Brendan, et al. 2008. "'They Did Not Have a Word': The Parental Quest to Locate a 'True Sex' for Their Intersex Children." *Psychology and Health* 23 (4): 493–507. https://doi.org/10.1080/14768320601176170.

Government of Canada. 2013. "Genetic Testing and Screening." February 5. https://www.canada.ca/en/public-health/services/fertility/genetic-testing-screening.html.

Government of Ontario. 2015. "Ontario to Expand Funding for Fertility Services." October 1. https://news.ontario.ca/mohltc/en/2015/10/ontario-to-expand-funding-for-fertility-services.html.

Grabham, Emily. 2007. "Citizen Bodies, Intersex Citizenship." *Sexualities* 10 (1): 29–48. https://doi.org/10.1177/1363460707072951.

Grand View Research. 2016. "Non-Invasive Prenatal Testing (NIPT) Market Worth $5.5 Billion by 2025." December. https://www.grandviewresearch.com/press -release/global-noninvasive-prenatal-testing-market.

Gray, Mary, Brian Gilley, and Colin Johnson, eds. 2016. *Queering the Countryside: New Frontiers in Rural Queer Studies.* New York: New York University Press.

Green, Fiona J. 2005. "From Clitoridectomies to 'Designer Vaginas': The Medical Construction of Heteronormative Female Bodies and Sexuality through Female Genital Cutting." *Sexualities, Evolution and Gender* 7 (2): 153–87. https://doi. org/10.1080/14616660500200223.

Green, Josephine, and Helen Statham. 1996. "Psychosocial Aspects of Prenatal Screening and Diagnosis." In *The Troubled Helix: Social and Psychological Implications of the New Human Genetics,* ed. Theresa Marteau and Martin Richards, 140–63. Cambridge, UK: Cambridge University Press.

Green, Stephen. 2016. "Sorry Caster Semenya, You Aren't a Woman." *Christian Voice,* August 17. http://www.christianvoice.org.uk/index.php/sorry-caster -semenya-you-arent-a-woman/.

Greenberg, Julie A. 2012. *Intersexuality and the Law.* New York: New York University Press.

Gregorio, I.W. 2017. "When Emergency Pediatric Surgery Is Anything But." *Scientific American,* May 17. https://blogs.scientificamerican.com/observations/ when-emergency-pediatric-surgery-is-anything-but/.

Grekul, Jana, Arvey Krahn, and Dave Odynak. 2004. "Sterilizing the 'Feeble-Minded': Eugenics in Alberta, Canada, 1929–1972." *Journal of Historical Sociology* 17 (4): 358–84. https://doi.org/10.1111/j.1467-6443.2004.00237.x.

Griffiths, David Andrew. 2018. "Diagnosing Sex: Intersex Surgery and 'Sex Change' in Britain 1930–1955." *Sexualities* 21 (3): 476–95. https://doi.org/10.1177/ 1363460717740339.

Grinspan, Mauro Cabral, and Morgan Carpenter. 2018. "Gendering the Lens: Critical Reflections on Gender, Hospitality and Torture." In *Gender Perspectives on Torture: Law and Practice,* ed. Center for Human Rights and Humanitarian Law, 183–96. Washington, DC: American University Washington College of Law.

Groveman, Sherri A. 1996. "Sex, Lies and Androgen Insensitivity Syndrome." *Canadian Medical Association Journal* 154 (12): 1829–30.

Grue, Jan. 2016. "The Problem with Inspiration Porn: A Tentative Definition and Provisional Critique." *Disability and Society* 31 (6): 838–49. https://doi.org/10.1 080/09687599.2016.1205473.

Gugala, Jon. 2014. "IAAF, IOC: Indian Woman Not Woman Enough to Compete in Track." *Deadspin,* July 10. https://deadspin.com/iaaf-ioc-indian-woman-not -woman-enough-to-compete-in-1643329298.

Guillot, Vincent, Markus Bauer, and Daniela Truffer. 2016. *Intersex Genital Mutilations: Human Rights Violations of Persons with Variations of Sex Anatomy: NGO Report to the 7th Periodic Report of France on the Convention against Torture.* Zurich: StopIGM.org.

Gunn, Joshua. 2004. "Mourning Speech: Haunting and the Spectral Voices of Nine-Eleven." *Text and Performance Quarterly* 24 (2): 91–114. https://doi.org/10. 1080/1046293042000288344.

Gupta, Kristina, and Sara M. Freeman. 2013. "Preimplantation Genetic Diagnosis for Intersex Conditions: Beyond Parental Decision Making." *American Journal of Bioethics* 13 (10): 49–51. https://doi.org/10.1080/15265161.2013.828124.

Gurney, Karen. 2007. "Sex and the Surgeon's Knife: The Family Court's Dilemma ... Informed Consent and the Specter of Iatrogenic Harm to Children with Intersex Characteristics." *American Journal of Law and Medicine* 33 (4): 625–61. https://doi.org/10.1177/009885880703300403.

Gush, Charlotte. 2015. "Casting Spells for a Female Future with 70s Lesbian Separatist Liza Cowan." *Dyke, A Quarterly,* December 8. Accessed March 15, 2022. https://www.dykeaquarterly.com/2015/12/in-recent-weeks-perhaps-thevery-first-truly-insta-famous-feminist-fashion-item-has-emerged-a-sweatshirt-worn-by-annie-c.html.

Hadidi, Ahmed T., and Amir F. Azmy, eds. 2004. *Hypospadias Surgery: An Illustrated Guide.* New York: Springer. doi:10.1007/978-3-662-07841-9.

Halberstam, Jack. 2005. *In a Queer Time and Place: Transgender Bodies, Subcultural Lives.* New York: New York University Press.

—. 2011. *The Queer Art of Failure.* Durham, NC: Duke University Press.

Hall, Kim Q. 2011. "Reimagining Disability and Gender through Feminist Studies." In *Feminist Disability Studies,* ed. Kim Q. Hall, 1–10. Bloomington: Indiana University Press.

Hamilton, Laura T., et al. 2019. "Hegemonic Femininities and Intersectional Domination." *Sociological Theory* 37 (4): 315–41. https://doi.org/10.1177/0735275119888248.

Hammer, Karen. 2014. "A Scar Is More Than a Wound: Rethinking Community and Intimacy through Queer and Disability Theory." *Rocky Mountain Review of Language and Literature* 68 (2): 159–76. doi:10.1353/rmr.2014.0044.

Hanisch, Carol. 2000. "The Personal Is Political." In *Radical Feminism: A Documentary Reader,* ed. Barbara A. Crow, 113–16. New York: New York University Press.

Hansen, Randall, and Desmond King. 2001. "Eugenic Ideas, Political Interests, and Policy Variance." *World Politics* 53 (2): 237–63. doi:10.1353/wp.2001.0003.

Hansen, Rick. 2010. "Mansbridge One on One." Interview with Peter Mansbridge. *CBC.* http://www.cbc.ca/player/play/1420156690.

Haramia, Chelsea. 2013. "PGD and Parental Obligations: What Parents Owe to Communities That Do Not Yet Exist." *American Journal of Bioethics* 13 (10): 41–42. https://doi.org/10.1080/15265161.2013.828130.

Haraway, Donna. 1988. "Situated Knowledges: The Science Question in Feminism and the Privilege of Partial Perspective." *Feminist Studies* 14 (3): 575–99. doi:10.2307/3178066.

—. 1990. "A Manifesto for Cyborgs: Science, Technology and Socialist Feminism in the 1980s." In *Feminism/Postmodernism,* ed. Linda Nicholson, 190–233. New York: Routledge.

—. 1991. *Simians, Cyborgs and Women: The Reinvention of Nature.* New York: Routledge.

—. 1992. "Ecce Homo, Ain't (Ar'n't) I a Woman, and Inappropriate/d Others: The Human in a Post-Humanist Landscape." In *Feminists Theorize the Political,* ed. Judith Butler and Joan W. Scott, 86–100. New York and London: Routledge.

–. 1997. *Modest_Witness@Second_Millenium.Femaleman©_Meets_OncoMouse^TM: Feminism and Technoscience.* New York: Routledge.

Harding, Sandra. 1986. *The Science Question in Feminism.* Ithaca, NY: Cornell University Press.

–. 1991. *Whose Science? Whose Knowledge? Thinking from Women's Lives.* Ithaca, NY: Cornell University Press.

Hargreaves, Jennifer. 2000. *Heroines of Sport: The Politics of Difference and Identity.* London: Routledge.

–. 2003. *Sporting Females: Critical Issues in the History and Sociology of Women's Sports.* 1994. Reprint, New York: Routledge.

Harper, Catherine. 2007. *Intersex.* Oxford: Berg.

Harris, Anita. 2004. *Future Girl: Young Women in the Twenty-First Century.* London: Routledge.

Harris, John. 2001. "One Principle and Three Fallacies of Disability Studies." *Journal of Medical Ethics* 27 (6): 383–87. https://jme.bmj.com/content/27/6/383.

Harrison, Giles, dir. 2011. *Me, My Sex, and I.* BBC and Top Documentary Films.

Harrison, Keith C., and Suzanne Malia Lawrence. 2004. "College Students' Perceptions, Myths, and Stereotypes about African American Athleticism: A Qualitative Investigation." *Sport, Education and Society* 9 (1): 33–52. https://doi.org/10.1080/1357332042000175809.

Hart, Simon. 2009. "Caster Semenya 'Is a Hermaphrodite,' Tests Show." *Telegraph* (London), September 11. https://www.telegraph.co.uk/sport/othersports/athletics/6170229/Caster-Semenya-is-a-hermaphrodite-tests-show.html.

Hartsock, Nancy. 1981. "Fundamental Feminism: Prospect and Perspective." In *Building Feminist Theory,* ed. Charlotte Bunch, 32–43. Harlow: Longman.

–. 1983. "The Feminist Standpoint: Developing the Ground for a Specifically Feminist Historical Materialism." In *Discovering Reality: Feminist Perspectives on Epistemology, Metaphysics, Methodology, and the Philosophy of Science,* ed. Sandra Harding and Merrill Hintikka, 283–310. New York: Kluwer Academic.

–. 1987. "Rethinking Modernism: Minority vs. Majority Theories." *Cultural Critique* (7): 187–206. doi:10.2307/1354155.

–. 1990. "Foucault on Power: A Theory for Women?" In *Feminism/Postmoderism,* ed. Linda Nicholson, 157–75. New York: Routledge.

Hayhurst, Lyndsay M.C. 2014. "Using Postcolonial Feminism to Investigate Cultural Difference and Neoliberalism in Sport, Gender and Development Programming in Uganda." In *Sport, Social Development and Peace,* ed. Kevin Young and Chiaki Okada, 45–65. Bingley, UK: Emerald Group. https://doi.org/10.1108/S1476-285420140000008002.

Heilpern, Will. 2016. "Why the Olympics and Paralympics Are Still Separate Events." *Business Insider,* August 17. https://www.businessinsider.com/why-the-olympics-and-paralympics-are-separate-events-2016-8.

Heisinger-Nixon, David. 2017. "On Crip Horizons." *Disability Studies Quarterly* 37 (3). http://dx.doi.org/10.18061/dsq.v37i3.5961.

Hellsten, S.K. 2004. "Rationalising Circumcision: From Tradition to Fashion, from Public Health to Individual Freedom – Critical Notes on Cultural Persistence of the Practice of Genital Mutilation." *Journal of Medical Ethics* 30 (3): 248–53. doi:10.1136/jme.2004.008888.

Henry, Elsa S. 2013. "Pro Choice Should NOT Mean Ableist." *Feminist Sonar,* July 9. http://feministsonar.com/2013/07/pro-choice-should-not-mean-ableist/.

Herdt, Gilbert. 1994. *Third Sex, Third Gender.* New York: Zone Books.

Hern, Matt. 2013. *One Game at a Time: Why Sports Matter.* Minneapolis, MN: AK Press.

Hesford, Wendy S., and Brenda Jo Brueggemann. 2007. *Rhetorical Visions: Reading and Writing in a Visual Culture.* London: Pearson/Prentice Hall.

Hester, J. David. 2006. "Intersex and the Rhetorics of Healing." In *Ethics and Intersex,* ed. Sharon E. Sytsma, 47–71. New York: Springer. doi:10.1007/1-4220-4314-7_3.

Hevey, David. 2013. "The Enfreakment of Photography." In *The Disability Studies Reader,* 4th ed., ed. Lennard J. Davis, 432–47. New York: Routledge.

Hinkle, Curtis E., and Hida Viloria. 2012. "Ten Misconceptions about Intersex." Intersex Campaign for Equality, January 17. https://www.intersexequality.com/ten-misconceptions-intersex/.

Hird, Myra J. 2000. "Gender's Nature: Intersexuality, Transsexualism and the 'Sex'/'Gender' Binary." *Feminist Theory* 1 (3): 347–64. https://doi.org/10.1177/146470010000100305.

Hirschberg, Angelica Linden, Richard Auchus, and Stéphane Bermon. 2019. "IAAF Letter to the World Medical Association." *World Athletics,* May 7. https://www.worldathletics.org/news/press-release/iaaf-letter-wma.

Hoag, Trevor L. 2014. "Ghosts of Memory: Mournful Performance and the Rhetorical Event of Haunting (Or: Spectres of Occupy)." *Liminalities: A Journal of Performance Studies* 10 (3–4): 1–22. http://liminalities.net/10-3/ghosts.pdf.

Hobson, Janell. 2003. "The 'Batty' Politic: Toward an Aesthetic of the Black Female Body." *Hypatia* 18 (4): 87–105. https://doi.org/10.1111/j.1527-2001.2003.tb01414.x.

Holbert, Nathan, Michael Dando, and Isabel Correa. 2020. "Afrofuturism as Critical Constructionist Design: Building Futures from the Past and Present." *Learning, Media and Technology* 45 (4): 328–44. https://doi.org/10.1080/17439884.2020.1754237.

Holland, Suzanne. 2002. "Selecting against Difference: Assisted Reproduction, Disability and Regulation." *Florida State University Law Review* 30 (2): 401–10.

Holmes, Morgan. 2000. "Queer Cut Bodies." In *Queer Frontiers: Millennial Georg raphies, Gender, and Generations,* ed. Joseph A. Boone et al., 84–110. Madison: University of Wisconsin Press.

–. 2002. "Rethinking the Meaning and Management of Intersexuality." *Sexualities* 5 (2): 159–80. https://doi.org/10.1177/1363460702005002002.

–. 2008a. *Intersex: A Perilous Difference.* Selinsgrove, PA: Susquehanna University Press.

–. 2008b. "Mind the Gaps: Intersex and (Re-productive) Spaces in Disability Studies and Bioethics." *Journal of Bioethical Inquiry* 5 (2): 169–81. doi:10.1007/s11673-007-9073-2.

–, ed. 2009a. *Critical Intersex.* Farnham, UK: Ashgate.

–. 2009b. "Introduction: Straddling Past, Present and Future." In *Critical Intersex*, ed. Morgan Holmes, 1–14. Farnham, UK: Ashgate.

–. 2011. "Intersex Enchiridion: Naming and Knowledge." *Somatechnics* 1 (2): 388–411.

Holzer, Lena. 2019. "Sexually Dimorphic Bodies: A Production of Birth Certificates." *Australian Feminist Law Journal* 45 (1): 91–110. https://doi.org/10.1080/132009 68.2019.1649002.

Horne, John. 2012. "The Four 'Cs' of Sports Mega-Events: Capitalism, Connections, Citizenship, and Contradictions." In *Olympic Games, Mega-Events and Civil Societies*, ed. Graeme Hayes and John Karamichas, 31–45. New York: Palgrave Macmillan.

Hossain, Adnan. 2018. "De-Indianizing Hijra: Intraregional Effacements and In-equalities on South Asian Queer Space." *TSQ* 5 (3): 321–31. https://doi.org/ 10.1215/23289252-6900710.

Howe, David P. 2008. *The Cultural Politics of the Paralympic Movement: Through an Anthropological Lens*. New York: Routledge.

–. 2011. "Cyborg and Supercrip: The Paralympics Technology and the (Dis)em-powerment of Disabled Athletes." *Sociology* 45 (5): 868–82. https://doi.org/ 10.1177/0038038511413421.

Hraba, Joseph, and Geoffrey Grant. 1970. "Black Is Beautiful: A Reexamination of Racial Preference and Identification." *Journal of Personality and Social Psych-ology* 16 (3): 398–402. https://doi.org/10.1037/h0030043.

Hrabovszky, Zoltan, and John M. Huston. 2002. "Surgical Treatment of Intersex Abnormalities: A Review." *Surgery* 131 (1): 92–104. https://doi.org/10.1067/msy. 2002.115840.

Hubbard, Ruth. 2013. "Abortion and Disability: Who Should and Should Not Inhabit the World?" In *The Disability Studies Reader*, 4th ed., ed. Lennard J. Davis, 74–86. New York: Routledge.

Hughes, Bill. 2000. "Medicine and the Aesthetic Invalidation of Disabled People." *Disability and Society* 15 (4): 555–68. https://doi.org/10.1080/09687590050058170.

Hughes, Ieuan A., et al. 2006. "Consensus Statement on Management of Intersex Disorders." *Archives of Disease in Childhood* 91 (7): 554–63. http://dx.doi.org/ 10.1136/adc.2006.098319.

Hull, Richard. 2009. "Projected Disability and Parental Responsibilities." In *Disability and Disadvantage*, ed. Kimberley Brownlee and Adam Cureton, 369–84. Oxford: Oxford University Press. doi:10.1093/acprof:osobl/9780199234509.003.0014.

Human Rights Watch and interACT: Advocates for Intersex Youth. 2017. "'I Want to Be Like Nature Made Me': Medically Unnecessary Surgeries on Intersex Children in the US." July 25. https://www.hrw.org/report/2017/07/25/i-want-be-nature -made-me/medically-unnecessary-surgeries-intersex-children-us#page.

Hume, David. 1894. *Essays: Moral, Political, and Literary.* Ed. Eugene F. Miller. Original 1757. New York: George Routledge and Sons.

–. 1988. *A Treatise of Human Nature.* 1740. Reprint, Oxford: Oxford University Press.

Hurst, Mike. 2009. "Caster Semenya Has Male Sex Organs and No Womb or Ovaries." *Daily Telegraph* (London), September 11. Accessed July 20, 2020.

http://www.dailytelegraph.com.au/sport/semenya-has-no-womb-or-ovaries/story-e6frexni-1225771672245.

Hyder, Nishat. 2011. "Germany Allows PGD for Life-Threatening Genetic Defects." *BioNews,* January 25. https://www.bionews.org.uk/page_93058.

Inacio, Marlene, et al. 2011. "46,XY DSD Due to 17β-HSD3 Deficiency and 5α-Reductase Type 2 Deficiency." In *Hormonal and Genetic Basis of Sexual Differentiation Disorders and Hot Topics in Endocrinology: Proceedings of the 2nd World Conference,* ed. Maria I. New and Joe Leigh Simpson, 9–14. New York: Springer.

Ingle, Sean. 2019. "Semenya Loses Landmark Legal Case against IAAF over Testosterone Levels." *Guardian* (London), May 1. https://www.theguardian.com/sport/2019/may/01/caster-semenya-loses-landmark-legal-case-iaaf-athletics.

Inhorn, Marcia, et al., eds. 2009. *Reconceiving the Second Sex: Men, Masculinity, and Reproduction.* New York: Berghahn Books.

Inter, Laura (pseud.). 2015. "Finding My Compass." *Narrative Inquiry in Bioethics* 5 (2): 95–98. doi:10.1353/nib.2015.0039.

Inter/Act. n.d. "What Is Intersex? An Intersex FAQ by Inter/Act." AIS-DSD Support Group. http://aisdsdhistorical.interconnect.support/intersex-faq-interact-mtvs-faking/.

International Association of Athletics Federations (IAAF). 2011. *IAAF Regulations Governing Eligibility of Females with Hyperandrogenism to Compete in Women's Competition.* https://www.worldathletics.org/search/?q=IAAF+Regulations+Governing+Eligibility+of+Females+with+Hyperandrogenism+to+Compete+in+Women%27s+Competition.

—. 2015. *Code of Ethics: In Force as from 1 May 2015 until and Including 2 April 2017.* https://www.worldathletics.org/download/download?filename=aece54d4-d019-4a8c-8ea5-ee07ff76114c.pdf&urlslug=D6.1%20-%20Former%20Code%20of%20Ethics.

—. 2018. *Eligibility Regulations for the Female Classification (Athletes with Differences of Sex Development).* https://www.worldathletics.org/search/?q=Eligibility+Regulations+for+the+Female+Classification.

—. 2019. *Eligibility Regulations for the Female Classification (Athletes with Differences of Sex Development).* https://www.worldathletics.org/search/?q=Eligibility+Regulations+for+the+Female+Classification.

International Paralympic Committee (IPC). n.d. "Paralympics History." https://www.paralympic.org/ipc/history.

—. 2015. *Explanatory Guide to Paralympic Classification: Paralympic Summer Sports.* Bonn, Germany: International Paralympic Committee.

—. 2016. *Explanatory Guide to Paralympic Classification: Paralympic Winter Sports.* Bonn, Germany: International Paralympic Committee.

Intersex Society of North America. n.d. "What Is Intersex?" http://www.isna.org/faq/what_is_intersex.

Iuvone, Laura, et al. 2011. "Pretreatment Neuropsychological Deficits in Children with Brain Tumors." *Neuro-oncology* 13 (5): 517–24. https://doi.org/10.1093/neuonc/nor013.

Ives, Mike. 2019. "Sprinter Dutee Chand Becomes India's First Openly Gay Athlete." *New York Times,* May 20. https://www.nytimes.com/2019/05/20/world/asia/india-dutee-chand-gay.html.

Jain, Tarun, and Mark D. Hornstein. 2005. "Disparities in Access to Infertility Services in a State with Mandated Insurance Coverage." *Fertility and Sterility* 84 (1): 221–23. https://doi.org/10.1016/j.fertnstert.2005.01.118.

Jamieson, Alastair. 2009. "Caster Semenya Gender Row: What Is a Hermaphrodite?" *Telegraph* (London), August 20. http://www.telegraph.co.uk/news/health/news/6060027/Caster-Semenya-gender-row-what-is-a-hermaphrodite.html.

Jarmakani, Amira. 2008. *Imagining Arab Womanhood: The Cultural Mythology of Veils, Harems, and Belly Dancers in the U.S.* New York: Palgrave Macmillan. doi:10.1057/9780230612112.

Jerreat-Poole, Adan. 2020. "Sick, Slow, Cyborg: Crip Futurity in Mass Effect." *Game Studies* 20 (1). http://gamestudies.org/2001/articles/jerreatpoole.

Johari, Aarefa. 2014. "Hijra, Kothi, Aravani: A Quick Guide to Transgender Terminology." *Scroll.in,* April 17. https://scroll.in/article/662023/hijra-kothi-aravani-a-quick-guide-to-transgender-terminology.

Johnson, Austin H. 2016. "Transnormativity: A New Concept and Its Validation through Documentary Film about Transgender Men." *Sociological Inquiry* 86 (4): 465–91. doi:10.1111/soin.12127.

Jones, Tiffany, et al. 2016. *Intersex: Stories and Statistics from Australia.* Cambridge, UK: Open Book Publishers. https://doi.org/10.11647/OBP.0089.

Jordan-Young, Rebecca M. 2010. *Brain Storm: The Flaws in the Science of Sex Differences.* Cambridge, MA: Harvard University Press.

—. 2012. "Hormones, Context, and 'Brain Gender': A Review of Evidence from Congenital Adrenal Hyperplasia." *Social Science and Medicine* 74 (11): 1738–44. doi:10.1016/j.socscimed.2011.08.026.

Jordan-Young, Rebecca M., and Katrina Karkazis. 2012. "You Say You're a Woman? That Should Be Enough." *New York Times,* June 17. https://www.nytimes.com/2012/06/18/sports/olympics/olympic-sex-verification-you-say-youre-a-woman-that-should-be-enough.html.

—. 2019. *Testosterone: An Unauthorized Biography.* Cambridge, MA: Harvard University Press.

Jordan-Young, Rebecca M., Peter H. Sönksen, and Katrina Karkazis. 2014. "Sex, Health, and Athletes." *British Medical Journal* 348 (7957): 1–3. https://doi.org/10.1136/bmj.g2926.

Joseph, Sadé Clacken, and River Gallo, dirs. 2019. *Ponyboi.* GapToof Entertainment.

Jung, Eun Jung, et al. 2017. "Female with 46, XY Karyotype." *Obstetrics and Gynecology Science* 60 (4): 378–83. https://doi.org/10.5468/ogs.2017.60.4.378.

JVW Football Club. 2019. "Olympic Champion Caster Semenya Joins JVW FC." September 5. https://www.jvw5.co.za/olympic-champion-caster-semenya-joins-jvw-fc/.

Kafer, Alison. 2003. "Compulsory Bodies: Reflections on Heterosexuality and Able-Bodiedness." *Journal of Women's History* 15 (3): 77–89. doi:10.1353/jowh.2003.0071.

—. 2013. *Feminist, Queer, Crip.* Bloomington: Indiana University Press.

Kalra, Sanjay, Bindu Kulshreshtha, and Ambika Gopalakrishnan Unnikrishnan. 2012. "We Care for Intersex: For Pinky, for Santhi, and for Anamika." *Indian Journal of Endocrinology and Metabolism* 16 (6): 873–75. doi:10.4103/2230 -8210.102980.

Kampantais, Spyridon, et al. 2012. "Urethral Hairballs as a Long-Term Complication of Hypospadias Repairs: Two Case Reports." *Case Reports in Urology* 2012 (2012): 1–3. https://doi.org/10.1155/2012/769706.

Kanayama, Kelly. 2016. "British Runner Lynsey Sharp's Comments about Gold Medalist Caster Semenya Are Just Racist and Sexist." *The Frisky,* August 22. Accessed January 17, 2017. http://www.thefrisky.com/2016-08-22/british-runner -lynsey-sharps-comments-about-gold-medalist-caster-semenya-are-just-racist -and-sexist/.

Kane, Mary Jo. 1995. "Resistance/Transformation of the Oppositional Binary: Exposing Sport as a Continuum." *Journal of Sport and Social Issues* 19 (2): 191–218. https://doi.org/10.1177/019372395019002006.

Kant, Immanuel. 1997. *Groundwork of the Metaphysics of Morals.* Ed. and trans. Mary J. Gregor. Original 1785. Cambridge, UK: Cambridge University Press.

Kaplan, Deborah J.D. 1993. "Prenatal Screening and Its Impacts on Persons with Disabilities." *Clinical Obstetrics and Gynecology* 36 (3): 605–12. doi:10.1159/ 000263874.

Kaposy, Chris. 2013. "A Disability Critique of the New Prenatal Test for Down Syndrome." *Kennedy Institute of Ethics Journal* 23 (4): 299–324. doi:10.1353/ ken.2013.0017.

–. 2014. "The Big Business of Prenatal Testing for Down Syndrome." *Impact Ethics,* January 2. https://impactethics.ca/2014/01/02/the-big-business-of-prenatal -testing-for-down-syndrome/.

–. 2015. "Do We Really Need an Even Better Prenatal Test for Down Syndrome?" *Impact Ethics,* May 19. https://impactethics.ca/2015/05/19/do-we-really-need -an-even-better-prenatal-test-for-down-syndrome/.

–. 2018. *Choosing Down Syndrome: Ethics and New Prenatal Technologies.* Cambridge, MA: MIT Press.

Karkazis, Katrina. 2008. *Fixing Sex: Intersex, Medical Authority, and Lived Experience.* Durham, NC: Duke University Press. https://doi.org/10.1215/9780 822389217.

–. 2016a. "The Ignorance Aimed at Caster Semenya Flies in the Face of the Olympic Spirit." *Guardian* (London), August 23. https://www.theguardian.com/ commentisfree/2016/aug/23/caster-semenya-olympic-spirit-iaaf-athletes -women.

–. 2016b. "One-Track Minds: Semenya, Chand & the Violence of Public Scrutiny." *Medium,* July 19. https://medium.com/@Karkazis/medias-one-track-mind -semenya-chand-the-violence-of-public-scrutiny-1aa6d1a08454#.q36uqmxqv.

Karkazis, Katrina, and Gideon Meyerowitz-Katz. 2017. "Why the IAAF's Latest Testosterone Study Won't Help Them at CAS." *World Sports Advocate.*

Kazyak, Emily. 2011. "Disrupting Cultural Selves: Constructing Gay and Lesbian Identities in Rural Locales." *Qualitative Sociology* 34 (4): 561–81. https://doi. org/10.1007/s11133-011-9205-1.

–. 2012. "Midwest or Lesbian? Gender, Rurality, and Sexuality." *Gender and Society* 26 (6): 825–48. https://doi.org/10.1177/0891243212458361.

Keeling, Kara. 2019. *Queer Times, Black Futures.* New York: New York University Press.

Kelly, Christine. 2018. "A Future for Disability: Perceptions of Disabled Youth and Nonprofit Organizations." *Social Theory and Health* 16 (1): 44–59. https://doi.org/10.1057/s41285-017-0042-5.

Kelly, Christine, and Michael Orsini, eds. 2016. *Mobilizing Metaphor: Art, Culture, and Disability Activism in Canada.* Vancouver: UBC Press.

Kerr, Anne, and Tom Shakespeare. 2002. *Genetic Politics: From Eugenics to Genome.* Cheltenham, UK: New Clarion.

Kerry, Stephen Craig. 2014. "Hypospadias, the 'Bathroom Panopticon,' and Men's Psychological and Social Urinary Practices." In *Masculinities in a Global Era,* ed. Joseph Gelfer, 215–28. New York: Springer. https://doi.org/10.1007/978-1-4614-6931-5_12.

Kessler, Suzanne J. 1998. *Lessons from the Intersexed.* New Brunswick, NJ: Rutgers University Press.

Kevles, Daniel J. 1985. *In the Name of Eugenics: Genetics and the Uses of Human Heredity.* Berkeley: University of California Press.

Khaleeli, Homa. 2016. "'We're the Superhumans: Meet the Stars of Channel 4's Paralympic Trailer." *Guardian* (London), July 20. https://www.theguardian.com/tv-and-radio/2016/jul/19/meet-the-superhumans-stars-of-channel-4s-paralympics-trailer.

Khan, Sharful Islam, et al. 2009. "Living on the Extreme Margin: Social Exclusion of the Transgender Population (Hijra) in Bangladesh." *Journal of Health, Population and Nutrition* 27 (4): 441–51. doi:10.3329/jhpn.v27i4.3388.

Kids Helpline. 2020. "LGBTIQ+: The Ultimate Dictionary." https://kidshelpline.com.au/teens/issues/lgbtiqa-ultimate-dictionary.

Kim, Eunjung. 2017. *Curative Violence: Rehabilitating Disability, Gender, and Sexuality in Modern Korea.* Durham, NC: Duke University Press. https://doi.org/10.1215/9780822373513.

Kimmel, Michael. 1996. *Manhood in America: A Cultural History.* New York: Free Press.

King, Samantha. 2010. "Pink Diplomacy: On the Uses and Abuses of Breast Cancer Awareness." *Health Communication* 15 (3): 286–89. https://doi.org/10.1080/10410231003698960.

Kingston, Anne. 2018. "An Explosive Gender Revolution Is Under Way. So Why Isn't It Changing Anything?" *Maclean's,* November 14. https://www.macleans.ca/society/an-explosive-gender-revolution-is-under-way-so-why-isnt-it-changing-anything/.

Klein, Alyssa. 2016. "South Africans on Twitter Defend Caster Semenya against U.S. Media." *okayafrica,* August 13. https://www.okayafrica.com/rio2016-olympics-caster-semenya-south-african-twitter/.

Klöppel, Ulrike. 2009. "Who Has the Right to Change Gender Status? Drawing Boundaries between Inter- and Transsexuality." In *Critical Intersex,* ed. Morgan Holmes, 171–90. Farnham, UK: Ashgate. https://doi.org/10.4324/9781315575018.

—. 2016. "Zur Aktualität kosmetischer Operationen ,uneindeutiger' Genitalien im Kindesalter." Zentrum für transdisziplinäre Geschlechterstudien, *Bulletin Texte* (42): 1–85. http://dx.doi.org/10.25595/12.

Knight, Amber. 2017. "Disability and the Meaning of Reproductive Liberty." *Politics, Groups, and Identities* 5 (1): 1–17. https://doi.org/10.1080/21565503.2016.1273120.

Koedt, Anne. 2000. "The Myth of the Vaginal Orgasm." 1970. Reprinted in *Radical Feminisms: A Documentary Reader,* ed. Barbara A. Crow, 371–77. New York: New York University Press.

Kokozos, Michael, and Nora Gross. 2015. "Opening Up a Dialogue about the Boy Code." *Boyhood Studies: An Interdisciplinary Journal* 8 (2): 130–34. https://doi.org/10.3167/bhs.2015.080215.

Koomah. 2017. "Desirability Politics: Sex and the Intersex Body." *Intersex Day,* October 23. http://intersexday.org/en/desirability-politics-koomah/.

Korsgaard, Christine M. 2013. "Kantian Ethics, Animals, and the Law." *Oxford Journal of Legal Studies* 33 (4): 629–48. https://doi.org/10.1093/ojls/gqt028.

Koyama, Emi. 2003. *Introduction to Intersex Activism: A Guide for Allies.* 2nd ed. Portland, OR: Intersex Initiative Portland.

—. 2006. "From 'Intersex' to 'DSD': Toward a Queer Disability Politics of Gender." Intersex Initiative, February. http://www.intersexinitiative.org/articles/intersextodsd.html.

—. 2016. "The Transfeminist Manifesto." In *Feminist Theory Reader: Local and Global Perspectives,* 4th ed., ed. Carole McCann and Seung-Kyung Kim, 150–60. New York: Routledge.

Krane, Vikki. 2001. "We Can Be Athletic and Feminine, but Do We Want To? Challenging Hegemonic Femininity in Women's Sport." *Quest* 53 (1): 115–33. https://doi.org/10.1080/00336297.2001.10491733.

Krauzo, Daria. 2018. "The Problem with 'The Future Is Female': Because Is It Really?" *Scribe,* September 26. https://medium.com/scribe/the-problem-with-the-future-is-female-f3dd25d47d05.

Kristeva, Julia. 1982. *Powers of Horror: An Essay on Abjection.* Trans. Leon S. Roudiez. New York: Columbia University Press.

Kumar, Jatinder, et al. 2012. "Managing Disorder of Sexual Development Surgically: A Single Center Experience." *Indian Journal of Urology* 28 (3): 286–91. doi: 10.4103/0970-1591.102703.

Kumar, Sanjay, et al. 2016. "Fertility Potential in Adult Hypospadias." *Journal of Clinical and Diagnostic Research* 10 (8): PC01–5. doi:10.7860/JCDR/2016/21307.8276.

Kvam, Marit Hoem. 2008. "Is Sexual Abuse of Children with Disabilities Disclosed? A Retrospective Analysis of Child Disability and the Likelihood of Sexual Abuse among Those Attending Norwegian Hospitals." *Child Abuse and Neglect* 24 (8): 1073–84. https://doi.org/10.1016/S0145-2134(00)00159-9.

Lahood, Grant, dir. 2012. *Intersexion.* Wellington, New Zealand: Ponsonby Productions.

Laios, Konstantinos, et al. 2014. "Hypospadias and Sex Change in Ancient Greece." *Journal of Sexual Medicine* 11 (5): 1343–44. https://doi.org/10.1111/jsm.12475.

Laios, Konstantinos, Marianna Karamanou, and George Androutsos. 2012. "A Unique Representation of Hypospadias in Ancient Greek Art." *Canadian Urological Association Journal* 6 (1): E1–2. doi:10.5489/cuaj.11155.

Laqueur, Thomas. 1992. *Making Sex: Body and Gender from the Greeks to Freud.* Cambridge, MA: Harvard University Press.

Latour, Bruno, et al. 2015. "A Question from Bruno Latour." Society for Cultural Anthropology, Theorizing the Contemporary, *Fieldsights*, July 21. https://culanth.org/fieldsights/a-question-from-bruno-latour.

Layden, Tim. 2016. "Is It Fair for Caster Semenya to Compete against Women at the Rio Olympics." *Sports Illustrated,* August 11. https://www.si.com/olympics/2016/08/11/caster-semenya-2016-rio-olympics-track-and-field.

Lee, Peter A., et al. 2016. "Global Disorders of Sex Development Update since 2006: Perceptions, Approach and Care." *Hormone Research in Paediatrics* 85 (3): 158–80. doi:10.1159/000442975.

LeFrançois, Brenda A., Robert Menzies, and Geoffrey Reaume, eds. 2013. *Mad Matters: A Critical Reader in Canadian Mad Studies.* Toronto: Canadian Scholars' Press.

Levant, Ronald F. 2005. "The Crises of Boyhood." In *The New Handbook of Psychotherapy and Counseling with Men: A Comprehensive Guide to Settings, Problems and Treatment Approaches,* ed. Gary E. Good and Gleen R. Brooks, 161–71. San Francisco, CA: Jossey-Bass.

Levine, Ethan. 2014. "United Nations Policy and the Intersex Community." In *Disability, Human Rights and the Limits of Humanitarianism,* ed. Michael Gill and Cathy J. Schlund-Vials, 179–94. New York: Routledge.

Liao, Lih Mei, and Sarah Creighton. 2007. "Requests for Cosmetic Genitoplasty: How Should Healthcare Providers Respond?" *British Medical Journal* 334 (7603): 1090–92. https://doi.org/10.1136/bmj.39206.422269.BE.

Lightman, Ernie, et al. 2009. "'Not Disabled Enough': Episodic Disabilities and the Ontario Disability Support Program." *Disabilities Studies Quarterly* 29 (3). http://dx.doi.org/10.18061/dsq.v29i3.932.

Lind, Amy, and Stephanie Brzuzy. 2008. *Battleground: Women, Gender, and Sexuality.* Vol. 1, *A–L.* Westport, CT: Greenwood.

Lindblom, Jonas, and Kerstin Jacobsson. 2014. "A Deviance Perspective on Social Movements: The Case of Animal Rights Activism." *Deviant Behavior* 35 (2): 133–51. https://doi.org/10.1080/01639625.2013.834751.

Lindahl, Hans. 2017. "A Conversation with David Strachan, Intersex and Non-Binary Pioneer." interACT: Advocates for Intersex Youth, March 8. https://interactadvocates.org/a-conversation-with-david-strachan-intersex-and-non-binary-pioneer/.

–. 2019. "Intersex Youth React to the Discriminatory Ruling against Caster Semenya." *Them,* May 2. https://www.them.us/story/caster-semenya?fbclid=IwAR2snrLkWkw4x_lxJMoNRxOh-1yeElGk1ueZy0ixZKogC9NUOxkHxz7g90E.

Linton, Simi. 1998. *Claiming Disability: Knowledge and Identity.* New York: New York University Press.

Loftin, Craig M. 2007. "Unacceptable Mannerisms: Gender Anxieties, Homosexual Activism, and Swish in the United States, 1945–1965." *Journal of Social History* 40 (3): 577–96. doi:10.1353/jsh.2007.0053.

Lohr, Barbara, dir. 2016. *France: Not a Girl, Not a Boy.* ARTE Reportage.

Long, Christopher J., et al. 2017. "Intermediate-Term Followup of Proximal Hypospadias Repair Reveals High Complication Rate." *Journal of Urology* 197 (3): 852–58. https://doi.org/10.1016/j.juro.2016.11.054.

Long, Lynnell Stephani. 2015. "Still I Rise." *Narrative Inquiry in Bioethics* 5 (2): 100–3. doi:10.1353/nib.2015.0048.

Long, Lynnell Stephani, Sean Saifa M. Wall, and Pidgeon Pagonis. 2016. "A Statement from Intersex People of Color on the 20th Anniversary of Intersex Awareness Day." *Pidgeon: Your Local Hermaphrodite,* October 26. http://www.pidgeonismy.name/blog/2016/10/26/a-statement-from-intersex-people-of-color-on-the-20th-anniversary-of-intersex-awareness-day.

Longman, Jeré. 2019. "Caster Semenya Plans to Run 3,000-Meter Race, Which Doesn't Require Her to Limit Testosterone." *New York Times,* May 21. https://www.nytimes.com/2019/05/21/sports/caster-semenya-enters-3000-meter-race-which-doesnt-require-her-to-limit-testosterone.html.

Longmore, Paul K. 2005. "The Cultural Framing of Disability: Telethons as a Case Study." *PMLA* 120 (2): 502–8.

Lugones, María. 2007. "Heterosexualism and the Colonial/Modern Gender System." *Hypatia* 22 (1): 186–209. https://doi.org/10.1111/j.1527-2001.2007.tb01156.x.

Luk, Small. 2015. "Beyond Boundaries." *Intersex Day,* October 20. http://intersexday.org/en/beyond-boundaries-intersex-hk-china/.

Maccartney, Jane, and Hattie Garlick. 2008. "Girls Will Be Girls at the Beijing Olympics – Sex Tests Will Prove It." *Times* (London), July 29. https://www.thetimes.co.uk/article/girls-will-be-girls-at-the-beijing-olympics-sex-tests-will-prove-it-7gm5l0jfgrt.

Mackey, Peter Joseph. 2009. "Crip Utopia and the Future of Disability." *Critical Disability Discourses/Discours critiques dans le champ du handicap* 1: 1–29. https://cdd.journals.yorku.ca/index.php/cdd/article/view/23383.

MacLean, Malcolm. 2019. "Engaging (with) Indigeneity: Decolonization and Indigenous/Indigenizing Sport History." *Journal of Sport History* 46 (2): 189–207. doi:10.5406/jsporthistory.46.2.0189.

Magnet, Shoshana. 2013. "Identity and the New Eugenics in the Newborn Screening Saves Lives Act." *Media, Culture, and Society* 35 (1): 71–77. https://doi.org/10.1177/0163443712464560.

Magubane, Zine. 2001. "Which Bodies Matter? Feminism, Poststructuralism, Race, and the Curious Odyssey of the 'Hottentot Venus.'" *Gender and Society* 15 (6): 816–35. https://doi.org/10.1177/089124301015006003.

–. 2014. "Spectacles and Scholarship: Caster Semenya, Intersex Studies, and the Problem of Race in Feminist Theory." *Signs: Journal of Women's History* 39 (3): 761–85. https://doi.org/10.1086/674301.

Mahar, Elizabeth A., Laurie B. Mintz, and Brianna M. Akers. 2020. "Orgasm Equality: Scientific Findings and Societal Implications." *Current Sexual Health Reports* 12 (1): 24–32. https://doi.org/10.1007/s11930-020-00254-8.

Maika, Melinda, and Karen Danylchuk. 2016. "Representing Paralympics: The 'Other' Athletes in Canadian Print Media Coverage of London 2012." *International Journal of the History of Sport* 33 (4): 401–17. https://doi.org/10.1080/09523367.2016.1160061.

Mansfield, Caroline, Suellen Hopfer, and Theresa M. Matrau. 1999. "Termination Rates after Prenatal Diagnosis of Down Syndrome, Spina Bifida, Anencephaly, and Turner and Klinefelter Syndromes: A Systematic Literature Review." *Prenatal Diagnosis* 19 (9): 808–12. https://doi.org/10.1002/(SICI)1097-0223 (199909)19:9<808::AID-PD637>3.0.CO;2-B.

Marquez, Anunnaki Ray. 2019a. "Biological and Anatomical Sex: Endosex, Intersex & Altersex." *Mx. Anunnaki Ray Marquez,* December 12. https://anunnakiray.com/2019/12/12/biological-and-anatomical-sex-endosex-intersex-altersex/.

–. 2019b. "'Intersex' Can Not Be an Endosex Person's Gender Identity." *Mx. Anunnaki Ray Marquez,* September 9. https://anunnakiray.com/2019/09/20/intersex-can-not-be-an-endosex-persons-gender-identity/.

Martin, Jeffery J. 2017. *Handbook of Disability Sport and Exercise Psychology.* Oxford: Oxford University Press. doi:10.1093/oso/9780190638054.001.0001.

Martínez-Patiño, María José, et al. 2010. "An Approach to the Biological, Historical and Psychological Repercussions of Gender Verification in Top Level Competitions." *Journal of Human Sport and Exercise* 5 (3): 307–21. doi:10.4100/jhse.2010.53.01.

Mastenbroek, Sebastiaan, et al. 2007. "In Vitro Fertilization with Preimplantation Genetic Screening." *New England Journal of Medicine* 357 (17): 1769–70. doi:10.1056/NEJMoa067744.

Mazur, Tom, et al. 2004. "Male Pseudohermaphroditism: Long-Term Quality of Life Outcome in Five 46,XY Individuals Reared Female." *Journal of Pediatric Endocrinology and Metabolism* 17 (6): 809–23. https://doi.org/10.1515/JPEM.2004.17.6.809.

McCaskell, Tim. 2016. *Queer Progress: From Homophobia to Homonationalism.* Toronto: Between the Lines.

McClintock, Anne. 1995. *Imperial Leather: Race, Gender and Sexuality in the Colonial Context.* New York: Routledge.

McClintock, Anne, Aamir Mufti, and Ella Shohat, eds. 1997. *Dangerous Liaisons: Gender, Nation, and Postcolonial Perspectives.* Minneapolis: University of Minnesota Press.

McCullough, Laurence B. 2013. "Critically Appraising Prenatal Genetic Diagnosis to Prevent Disorders of Sexual Development: An Opportunity Missed." *American Journal of Bioethics* 13 (10): 1–3. https://doi.org/10.1080/15265161.2013.832823.

McDermott, Nick. 2015. "Wonder Womb Man." *Sun* (London), February 7. https://www.thesun.co.uk/archives/news/23511/wonder-womb-man/.

McDonagh, Eileen, and Laura Pappano. 2008. *Playing with Boys: Why Separate Is Not Equal in Sports.* Oxford: Oxford University Press.

McLaren, Angus. 2014. *Our Own Master Race: Eugenics in Canada, 1885–1945.* 1990. Reprint, Toronto: University of Toronto Press.

McNamara, Erin R., et al. 2015. "Management of Proximal Hypospadias with 2-Stage Repair: 20-Year Experience." *Journal of Urology* 194 (4): 1080–85. https://doi.org/10.1016/j.juro.2015.04.105.

McRuer, Robert. 2006. *Crip Theory: Cultural Signs of Queerness and Disability.* New York: New York University Press.

–. 2009. "The Future of Critical Intersex." In *Critical Intersex,* ed. Morgan Holmes, 245–50. Farnham, UK: Ashgate. https://doi.org/10.4324/9781315575018.

–. 2011. "Disabling Sex: Notes for the Crip Theory of Sexuality." *GLQ* 17 (1): 107–17. https://doi.org/10.1215/10642684-2010-021.

–. 2013. "Compulsory Able-Bodiedness and Queer/Disabled Existence." In *The Disability Studies Reader,* 4th ed., ed. Lennard J. Davis, 369–80. New York: Routledge.

McRuer, Robert, and Anna Mollow, eds. 2012. *Sex and Disability.* Durham, NC: Duke University Press. https://doi.org/10.1215/9780822394877.

McWade, Brigit, Damian Milton, and Peter Beresford. 2015. "Mad Studies and Neurodiversity: A Dialogue." *Disability and Society* 30 (2): 305–9. https://doi.org/10.1080/09687599.2014.1000512.

McWhorter. 1999. *Bodies and Pleasure: Foucault and the Politics of Sexual Normalization.* Bloomington: Indiana University Press.

Mei, Gina. 2016. "This Commentator Is in Hot Water after Crediting This Swimmer's World Record to Her Husband." *Cosmopolitan,* August 7. http://www.cosmopolitan.com/entertainment/news/a62457/katinka-hosszu-world-record-shane-tusup-credit-commentator-olympics/.

Méndez, Juan E. 2016. *Report of the Special Rapporteur on Torture and Other Cruel, Inhuman or Degrading Treatment or Punishment.* A/HRC/31/57, Human Rights Council, General Assembly, United Nations. https://undocs.org/A/HRC/31/57.

Mendonca, Berenice Bilharinho, et al. 2009. "46,XY Disorders of Sex Development (DSD)." *Clinical Endocrinology* 70 (2): 173–87. https://doi.org/10.1111/j.1365-2265.2008.03392.x.

Menon, Nivedita. 2011. "The Disappearing Body and Feminist Thought." *Critical Encounters,* February 18. https://kafila.online/2011/02/18/the-disappearing-body-and-feminist-thought/.

Menon, Yamuna. 2011. "The Intersex Community and the Americans with Disabilities Act." *Connecticut Law Review* 43 (4): 1221–51.

Messner, Michael. 2002. *Taking the Field: Women, Men, and Sport.* Minneapolis: University of Minnesota Press.

Meyerowitz-Katz, Gideon. 2017. "Testing Testosterone Is a Waste of Time: Delineating Gender in Sport Is Not That Easy." *Medium,* July 4. https://medium.com/@gidmk/testing-testosterone-is-a-waste-of-time-684917805957.

Michalko, Rod, and Tanya Titchkosky. 2001. "Putting Disability in Its Place." In *Embodied Rhetorics: Disability in Language and Culture,* ed. James C. Wilson and Cynthia Lewiecki-Wilson, 200–28. Carbondale: Southern Illinois University Press.

Migneault, Jonathan. 2016. "Get Rid of the Paralympics, Says Rick Hansen." *Sudbury,* September 14. https://www.sudbury.com/local-news/get-rid-of-the -paralympics-says-rick-hansen-414284.

Miller, Patrick B. 2015. "The Anatomy of Scientific Racism: Racialist Responses to Black Athletic Achievement." In *Sociological Perspectives on Sport: The Games Outside the Games,* ed. David Karen and Robert E. Washington, 70–81. New York: Routledge.

Milner, Adrienne N., and Jomills Henry Braddock II. 2016. *Sex Segregation in Sports: Why Separate Is Not Equal.* Santa Barbara, CA: Praeger.

Misener, Laura, et al. 2019. *Leveraging Disability Sport Events: Impacts, Promises, and Possibilities.* London: Routledge.

Mitchell, David, and Sharon Snyder. 2000. *Narrative Prosthesis: Disability and the Dependencies of Discourse.* Ann Arbor: University of Michigan Press. doi: 10.3998/mpub.11523.

Mitra, Payoshni. 2014a. "Male/Female or Other: The Untold Stories of Female Athletes with Intersex Variations in India." In *Routledge Handbook of Sport, Gender and Sexuality,* ed. Jennifer Hargreaves and Eric Anderson, 384–94. London: Routledge.

–. 2014b. "No Games for Women with 'Too Much' Testosterone." Interview with Malika Bilal. *Al Jazeera,* September 3. https://www.aljazeera.com/program/ the-stream/2014/9/3/no-games-for-women-with-too-much-testosterone.

Mollow, Anna, and Robert McRuer. 2012. "Introduction." In *Sex and Disability,* ed. Robert McRuer and Anna Mollow, 1–36. Durham, NC: Duke University Press. https://doi.org/10.1215/9780822394877-001.

Money, John. 1968. *Sex Errors of the Body and Related Syndromes: A Guide to Counseling Children, Adolescents and Their Families.* Baltimore, MD: Paul H. Brooks.

Money, John, and Anke A. Ehrhardt. 1972. *Man and Woman, Boy and Girl.* Baltimore, MD: Johns Hopkins University Press.

Monro, Surya. 2019. "Non-binary and Genderqueer: An Overview of the Field." *International Journal of Transgenderism* 20 (2–3): 126–31. https://doi.org/ 10.1080/15532739.2018.1538841.

Monro, Surya, Daniela Crocetti, and Tray Yeadon-Lee. 2019. "Intersex/Variations of Sex Characteristics and DSD Citizenship in the UK, Italy and Switzerland." *Citizenship Studies* 23 (8): 780–97. http://doi/10.1080/13621025.2019.1645813.

Morgan, Kathryn Pauly. 2005. "Gender Police." In *Foucault and the Government of Disability,* ed. Shelley Tremain, 298–328. Ann Arbor: University of Michigan Press. doi:10.3998/mpub.8265343.

Morgan, Tom. 2016. "Caster Semenya Wins 800m: Beaten GB Finalist Lynsey Sharp Criticises Rule Changes over 'Obvious' Hyperandrogenous Women." *Telegraph* (London), August 21. http://www.telegraph.co.uk/news/2016/08/21/lynsey-sharp -criticises-obvious-hypoadrogenous-women-having-bein/.

–. 2019. "Female Athletes Claim Careers Ruined after Being 'Coerced' into Surgery to Curb Testosterone Levels." *Telegraph* (London), September 27. https://www.

telegraph.co.uk/athletics/2019/09/27/female-athletes-claim-careers-ruined
-coerced-surgery-curb-testosterone/.

Morland, Iain. 2009. "What Can Queer Theory Do for Intersex?" *GLQ* 15 (2): 285–312. https://doi.org/10.1215/10642684-2008-139.

Mount Sinai Fertility. 2019. "Supplementary Services for Funded Patients." November 17. https://mountsinaifertility.com/wp-content/uploads/2019/11/Fee-Schedule-Funded-WEBSITE-Nov-17-2019-1.pdf.

Mposo, Paulina S. 2017. "Alternative Sexualities in India." MA thesis, University of Leiden.

Mulgan, Tim. 2001. *The Demands of Consequentialism.* Oxford: Clarendon.

Müller, Johannes. 1834. "Über die äusseren Geschlechtstheile der Buschmänninnen." In *Archiv für Anatomie, Physiologie und Wissenschaftliche Medizin,* ed. Carl Bogislaus Reichert and Emil du Bois-Reymond, 319–45. Leipzig: Verlag von Veit et Comp.

Munro, Brenna. 2010. "Caster Semenya: Gods and Monsters." *Safundi* 11 (4): 383–96. https://doi.org/10.1080/17533171.2010.511782.

Nabhan, Zeina M., Richard C. Rink, and Erica A. Eugster. 2006. "Urinary Tract Infections in Children with Congenital Adrenal Hyperplasia." *Journal of Pediatric Endocrinology and Metabolism* 19 (6): 815–20. https://doi.org/10.1515/JPEM.2006.19.6.815.

Natarajan, Anita. 1996. "Medical Ethics and Truth Telling in the Case of Androgen Insensitivity Syndrome." *Canadian Medical Association Journal* 154 (4): 568–70.

Natoli, Jaime L., et al. 2012. "Prenatal Diagnosis of Down Syndrome: A Systematic Review of Termination Rates (1995–2011)." *Prenatal Diagnosis* 32 (2): 142–53. https://doi.org/10.1002/pd.2910.

Nelson, Jennifer. 2003. *Women of Color and the Reproductive Rights Movement.* New York: New York University Press.

Nelson, Katherine, and Robyn Fivush. 2004. "The Emergence of Autobiographical Memory: A Social Cultural Developmental Theory." *Psychological Review* 111 (2): 486–511. https://doi.org/10.1037/0033-295X.111.2.486.

Nguyen, Viet. 2018. "A Critical Analysis of the Impact of Participation Trophies in Youth Sports." PhD diss., Kalamazoo College.

Nielsen-Bohlman, Lynn, Allison M. Panzer, and David A. Kindig. 2004. *Health literacy: A Prescription to End Confusion.* Washington: National Academies Press.

Nisker, Jeff. 2013. "Informed Choice and PGD to Prevent 'Intersex Conditions.'" *American Journal of Bioethics* 13 (10): 47–49. https://doi.org/10.1080/15265161.2013.828125.

Noddings, Nel. 1984. *Caring: A Feminine Approach to Ethics and Moral Education.* Berkeley: University of California Press.

Nordenvall, Anna Skarin, et al. 2020. "Fertility in Adult Men Born with Hypospadias: A Nationwide Register-Based Cohort Study on Birthrates, the Use of Assisted Reproductive Technologies and Infertility." *Andrology* 8 (2): 372–801. https://doi.org/10.1111/andr.12723.

Nyong'o, Tavia. 2010. "The Unforgivable Transgression of Being Caster Semenya." *Women and Performance: A Journal of Feminist Theory* 20 (1): 95–100. https://doi.org/10.1080/07407701003589501.

O'Keefe, James. 2016. "Homosexuality: It's about Survival – Not Sex." *YouTube*, November 15. https://www.youtube.com/watch?v=4Khn_z9FPmU.

Oliver, Michael. 2004. "The Social Model in Action: If I Had a Hammer." In *Implementing the Social Model of Disability: Theory and Research*, ed. Colin Barnes and Geof Mercer, 18–31. Leeds, UK: Disability Press.

O'Neill, Onora. 2013. *Acting on Principle: An Essay on Kantian Ethics*. 2nd ed. Cambridge, UK: Cambridge University Press. https://doi.org/10.1017/CBO97 81139565097.

O'Neill, Shannon, and Jeff Blackmer. 2015. *Assisted Reproduction in Canada: An Overview of Ethical and Legal Issues and Recommendations for the Development of National Standards*. Ottawa: Canadian Medical Association. https://docplayer.net/18332642-Assisted-reproduction-in-canada.html.

O'Sullivan, Sandy. 2021. "The Colonial Project of Gender (and Everything Else)." *Genealogy* 5 (3): 67. https://doi.org/10.3390/genealogy5030067.

Ontario Ministry of Health and Long-Term Care. 1998. "Fact Sheet: Ultrasound for Pregnancy." http://health.gov.on.ca/en/pro/programs/ohip/bulletins/4317/bul4317c.aspx.

O'Rourke, Michael, and Noreen Giffney. 2009. "Preface." In *Critical Intersex*, ed. Morgan Holmes, ix-xii. Farnham, UK: Ashgate. https://doi.org/10.4324/9781315575018.

Orr, Celeste E. 2018. "Sexual Assault in Medical Contexts." *Impact Ethics*, February 16. https://impactethics.ca/2018/02/16/sexual-assault-in-medical-contexts/.

–. 2019. "Resisting the Demand to Stand: Boys, Bathrooms, Hypospadias, and Interphobic Violence." *Boyhood Studies: An Interdisciplinary Journal* 12 (2): 89–113. https://doi.org/10.3167/bhs.2019.120206.

Orr, Celeste E., and Meg Peters. "Introducing Mad Intersex Studies" (working paper, Institute of Feminist and Gender Studies, Faculty of Social Sciences, University of Ottawa).

Orr, Celeste E., and Amanda D. Watson. 2018. "'We Changed Her Nappies. We Saw That She Was a Girl'': Caster Semenya's Femininity and the Power of Maternal Testimony." In *Mothering, Mothers, and Sport: Experiences, Representations, Resistances*, ed. Judy Battaglia, Rebecca Bromwich, and Pamela Redela, 15–48. Bradford, ON: Demeter.

–. 2021. "'Usually the Mother': Dilation and the Medical Management of Intersex Children." In *From Band-Aids to Scalpels: Motherhood Experiences in/of Medicine*, ed. Rohini Bannerjee and Karim Mukhida, 65–83. Bradford, ON: Demeter.

Orsini, Michael. 2009. "Contesting the Autistic Subject: Biological Citizenship and the Autism/Autistic Movement." In *Critical Interventions in the Ethics of Healthcare: Challenging the Principle of Autonomy in Bioethics*, ed. Stuart J. Murray and Dave Holmes, 115–30. Farnham, UK: Ashgate.

Örtqvist, Lisa, et al. 2017. "Sexuality and Fertility in Men with Hypospadias: Improved Outcome." *Andrology* 5 (2): 286–93. https://doi.org/10.1111/andr.12309.

Ostertag, Stephen F. 2020. "Antiracism Movements and the US Civil Sphere: The Case of Black Lives Matter." In *Breaching the Civil Order: Radicalism and the*

Civil Sphere, ed. Jeffrey C. Alexander, Trevor Stack, and Ferhad Khosrokhavar, 70–91. Cambridge, UK: Cambridge University Press.

Ottawa Fertility Centre. n.d. "Fees." https://conceive.ca/fees/#Additional-Fees-For -Non-OHIP-Insured-Patients.

—. n.d. "Fertility Treatments." https://conceive.ca/fertility-treatments/pgta-pgtm/.

Otto, Adolf Wilhelm. 1816. *Seltene Beobachtungen zur Anatomie, Physiologie und Pathologie gehörig.* Breslau, Germany: Wilibald Holäafer.

Oudshoorn, Nelly. 1994. *Beyond the Natural Body: An Archaeology of Sex Hormones.* New York: Routledge.

Owen, Gibson. 2016. "Paralympic Games: Countries Still Waiting for Vital Travel Grants." *Guardian* (London), August 14. https://www.theguardian.com/sport/ 2016/aug/14/paralympic-committee-to-hold-budget-crisis-talks-with-brazil.

Paduch, Darius A., et al. 2008. "New Concepts in Klinefelter Syndrome." *Current Opinion in Urology* 19 (6): 621–27. doi:10.1097/MOU.0b013e32831367c7.

Paget, Marianne A. 2004. *The Unity of Mistakes: A Phenomenological Interpretation of Medical Work.* 1988. Reprint, Philadelphia: Temple University Press.

Pagonis, Pidgeon. 2015a. "9 Damaging Lies Doctors Told Me When I Was Growing Up Intersex." *Everyday Feminism,* December 3. https://everydayfeminism.com/ 2015/12/lies-from-doctors-intersex/.

—. 2015b. "The Son They Never Had." *Narrative Inquiry in Bioethics* 5 (2): 103–6. doi:10.1353/nib.2015.0053.

—. 2015c. "The Future is Intersex." Digital. Chicago.

—. 2016. "6 Things Intersex Folks Need to Know about How We Perpetuate Anti-Black Racism." *Everyday Feminism,* June 3. https://everydayfeminism.com/ 2016/06/intersex-anti-black-racism/.

—. 2017a. "Episode 7." Interview with Tai Jacob and Cary Gabriel Costello. *Gender Blender,* August 28. https://soundcloud.com/gender-blender-podcast/episode -7-pidgeon-ft-dr-cary-costello.

—. 2017b. "First Do No Harm: How Intersex Kids Are Hurt by Those Who Have Taken the Hippocratic Oath." *Griffith Journal of Law and Human Dignity,* special issue: 40–51. https://griffithlawjournal.org/index.php/gjlhd/issue/view/94.

Pai, A.L.H., et al. 2008. "The Psychological Assessment Tool (PAT2.0): Psychometric Properties of a Screener for Psychosocial Distress in Families of Children Newly Diagnosed with Cancer." *Journal of Pediatric Psychology* 33 (1): 50–62. doi: 10.1093/jpepsy/jam053.

Pape, Madeleine. 2016. "The Way Out of This Mess: Taking Caster Semenya with Us." *SBS,* August 23. https://www.sbs.com.au/topics/zela/article/2016/08/23/ way-out-mess-taking-caster-semenya-us.

—. 2019. "I Was Sore about Losing to Caster Semenya. But This Decision against Her Is Wrong." *Guardian* (London), May 1. https://www.theguardian.com/ commentisfree/2019/may/01/losing-caster-semenya-decision-wrong-women -testosterone-iaaf.

Park, Madison. 2016. "Is Olympic Coverage Undercutting Women's Achievements?" *CNN,* August 9. http://www.cnn.com/2016/08/09/sport/olympics-women-sexism -trnd/index.html.

Parker, Jim. 2016. "'I Didn't Run Fast Enough': Melissa Bishop Won't Wallow in Disappointment of Missing 800m Podium in Rio." *National Post,* August 24. http://

nationalpost.com/sports/olympics/i-didnt-run-fast-enough-canadas-melissa
-bishop-wont-wallow-in-disappointment-of-missing-800m-podium-in-rio.

Pasche Guignard, Florence. 2015. "A Gendered Bun in the Oven: The Gender-Reveal Party as a New Ritualization during Pregnancy." *Studies in Religion/Sciences Religieuses* 44 (4): 470–500. https://doi.org/10.1177/0008429815599802.

Pasterski, Vickie, et al. 2014. "Predictors of Posttraumatic Stress in Parents of Children Diagnosed with a Disorder of Sex Development." *Archives of Sexual Behavior* 43 (2): 369–75. https://doi.org/10.1007/s10508-013-0196-8.

Paterson, Paul, et al. 2011. "Cleft Lip/Palate: Incidence of Prenatal Diagnosis in Glasgow, Scotland, and Comparison with Other Centers in the United Kingdom." *Cleft Palate-Craniofacial Journal* 43 (5): 608–13. https://doi.org/10. 1597/09-238.

Peers, Danielle. 2009. "(Dis)empowering Paralympic Histories: Absent Athletes and Disabling Discourses." *Disability and Society* 24 (5): 653–65. https://doi. org/10.1080/09687590903011113.

–. 2012. "Interrogating Disability: The (De)composition of a Recovering Paralympian." *Qualitative Research in Sport, Exercise and Health* 4 (2): 175–88. https:// doi.org/10.1080/2159676X.2012.685101.

–. 2015. "From Inhalation to Inspiration: A Genealogical Auto-ethnography of a Supercrip." In *Foucault and the Government of Disability*, ed. Shelley Tremain, 331–49. Ann Arbor: University of Michigan Press. doi:10.3998/mpub.8265343.

Phala, Mbali. 2016. "South Africa: Who Is Caster Semenya and Why Does She Matter?" *All Africa*, August 26. http://allafrica.com/stories/201608270017.html.

Picq, Manuela L. 2020. "Decolonizing Indigenous Sexualities: Between Erasure and Resurgence." In *The Oxford Handbook of Global LGBT and Sexual Diversity Politics*, ed. Michael J. Bosia, Sandra M. McEvoy, and Momin Rahman, 169–84. Oxford: Oxford University Press.

Pieper, Lindsay Parks. 2014. "Sex Testing and the Maintenance of Western Femininity in International Sport." *International Journal of the History of Sport* 31 (13): 1557–76. https://doi.org/10.1080/09523367.2014.927184.

–. 2016. *Sex Testing: Gender Policing in Women's Sports*. Champaign: University of Illinois Press.

Pizot, Cécile, et al. 2016. "Physical Activity, Hormone Replacement Therapy and Breast Cancer Risk: A Meta-analysis of Prospective Studies." *European Journal of Cancer* 52: 138–54. https://doi.org/10.1016/j.ejca.2015.10.063.

Plato. 1962. *Dialogues*. Ed. Edith Hamilton and Huntington Cairns. Original 4th century BCE. Princeton, NJ: Princeton University Press.

Plattner, Karin. 2011. "Intersex and ISGD: Yet Another Attempt to Co-opt Intersex?" *Intersex Human Rights Australia*, May 21. https://ihra.org.au/13588/ isgd-attempts-colonize-intersex/.

Plotinus. 1952. *The Six Enneads*. Ed. Stephen McKenna and B.S. Page. Original 3rd century CE. London: Encyclopedia Britannica.

Porter, Roy. 1998. *The Greatest Benefit to Mankind: A Medical History of Humanity*. New York: W.W. Norton and Company.

Potter, Elizabeth. 2006. *Feminism and Philosophy of Science: An Introduction*. New York: Routledge.

Preciado, Paul B. 2005. "The Intersextional Darkroom." In *Sex Works: 1978–2005,* ed. Del LaGrace Volcano, 155–59. Tübingen, Germany: Konkursbuchverlag Verlag.

–. 2013. *Testo Junkie: Sex, Drugs, and Biopolitics in the Pharmacopornographic Era.* New York: Feminist Press.

Prest, Dayna. 2016. "Lesbians and Space: An Interpretive Phenomenological Analysis." MA thesis, University of Ottawa.

Preves, Sharon E. 1999. "For the Sake of the Children: Destigmatizing Intersexuality." In *Intersex in the Age of Ethics,* ed. Alice Domurat Dreger, 51–65. Hagerstown, MD: University Publishing Group.

–. 2003. *Intersex and Identity.* New Brunswick, NJ: Rutgers University Press.

Preves, Sharon E., and A. Evan Eyler. 1999. "Belief in Having Been Born Intersexed as a Psychological Defense among 'Transphobic' Transsexuals: Report of Three Cases." Paper presented at "XVI Harry Benjamin International Gender Dysphoria Association Symposium," London, England, August 17–21.

Puar, Jasbir K. 2007. *Terrorist Assemblages: Homonationalism in Queer Times.* Durham, NC: Duke University Press. https://doi.org/10.1215/9780822390442.

–. 2009. "Prognosis Time: Towards a Geopolitics of Affect, Debility and Capacity." *Women & Performance: a journal of feminist theory* 19 (2): 161–72. https://doi.org/10.1080/07407700903034147.

–. 2013. "Rethinking Homonationalism." *International Journal of Middle East Studies* 45 (2): 336–39. https://doi.org/10.1017/S002074381300007X.

–. 2017. *The Right to Maim: Debility, Capacity, Disability.* Durham, NC: Duke University Press. https://doi.org/10.1215/9780822372530.

Putnam, Frank W. 2003. "Ten-Year Research Update Review: Child Sexual Abuse." *Journal of the American Academy of Child and Adolescent Psychiatry* 42 (3): 269–78. https://doi.org/10.1097/00004583-200303000-00006.

Queer Nation NY. 2016. "Queer Nation NY History." https://queernationny.org/history.

Quinn, Emily. 2015. "Standing Up." *Narrative Inquiry into Bioethics* 5 (2): 109–11. doi:10.1353/nib.2015.0032.

–. 2016. "Intersex Surgeries | Vaginoplasty & Clitorectomy." *YouTube,* November 17. https://www.youtube.com/watch?v=uNjBKdACu50.

Quinton, Anthony. 1973. *Utilitarian Ethics.* London: Palgrave Macmillan.

Railton, Peter. 1984. "Alienation, Consequentialism, and the Demands of Morality." *Philosophy and Public Affairs* 13 (2): 134–71.

Rainbow Fertility. 2020. "Additional Options with IVF." https://www.rainbowfertility.com.au/family-building-for-gay-men/fertility-services-for-gay-men/additional-treatment-options-with-ivf/.

Rainbow Health Ontario. 2011. *Evidence Brief: Inform Your Practice Because LGBTQ Health Matters.* https://www.rainbowhealthontario.ca/wp-content/uploads/2011/08/RHO_FactSheet_INTERSEXHEALTH_E.pdf.

Ramasamy, Ranjith, et al. 2009. "Successful Fertility Treatment for Klinefelter's Syndrome." *Journal of Urology* 182 (3): 1108–13. https://doi.org/10.1016/j.juro.2009.05.019.

Ramsay, Michèle, et al. 1988. "XX True Hermaphroditism in Southern Africa Blacks: An Enigma of Primary Sexual Differentiation." *American Journal of Human Genetics* 43 (1): 4–13.

Rapp, Rayna. 1999. *Testing Women, Testing the Fetus: The Social Impact of Amniocentesis in America.* New York: Routledge.

Real, Terrence. 1998. *I Don't Want to Talk about It: Overcoming the Secret Legacy of Male Depression.* New York: Scribner.

Reaume, Geoffrey. 2002. "Lunatic to Patient to Person: Nomenclature in Psychiatric History and the Influence of Patients' Activism in North America." *International Journal of Law and Psychiatry* 25 (4): 405–26. https://doi.org/10.1016/S0160 -2527(02)00130-9.

Reddy, Gayatri. 2005. *With Respect to Sex: Negotiating Hijra Identity in South India.* Chicago: University of Chicago Press.

Reichert, Michael, et al. 2012. "'A Place to Be Myself': The Critical Role of Schools in Boys' Emotional Development." *Boyhood Studies: An Interdisciplinary Journal* 6 (1): 55–75. https://doi.org/10.3149/thy.0601.55.

Reimers, Tonny Solveig, et al. 2009. "Health-Related Quality of Life in Long-Term Survivors of Childhood Brain Tumors." *Pediatric Blood and Cancer* 53 (6): 1086–91. https://doi.org/10.1002/pbc.22122.

Reis, Elizabeth. 2005. "Impossible Hermaphrodites: Intersex in America, 1620– 1960." *Journal of American History* 92 (2): 411–41. https://doi.org/10.2307/ 3659273.

–. 2009. *Bodies in Doubt: An American History of Intersex.* Baltimore, MD: Johns Hopkins University Press.

Reis, Elizabeth, and Suzanne Kessler. 2010. "Why History Matters: Fetal Dex and Intersex." *American Journal of Bioethics* 10 (9): 58–59. https://doi.org/10.1080/ 15265161.2010.499586.

Reitman, Ivan, dir. 1994. *Junior.* Northern Lights Entertainment.

Rice, Carla, et al. 2017. "Imagining Disability Futurities." *Hypatia* 32 (2): 213–29. https://doi.org/10.1111/hypa.12321.

Rice, Condoleezza. 2000. "Promoting the National Interest." *Foreign Affairs* 79 (1): 45–62. doi:10.2307/20049613.

Rich, Adrienne. 1980. "Compulsory Heterosexuality and Lesbian Existence." *Signs: Journal of Women's History* 15 (3): 11–48. https://doi.org/10.1086/493756.

Richards, Deborah, et al. 2009. "Sexuality and Human Rights of Persons with Intellectual Disabilities." In *Challenges to the Human Rights of People with Intellectual Disabilities,* ed. Frances Owen and Dorothy Griffiths, 184–218. London: Jessica Kingsley.

Richards, Stephanie. 2018. "The No Longer Silent 'I' in LGBTIQ." *InDaily,* August 1. https://indaily.com.au/news/2018/08/01/the-no-longer-silent-i-in-lgbtiq/.

Riggs, Damien, and Elizabeth Peel. 2016. *Critical Kinship Studies.* London: Palgrave Macmillan. doi:10.1057/978-1-137-50505-7.

Rinaldi, Jen, and nancy viva davis halifax. 2016. "Challenging Rhetorical Indifference with a Cripped Poetry of Witness." In *Mobilizing Metaphor: Art, Culture, and*

Disability Activism in Canada, ed. Christine Kelly and Michael Orsini, 241–59. Vancouver: UBC Press.

Ristock, Janice, et al. 2019. "Impacts of Colonization on Indigenous Two-Spirit/ LGBTQ Canadians" Experiences of Migration, Mobility and Relationship Violence." *Sexualities* 22 (5–6): 767–84. https://doi.org/10.1177/1363460716681474.

Roen, Katrina. 2005. "Queer Kids: Toward Ethical Clinical Interactions with Intersex People." In *Ethics of the Body: Postconventional Challenges,* ed. Margrit Shildrick and Roxanne Mykitiuk, 259–78. Cambridge, MA: MIT Press.

–. 2009. "Clinical Intervention and Embodied Subjectivity: Atypically Sexed Children and Their Parents." In *Critical Intersex,* ed. Morgan Holmes, 15–40. Farnham, UK: Ashgate. https://doi.org/10.4324/9781315575018.

Roscoe, Will. 1992. *The Zuni Man-Woman.* Albuquerque: University of New Mexico Press.

–. 1998. *Changing Ones: Third and Fourth Genders in Native North America.* New York: St. Martin's Press.

Rose, Damon. 2012. "Paralympics and Olympics Merger 'Possible after 2020.'" *BBC,* May 23. https://www.bbc.com/news/uk-18174501.

Rose, Rebecca. 2015. "Man Shocked to Discover He Has a Fully Functioning Womb." *Cosmopolitan,* February 10. http://www.cosmopolitan.com/lifestyle/news/ a36344/man-discovers-he-has-a-working-womb-and-uterus/.

Ross, Ronald K., et al. 2000. "Effect of Hormone Replacement Therapy on Breast Cancer Risk: Estrogen versus Estrogen Plus Progestin." *Journal of the National Cancer Institute* 92 (4): 328–32. https://doi.org/10.1093/jnci/92.4.328.

Rosenwohl-Mack, Amy, et al. 2020. "A National Study on the Physical and Mental Health of Intersex Adults in the US." *PloS one* 15 (10): 1–16. https://doi.org/ 10.1371/journal.pone.0240088.

Rubin, Gayle. 1998. "Thinking Sex: Notes for a Radical Theory of Politics of Sexuality." 1984. Reprinted in *Social Perspectives in Lesbian and Gay Studies: A Reader,* ed. Peter M. Nardi and Beth E. Schneider, 100–33. New York: Routledge.

Safwat, Ahmed S., Ahmad Elderwy, and Hisham M. Hammouda. 2013. "Which Type of Urethroplasty in Failed Hypospadias Repair? An 8-Year Follow Up." *Journal of Pediatric Urology* 9 (6): 1150–54. https://doi.org/10.1016/j.jpurol. 2013.04.015.

Saleeby, Caleb Williams. 1911. *Parenthood and Race Culture: An Outline of Eugenics.* New York: Moffat, Yard and Company.

Salle, J.L. Pippi, et al. 2016. "Proximal Hypospadias: A Persistent Challenge: Single Institution Outcome Analysis of Three Surgical Techniques over a 10-Year Period." *Journal of Pediatric Urology* 12 (1): 28.e1–7. https://doi.org/10.1016/j. jpurol.2015.06.011.

Salleh, Anna. 2010. "Cyborg Rights 'Need Debating Now.'" *ABC Science,* June 4. https://www.abc.net.au/science/articles/2010/06/04/2916443.htm.

Samuels, Ellen. 2003. "My Body, My Closet: Invisible Disability and the Limits of Coming-Out Discourse." *GLQ* 9 (1): 233–55. https://doi.org/10.1215/ 10642684-9-1-2-233.

Sandberg, David E., and Tom Mazur. 2014. "A Noncategorical Approach to the Psychosocial Care of Persons with DSD and Their Families." In *Gender Dysphoria and Disorders of Sex Development: Progress in Care and Knowledge*, ed. Baudewijntje P.C. Kreukels, Thomas D. Steensma, and Annelou L.C. de Vries, 93–114. New York: Springer. doi:10.1007/978-1-4614-7441-8.

Sandeen, Autumn. 2014. "Ipso Gender: A Third Term for Intersex People." *LGBT Weekly*, September 18. Accessed December 13, 2017. http://lgbtweekly.com/2014/09/18/ipso-gender-a-third-term-for-intersex-people/.

Sandel, Michael J. 2007. *The Case against Perfection: Ethics in the Age of Genetic Engineering*. Cambridge, MA: Harvard University Press.

Sanders, Joel, and Susan Stryker. 2016. "Stalled: Gender-Neutral Public Bathrooms." *South Atlantic Quarterly* 115 (4): 779–88. https://doi.org/10.1215/00382876-3656191.

Savulescu, Julian. 2001. "Procreative Beneficence: Why We Should Select the Best Children." *Bioethics* 15 (5): 413–26. https://doi.org/10.1111/1467-8519.00251.

–. 2007. "In Defence of Procreative Beneficence." *Journal of Medical Ethics* 33 (5): 284–88. http://dx.doi.org/10.1136/jme.2006.018184.

–. 2012. "Procreative Beneficence: Why We Should Select the Best Children." In *Arguing about Bioethics*, ed. Stephen Holland, 74–82. London: Routledge.

Sawer, Patrick. 2015. "'Ordinary Bloke' Prepares for Hysterectomy after Doctors Discover Womb during Bladder Cancer Test." *National Post*, February 8. https://nationalpost.com/news/world/ordinary-bloke-prepares-for-hysterectomy-after-doctors-discover-he-has-womb-during-bladder-cancer-test.

Sawyer, Jeremy, and Anup Gampa. 2018. "Implicit and Explicit Racial Attitudes Changed during Black Lives Matter." *Personality and Social Psychology Bulletin* 44 (7): 1039–59. https://doi.org/10.1177/0146167218757454.

Saxton, Marsha. 1997. "Disability Rights and Selective Abortion." In *Abortion Wars: A Half Century of Struggle, 1950–2000*, ed. Rickie Solinger, 374–95. Berkeley: University of California Press.

–. 2017. "Disability Rights and Selective Abortion." In *The Disability Studies Reader*, 5th ed., ed. Lennard J. Davis, 73–86. New York: Routledge.

Scherer, Heidi L., and Bradford W. Reyns. 2019. "Visible Disabilities and Risk of Interpersonal Victimization." In *Appearance Bias and Crime*, ed. Bonnie Berry, 243–55. Cambridge, UK: Cambridge University Press.

Schiebinger, Londa L. 1993. *Nature's Body: Sexual Politics and the Making of Modern Science*. Boston: Beacon.

Schiff, Jonathan D., et al. 2005. "Success of Testicular Sperm Injection and Intracytoplasmic Sperm Injection in Men with Klinefelter Syndrome." *Journal of Clinical Endocrinology and Metabolism* 90 (11): 6263–67. https://doi.org/10.1210/jc.2004-2322.

Schlauderaff, Sav. 2020. "Re-imagining Futurity for Fat, Disabled and 'Unhealthy' Bodyminds: A Response to 23andMe's Health + Ancestry Genetic Testing Kits." *Fat Studies: An Interdisciplinary Journal of Body Weight and Society* 9 (3): 238–58. https://doi.org/10.1080/21604851.2019.1651124.

Schoenberg, Nara. 2018. "'It's Medically Sanctioned Violence and Torture': Intersex Patients Call for End to Genital Surgeries on Children." *Chicago Tribune*, November 1. https://www.chicagotribune.com/lifestyles/ct-life-intersex-surgeries-20181018-story.html.

Schor, Naomi. 1999. "Blindness as Metaphor." *Differences: A Journal of Feminist Cultural Studies* 11 (2): 76–105. https://doi.org/10.1215/10407391-11-2-76.

Schulter, Margo. 2017. "Owning Endosex Privilege, and Supporting the Intersex Community: WPATH, Intersex Genital Mutilation (IGM), and Sex Variant Bodies." *TransAdvocate*, January 9. http://transadvocate.com/owning-endosex -privilege-and-supporting-the-intersex-community-wpath-intersex-genital -mutilation-igm-and-sex-variant-bodies_n_18868.htm.

Schützmann, Karsten, et al. 2009. "Psychological Distress, Self-Harming Behavior, and Suicidal Tendencies in Adults with Disorders of Sex Development." *Archives of Sexual Behavior* 38 (1): 16–33. https://doi.org/10.1007/s10508-007-9241-9.

Scope. 2011. "Scope NDPP Survey August 2011." https://comresglobal.com/wp -content/themes/comres/poll/Scope_DPP_Discrimination_and_Paralympics_ data_tables_August_2011.pdf.

Segal, Lynne. 1987. *Is the Future Female? Troubled Thoughts on Contemporary Feminism.* London: Virago.

Serano, Julia. 2007. *Whipping Girl: A Transsexual Woman on Sexism and the Scape-goating of Femininity.* Berkeley, CA: Seal.

—. 2012. "Trans Feminism: There's No Conundrum about It." *Ms. Magazine*, April 18. https://msmagazine.com/2012/04/18/trans-feminism-theres-no-conundrum -about-it/.

Shakespeare, Tom. 1995. "Back to the Future? New Genetics and Disabled People." *Critical Social Policy* 15 (44–45): 22–35. https://doi.org/10.1177/0261018395 01504402.

—. 1998. "Choices and Rights: Eugenics, Genetics and Disability Equality." *Disability and Society* 13 (5): 665–81. https://doi.org/10.1080/09687599826452.

—. 2013. "The Social Model of Disability." In *The Disability Studies Reader*, 4th ed., ed. Lennard J. Davis, 214–21. New York: Routledge.

Shalala, Amanda. 2018. "IAAF Female Classification Rules Slammed as 'Blatantly Racist.'" *ABC*, April 27. http://www.abc.net.au/news/2018-04-28/critics-say-iaaf -testosterone-rules-blatantly-racist/9706744.

Sharp, Keith, and Sarah Earle. 2002. "Feminism, Abortion and Disability: Irrecon-cilable Differences?" *Disability and Society* 17 (2): 137–45. https://doi.org/10. 1080/09687590120122297.

Shaw, William. *Contemporary Ethics: Taking Account of Utilitarianism.* Malden: Blackwell Publishers.

Sheible, Lenzi. 2014. "How the Pro-Choice Movement Excludes People with Dis-abilities." *Rewire News Group*, October 17. https://rewire.news/article/2014/ 10/17/pro-choice-movement-excludes-people-disabilities/.

Sherbahn, Richard. n.d. "PGD and IVF Costs – What Is the Cost for Preimplanta-tion Genetic Diagnosis – PGD and PGS, Preimplantation Genetic Screening?" Advanced Fertility Center of Chicago. http://www.advancedfertility.com/pgd -costs.htm.

Sherbourne Health. n.d. "Parenting and Family Resources, LGBT2SQ Communi-ties." Accessed March 15, 2022. https://sherbourne.on.ca/primary-family-health

-care/lgbt-health/lgbt2sq-parenting-family-resources/?doing_wp_cron=146198
5253.3047549724578857421875.

Sher Fertility Institute. n.d. "An Update on Autism and IVF: Fact vs. Fiction."
Accessed November 15, 2016. http://haveababy.com/fertility-information/ivf
-authority/update-autism-ivf-fact-vs-fiction.

Shildrick, Margrit. 2002. *Embodying the Monster: Encounters with the Vulnerable
Self.* New York: Sage. http://dx.doi.org/10.4135/9781446220573.

—. 2005. "Beyond the Body of Bioethics: Challenging the Conventions." In *Ethics of
the Body: Postconventional Challenges,* ed. Margrit Shildrick and Roxanne
Mykitiuk, 1–29. Cambridge, MA: MIT Press.

Shildrick, Margrit, and Roxanne Mykitiuk, eds. 2005. *Ethics of the Body: Post-
conventional Challenges.* Cambridge, MA: MIT Press.

Shumka, Leah, Susan Strega, and Helga Kristin Hallgrimsdottir. 2017. "'I Wanted to
Feel Like a Man Again': Hegemonic Masculinity in Relation to the Purchase of
Street-Level Sex." *Frontiers in Sociology* 2 (15): 1–15. https://doi.org/10.3389/
fsoc.2017.00015.

Silvers, Anita. 1994. "'Defective' Agents: Equality, Difference and the Tyranny of
the Normal." *Journal of Social Philosophy* 25 (1): 154–75. https://doi.org/10.
1111/j.1467-9833.1994.tb00353.x.

Simolke, Duane. 2005. *Holding Me Together: Essays and Poems.* New York: iUniverse.

Simpson, Joe Leigh, et al. 2000. "Gender Verification in the Olympics." *Journal of the
American Medical Association* 284 (12): 1568–69. doi:10.1001/jama.284.12.1568.

Sircili, Maria Helena Palma, et al. 2006. "Anatomical and Functional Outcomes of
Feminizing Genitoplasty for Ambiguous Genitalia in Patients with Virilizing
Congenital Adrenal Hyperplasia." *Clinics* 61 (3): 209–14. https://doi.org/10.1590/
S1807-59322006000300005.

Smith, Dorothy. 1979. "A Sociology of Women." In *The Prism of Sex,* ed. Julia
Sherman and Evelyn Beck, 135–87. Madison: University of Wisconsin Press.

—. 1987. *The Everyday World as Problematic: A Feminist Sociology.* Toronto: University of Toronto Press.

—. 1990. *The Conceptual Practices of Power: A Feminist Sociology of Knowledge.* Toronto: University of Toronto Press.

Smith, Durham E. 1997. "The History of Hypospadias." *Pediatric Surgery International* 12 (2): 81–85. https://doi.org/10.1007/BF01349969.

Smith, Malcolm A., et al. 2010. "Outcomes for Children and Adolescents with
Cancer: Challenges for the Twenty-First Century." *Journal of Clinical Oncology*
28 (15): 2625–34. doi:10.1200/JCO.2009.27.0421.

Smith, Phil. 2004. "Whiteness, Normal Theory, and Disability Studies." *Disability
Studies Quarterly* 24 (2). http://dx.doi.org/10.18061/dsq.v24i2.491.

Smith, Valerie. 2013. *Not Just Race, Not Just Gender: Black Feminist Readings.* 1998.
Reprint, New York: Routledge. https://doi.org/10.4324/9780203699843.

Smith-Squire, Alison. 2015. "Man with a Womb Intersex Story in the Sun News-
paper." *Feature World,* February 7. http://www.featureworld.co.uk/man-finds-he
-has-a-working-womb/.

Snodgrass, Warren, et al. 1998. "Tubularized Incised Plate Hypospadias Repair for Proximal Hypospadias." *Journal of Urology* 159 (6): 2129–31. https://doi.org/10.1016/S0022-5347(01)63293-2.

Snyder, Sharon L., Brenda Jo Brueggemann, and Rosemarie Garland-Thomson. 2002. *Disability Studies: Enabling the Humanities.* New York: Modern Language Association of America.

Snyder, Sharon L., and David T. Mitchell. 2010. "Introduction: Ablenationalism and the Geo-politics of Disability." *Journal of Literary and Cultural Disability Studies* 4 (2): 113–26. https://doi.org/10.3828/jlcds.2010.10.

Sobo, E.J., Helen Lambert, and Corliss D. Heath. 2020. "More Than a Teachable Moment: Black Lives Matter." *Anthropology and Medicine* 27 (3): 243–48. https://doi.org/10.1080/13648470.2020.1783054.

Sobsey, Dick, and Tanis Doe. 1991. "Patterns of Sexual Abuse and Assault." *Sexuality and Disability* 9 (3): 243–59. https://doi.org/10.1007/BF01102395.

Solomos, John, ed. 2020. *Routledge International Handbook of Contemporary Racisms.* New York: Routledge. https://doi.org/10.4324/9781351047326.

Soloway, Joey, and Andrea Sperling, dirs. 2014–19. *Transparent.* Topple and Picrow.

Somerville, Siobhan B. 2000. *Queering the Color Line: Race and the Invention of Homosexuality in American Culture.* Durham, NC: Duke University Press.

Soucek, Brian. 2014. "Perceived Homosexuals: Looking Gay Enough for Title VII." *American University Law Review* 63 (3): 715–88.

Sparrow, Robert. 2005. "Defending Deaf Culture: The Case of Cochlear Implants." *Journal of Political Philosophy* 13 (2): 135–52. https://doi.org/10.1111/j.1467-9760.2005.00217.x.

–. 2007. "Procreative Beneficence, Obligation, and Eugenics." *Genomics, Society and Policy* 3 (3): 43–59. https://doi.org/10.1186/1746-5354-3-3-43.

–. 2010. "Should Human Beings Have Sex? Sexual Dimorphism and Human Enhancement." *American Journal of Bioethics* 10 (7): 3–12. https://doi.org/10.1080/15265161.2010.489409.

–. 2013. "Gender Eugenics? The Ethics of PGD for Intersex Conditions." *American Journal of Bioethics* 13 (10): 29–38. https://doi.org/10.1080/15265161.2013.828115.

Speechley, Kathy N., and Jeff Nisker. 2010. "Preimplantation Genetic Diagnosis." *Journal of Obstetrics and Gynaecology Canada* 32 (4): 341–47. https://doi.org/10.1016/S1701-2163(16)34479-6.

Springer, Shira. 2016. "Paralympics Should Be Held before Olympics, Not After." *Boston Globe,* September 6. https://www.bostonglobe.com/sports/olympics2016/2016/09/06/paralympics-should-held-before-not-after-olympics/Xf40cAnGLNxQmziTLWu5qO/story.html.

Spurgas, Alyson K. 2009. "(Un)Queering Identity: The Biosocial Production of Intersex/DSD." In *Critical Intersex,* ed. Morgan Holmes, 97–122. Farnham, UK: Ashgate. https://doi.org/10.4324/9781315575018.

Stanasel, Irina, et al. 2015. "Complications Following Staged Hypospadias Repair Using Transposed Preputial Skin Flaps." *Journal of Urology* 195 (2): 512–16. https://doi.org/10.1016/j.juro.2015.02.044.

Standring, Susan. 2016. *Gray's Anatomy: The Anatomical Basis of Clinical Practice.* 41st ed. Philadelphia: Elsevier.

Stapleford, Rebecca. 2014. "Justifications for Abortion Are Inherently Ableist." *Secular Pro-Life Perspectives,* October 22. http://blog.secularprolife.org/2014/10/justifications-for-abortion-are.html.

Stevens, Bethany. 2011. "Interrogating Transability: A Catalyst to View Disability as Body Art." *Disability Studies Quarterly* 31 (4). http://dx.doi.org/10.18061/dsq.v31i4.1705.

Stiglitz, Joseph E. 2006. *Making Globalization Work.* New York: W.W. Norton and Company.

Stockton, Kathryn Bond. 2009. *The Queer Child, or Growing Sideways in the Twentieth Century.* Durham, NC: Duke University Press. https://doi.org/10.1215/9780822390268.

StopIGM.org. 2017. "Trans Persons Posing as Intersex (and the Damage They Do to Intersex Rights)." June 3. http://stop.genitalmutilation.org/post/Intersex-Posers?fbclid=IwAR1ddl_6gVwvSk6MB2jFo28mLCTQd6-o1DBYygYBipAjDoJBwv3aoWcXxAY.

Strang, Heather, and John Braithwaite, eds. 2002. *Restorative Justice and Family Violence.* Cambridge, UK: Cambridge University Press.

Strudwick, Patrick. 2018. "This Woman Only Discovered She Was Intersex after Watching a Viral Video about It." *BuzzFeedNews,* December 29. https://www.buzzfeed.com/patrickstrudwick/this-woman-only-discovered-she-was-intersex-after-watching.

Sudbury, Julia. 2013. *Global Lockdown: Race, Gender, and the Prison-Industrial Complex.* New York: Routledge. https://doi.org/10.4324/9781315810812.

Sullivan, Nikki. 2006. "Transmogrification: (Un)Becoming Other(s)." In *The Transgender Studies Reader,* ed. Susan Stryker and Stephan Whittle, 552–64. New York: Routledge. https://doi.org/10.4324/9780203955055.

Sumerau, J.E. 2020. "A Tale of Three Spectrums: Deviating from Normative Treatments of Sex and Gender." *Deviant Behavior* 41 (7): 893–904. https://doi.org/10.1080/01639625.2020.1735030.

Sumerau, J.E., and Lain A.B. Mathers. 2019. *America through Transgender Eyes.* Lanham, MD: Rowman and Littlefield.

Swaab, Dick F. 2004. "Sexual Differentiation of the Human Brain: Relevance for Gender, Identity, Transsexualism and Sexual Orientation." *Gynecological Endocrinology* 19 (6): 301–12. https://doi.org/10.1080/09513590400018231.

Swartz, Leslie, and Brian Watermeyer. 2008. "Cyborg Anxiety: Oscar Pistorius and the Boundaries of What It Means to Be Human." *Disability and Society* 23 (2): 187–90. https://doi.org/10.1080/09687590701841232.

Sykes, Heather. 2017. *The Sexual and Gender Politics of Sport Mega-Events: Roving Colonialism.* London: Routledge. https://doi.org/10.4324/9781315776286.

Sykes, Heather, and Christopher Smith. 2016. "Trans*, Intersex, and Cisgender Issues in Physical Education and Sport." In *Social Justice in Physical Education: Critical Reflections and Pedagogies for Change,* ed. Daniel B. Robinson and Lynn Randall, 271–96. Toronto: Canadian Scholars' Press.

Sykes, Heather, and Manal Hamzeh. 2018. "Anti-Colonial Critiques of Sport Mega-Events." *Leisure Studies* 37 (6): 735–46. https://doi.org/10.1080/02614367.2018.1532449.

Sytsma, Sharon E. 2006. "The Ethics of Using Dexamethasone to Prevent Virilization of Female Fetuses." In *Ethics and Intersex*, ed. Sharon E. Sytsma, 241–58. Dordrecht: Springer. https://doi.org/10.1007/1-4220-4314-7_15.

TallBear, Kim. 2018. "Making Love and Relations Beyond Settler Sex and Family." In *Making Kin Not Population*, ed. Donna J. Haraway and Adele Clarke, 145–64. Chicago: Prickly Paradigm Press.

Tamar-Mattis, Anne. 2012. *Medical Treatment of People with Intersex Conditions as Torture and Cruel, Inhuman, or Degrading Treatment or Punishment.* Report to the UN Special Rapporteur on Torture. https://interactadvocates.org/wp-content/uploads/2017/03/interACT-Report-for-UNSRT-on-Intersex.pdf.

Tate, Shirley. 2007. "Black Beauty: Shade, Hair and Anti-racist Aesthetics." *Ethnic and Racial Studies* 30 (2): 300–19. https://doi.org/10.1080/01419870601143992.

Taylor, Paul C. 2016. *Black Is Beautiful: A Philosophy of Black Aesthetics.* Oxford: John Wiley and Sons. doi:10.1002/9781119118527.

Thomas, Carol. 2004. "Developing the Social Relational in the Social Model of Disability: A Theoretical Agenda." In *Implementing the Social Model of Disability: Theory and Research*, ed. Colin Barnes and Geof Mercer, 32–47. Leeds, UK: Disability Press.

Thomas, Nigel, and Andy Smith. 2008. *Disability, Sport and Society: An Introduction.* New York: Routledge. https://doi.org/10.4324/9780203099360.

Thompson, Charis. 2005. *Making Parents: The Ontological Choreography of Reproductive Technologies.* Cambridge, MA: MIT Press.

Thomsen, Carly. 2013. "From Refusing Stigmatization toward Celebration: New Directions for Reproductive Justice Activism." *Feminist Studies* 39 (1): 149–58. doi:10.1353/fem.2013.0006.

–. 2016. "In Plain(s) Sight: Rural LGBTQ Women and the Politics of Visibility." In *Queering the Countryside: New Frontiers in Rural Queer Studies*, ed. Mary Gray, Brian Gilley, and Colin Johnson, 244–65. New York: New York University Press.

Titchkosky, Tanya. 2005. "Looking Blind: A Revelation of Culture's Eye." In *Bodies in Commotion: Disability and Performance*, ed. Carrie Sandahl and Philip Auslander, 219–29. Ann Arbor: University of Michigan Press.

Tolarova, Marie M. 2015. "Pediatric Cleft Lip and Palate." *Medscape*, November 30. http://emedicine.medscape.com/article/995535-overview.

Topps, Sarah S. 2015. "Medical Photography of the Bodies of Intersex Individuals." In *Disturbing Argument: Selected Works from the 18th NCA/AFA Alta Conference on Argumentation*, ed. Catherine H. Palczewski, 117–23. London: Routledge.

Tosh, Jemma. 2016. *Psychology and Gender Dysphoria: Feminist and Transgender Perspectives.* New York: Routledge.

Trafimow, David. 2013. "The Ethics of PGD for Intersex Conditions: Problems with the Diversity Argument." *American Journal of Bioethics* 13 (10): 53–55. https://doi.org/10.1080/15265161.2013.828116.

Trans Brain FX. n.d. "Autism, PCOS & 'Intersex.'" https://transbrainfx.com/pcos
-dsds-intersex/.

Transgender, Non-Binary, Intersex: Support & Activism. n.d. "Kyriarchy and Discrimination." Accessed October 12, 2019. https://studentweb.bellevuecollege.
edu/transactivism/about/kyriarchy-and-discrimination/.

Transparency Market Research. 2016. "Preimplantation Genetic Diagnosis (PGD)
Market's Future Lies in PGD for Aneuploidy Screening, Expected to Reach
US$118.0 Mn by 2020." May 20. https://www.transparencymarketresearch.com/
pressrelease/global-preimplantation-genetic-diagnosis-market.htm.

–. 2020. "Preimplantation Genetic Testing Market – Global Industry Analysis, Size,
Share, Growth, Trends, and Forecast, 2019–2027." https://www.transparency
marketresearch.com/preimplantation-genetic-testing-market.html.

Travers, Ann. 2008. "The Sport Nexus and Gender Injustice." *Studies in Social Justice* 2 (1): 79–101. https://doi.org/10.26522/ssj.v2i1.969.

Tremain, Shelley. 2002. "On the Subject of Impairment." In *Disability/Postmodernity:
Embodying Disability Theory*, ed. Mirian Corker and Tom Shakespeare, 32–47.
London: Bloomsbury.

Triea, Kira. 1999. "Power, Orgasm, and the Psychohormonal Research Unit." In *Intersex in the Age of Ethics*, ed. Alice Domurat Dreger, 141–46. Hagerstown, MD:
University Publishing Group.

Truffer, Daniela. 2015. "It's a Human Rights Issue!" *Narrative Inquiry in Bioethics* 5
(2): 111–14. doi:10.1353/nib.2015.0037.

Truth, Sojourner. 1851. "Ain't I a Woman?" Paper presented at "Women's Convention," Akron, Ohio, May 29.

Tuana, Nancy. 1992. "The Radical Future of Feminist Empiricism." *Hypatia* 7 (1):
100–14. https://doi.org/10.1111/j.1527-2001.1992.tb00700.x.

Tuck, Eve, and K. Wayne Yang. 2012. "Decolonization Is Not a Metaphor." *Decolonization: Indigeneity, Education and Society* 1 (1): 1–40. https://jps.library.
utoronto.ca/index.php/des/article/view/18630.

Tucker, Ross. 2016. "Hyperandrogenism and Women vs Women vs Men in Sport: A
Q&A with Joanna Harper." *The Science of Sport*, May 23. http://sportsscientists.
com/2016/05/hyperandrogenism-women-vs-women-vs-men-sport-qa
-joanna-harper/.

–. 2017. "Testosterone, Performance & Intersex Athletes: Will the IAAF Evidence Be
Enough?" *The Science of Sport*, July 5. https://sportsscientists.com/2017/07/
testosterone-performance-intersex-athletes-will-iaaf-evidence-enough/.

Tynedal, Jeremy, and Gregor Wolbring. 2013. "Paralympics and Its Athletes through
the Lens of the New York Times." *Sports* 1 (1): 13–36. https://doi.org/10.3390/
sports1010013.

United Nations Human Rights. 2017. "Public Consultation on Protection against
Violence and Discrimination Based on Sexual Orientation and Gender Identity."
Geneva, Switzerland, January 24–25.

Valentine, David. 2015. "Autobiography, Queer Time, and the Future." Society for
Cultural Anthropology, Theorizing the Contemporary, *Fieldsights*, July 21.
https://culanth.org/fieldsights/autobiography-queer-time-and-the-future.

Valla, Jeffery M., and Stephan J. Ceci. 2011. "Can Sex Differences in Science Be Tied to the Long Reach of Prenatal Hormones? Brain Organization Theory, Digit Ratio (2D/4D), and Sex Difference in Preferences and Cognition." *Perspectives on Psychological Science* 6 (2): 134–46. https://doi.org/10.1177/1745691611400236.

Valle, Jan W., and David J. Connor. 2019. *Rethinking Disability: A Disability Studies Approach to Inclusive Practices.* 2nd ed. New York: Routledge.

van der Werff, John F.A., and Jacques C. van der Meulen. 2000. "Treatment Modalities for Hypospadias Cripples." *Plastic and Reconstructive Surgery* 105 (2): 600–8. doi:10.1097/00006534-200002000-00019.

van Dijck, José. 2005. *The Transparent Body: A Cultural Analysis of Medical Imaging.* Seattle: University of Washington Press.

Van Eeden-Moorefield, Brad, et al. 2011. "Same-Sex Relationships and Dissolution: The Connection between Heteronormativity and Homonormativity." *Family Relations* 60 (5): 563–71. https://doi.org/10.1111/j.1741-3729.2011.00669.x.

van Heesch, Margriet. 2009. "Do I Have XY Chromosomes?" In *Critical Intersex,* ed. Morgan Holmes, 123–46. Farnham, UK: Ashgate. https://doi.org/10.4324/9781315575018.

van Wormer, Katherine. 2009. "Restorative Justice as Social Justice for Victims of Gendered Violence: A Standpoint Feminist Perspective." *Social Work* 54 (2): 107–16. https://doi.org/10.1093/sw/54.2.107.

Velazquez, Jose L. Perez, Diego M. Mateos, and Ramon Guevara Erra. 2019. "On a Simple General Principle of Brain Organization." *Frontiers in Neuroscience* 13: 1–16. doi:10.3389/fnins.2019.01106.

Velpeau, Alfred A.L.M. 1845. *An Elementary Treatise on Midwifery; or, the Principles of Tokology and Embryology.* Trans. Charles D. Meigs. Philadelphia: Lindsay and Blakiston.

Vidali, Amy. 2010. "Seeing What We Know: Disability and Theories of Metaphor." *Journal of Literary and Cultural Disability Studies* 4 (1): 33–54. https://doi.org/10.1353/jlc.0.0032.

Vidya. 2010. "PCOS and Intersex?" Feministing. http://feministing.com/2009/07/23/pcos-and-intersex/.

Vigneault, Karen. 2011. "LGBTIQ History Starts Here: Indigenous/Native Terminology." In *Serving LGBTQI Library and Archives Users: Essays on Outreach, Service, Collections and Access,* ed. Ellen Greenblatt, 244–46. Jefferson, NC: McFarland and Company.

Vikander, Tessa. 2019. "Ruling against Olympic Sprinter Caster Semenya Angers Elite Transgender Athletes and Inclusion Experts." *Toronto Star,* May 2. https://www.thestar.com/vancouver/2019/05/02/ruling-against-olympic-sprinter-caster-semenya-angers-elite-transgender-athletes-and-inclusion-experts.html.

Vilain, Eric. 2012. "Gender Testing for Athletes Remains a Tough Call." *New York Times,* June 18. https://www.nytimes.com/2012/06/18/sports/olympics/the-line-between-male-and-female-athletes-how-to-decide.html.

Villarreal, Daniel. 2022. "Forget 'the Gay Gene,' Because Science Has a New Explanation for Homosexuality." *Hornet,* January 4. https://hornet.com/stories/gay-gene-explanation-3/.

Viloria, Hida. 2014. "Caught in the Gender Binary Blind Spot: Intersex Erasure in Cisgender Rhetoric." *Hida Viloria: Author and Human Rights Activist,* August 18. http://hidaviloria.com/caught-in-the-gender-binary-blind-spot-intersex-erasure -in-cisgender-rhetoric/.

–. 2015. "How Common Is Intersex? An Explanation of the Stats." Intersex Campaign for Equality, April 1. https://www.intersexequality.com/how-common-is-intersex -in-humans/.

–. 2017. *Born Both: An Intersex Life.* New York: Hachette Books.

Vogel, David L., et al. 2011. "'Boys Don't Cry': Examination of the Links between Endorsement of Masculine Norms, Self-Stigma, and Help-Seeking Attitudes for Men from Diverse Backgrounds." *Journal of Counseling Psychology* 58 (3): 368– 82. https://doi.org/10.1037/a0023688.

von Luschka, Hubert, et al. 1868. "Die äusseren geschlechtstheile eines Busch- weibes." *Monatsschrift für Geburtskunde* 32: 343–50.

Wackwitz, Laura A. 1996. "Sex Testing in International Women's Athletics: A His- tory of Silence." *Women in Sport and Physical Activity Journal* 5 (1): 51–68. https://doi.org/10.1123/wspaj.5.1.51.

–. 2003. "Verifying the Myth: Olympic Sex Testing and the Category 'Woman.'" *Women's Studies International Forum* 26 (6): 553–60. https://doi.org/10.1016/j. wsif.2003.09.009.

Waggoner, Miranda R. 2015. "Cultivating the Maternal Future: Public Health and the Prepregnant Self." *Signs* 40 (4): 939–62. https://doi.org/10.1086/680404.

Waitz, Theodor. 1863. *Introduction to Anthropology.* London: Longman.

Walcott, Rinaldo, and Idil Abdillahi. 2019. *BlackLife: Post-BLM and the Struggle for Freedom.* Winnipeg: Arp Books.

Waldschmidt, Anne. 2015. "Who Is Normal? Who Is Deviant? 'Normality' and 'Risk' in Genetic Diagnostics and Counseling." In *Foucault and the Government of Disability,* ed. Shelley Tremain, 191–207. Ann Arbor: University of Michigan Press. doi:10.3998/mpub.8265343.

Wall, Sean Saifa M. 2015a. "American Surgeons Are Still Mutilating Children Who Don't Look 'Normal.'" *Quartz,* April 26. https://qz.com/391209/american-surgeons -are-still-mutilating-children-who-dont-look-normal/.

–. 2015b. "Standing at the Intersections: Navigating Life as a Black Intersex Man." *Narrative Inquiry in Bioethics* 5 (2): 117–19. doi:10.1353/nib.2015.0046.

–. 2015c. "36 Revolutions of Change." *YouTube,* June 30. https://www.youtube.com/ watch?v=9mvNmRlpfaM.

–. 2016. "Love, Complexity and Inter-sectionality." *Intersex Day,* November 8. http:// intersexday.org/en/love-complexity-intersectionality/.

Wall, Sean Saifa M., et al. 2015. "What It's Like to Be Intersex." *YouTube,* March 28. https://www.youtube.com/watch?v=cAUDKEI4QKI&feature=emb_logo.

Walsh, Karen A. 2015. "'Normalizing' Intersex Didn't Feel Normal or Honest to Me." *Narrative Inquiry into Bioethics* 5 (2): 119–22. doi:10.1353/nib.2015.0051.

Walsh, Pat, et al. 2011. "In Search of Biomarkers for Autism: Scientific, Social and Ethical Challenges." *Nature Reviews Neuroscience* 12 (10): 603–12. https://doi. org/10.1038/nrn3113.

Ward, Michael R.M. 2019. "(Un)belonging in Higher Education: Negotiating Working-Class Masculinities Within and Beyond the University Campus." In *Identities, Youth and Belonging: International Perspectives,* ed. Sadia Habib and Michael R.M. Ward, 159–76. London: Palgrave Macmillan. https://doi.org/10.1007/978-3-319-96113-2_10.

Warne, Garry, et al. 2005. "A Long-Term Outcome Study of Intersex Conditions." *Journal of Pediatric Endocrinology and Metabolism* 18 (5): 555–68. https://doi.org/10.1515/JPEM.2005.18.6.555.

Warne, Garry, and Vijayalakshmi Bhatia. 2006. "Intersex, East and West." In *Ethics and Intersex,* ed. Sharon E. Sytsma, 183–205. New York: Springer. https://doi.org/10.1007/1-4220-4314-7_11.

Warnke, Georgia. 2011. *Debating Sex and Gender.* Oxford: Oxford University Press.

Warren, Andrew, Amanda J. Sutherland, and Radka Lenz. 1994. "Factitious Hermaphroditism." *Psychosomatics: Journal of Consultation and Liaison Psychiatry* 35 (6): 578–81. https://doi.org/10.1016/S0033-3182(94)71727-8.

Watson, Amanda D. 2020. *The Juggling Mother: Coming Undone in the Age of Anxiety.* Vancouver: UBC Press.

Watson, Nick, and Simo Vehmas, eds. 2019. *Routledge Handbook of Disability Studies.* 2nd ed. New York: Routledge.

Way, Niobe, et al. 2014. "'It Might Be Nice to Be a Girl ... Then You Wouldn't Have to Be Emotionless': Boys' Resistance to Norms of Masculinity during Adolescence." *Psychology of Men and Masculinity* 15 (3): 241–52. https://doi.org/10.1037/a0037262.

Weiss, Linda K., et al. 2002. "Hormone Replacement Therapy Regimens and Breast Cancer Risk." *Obstetrics and Gynecology* 100 (6): 1148–58. https://doi.org/10.1016/S0029-7844(02)02502-4.

Weiss, Rachel. 2019. "She Sent 23andMe Her DNA. They Told Her She's Intersex." *Newsday,* December 31. https://www.newsday.com/news/health/dawn-covino-intersex-solidarity-day-1.38037837.

Wendell, Susan. 1996. *The Rejected Body: Feminist Philosophical Reflections on Disability.* New York: Routledge.

Whelan, Joan. 2002. "Joan Whelan Address to Robert Wood Johnson." Intersex Society of North America. https://isna.org/articles/whelan2002/.

Wikström, Anne M., et al. 2006. "Genetic Features of the X Chromosome Affect Pubertal Development and Testicular Degeneration in Adolescent Boys with Klinefelter Syndrome." *Clinical Endocrinology* 65 (1): 92–97. https://doi.org/10.1111/j.1365-2265.2006.02554.x.

Wilkerson, Abby L. 2002. "Disability, Sex Radicalism, and Political Agency." *Feminist Disability Studies* 14 (3): 33–57.

–. 2012. "Normate Sex and Its Discontents." In *Sex and Disability,* ed. Robert McRuer and Anna Mollow, 183–207. Durham, NC: Duke University Press. https://doi.org/10.1215/9780822394877-010.

Williams, Clare, Priscilla Alderson, and Bobbie Farsides. 2002. "'Drawing the Line' in Prenatal Screening and Testing: Health Practitioners' Discussions." *Health, Risk and Society* 4 (1): 61–75. https://doi.org/10.1080/13698570210294.

Williams, Walter L. 1992. *The Spirit of the Flesh: Sexual Diversity in American Indian Culture.* Boston: Beacon.

Willis, Deborah, ed. 2010. *Black Venus 2010: They Called Her "Hottentot."* Philadelphia: Temple University Press.

Wilson, Gina. 2012. "Intersex Domestic Violence: The Fourteen Days of Intersex." OII Intersex Network, February 25. http://oiiinternational.com/2568/intersex-domestic-violence-fourteen-days-intersex/.

Wilson, James C. 2000. "Making Disability Visible: How Disability Studies Might Transform the Medical and Science Writing Classroom." *Technical Communication Quarterly* 9 (2): 149–61. https://doi.org/10.1080/10572250009364691.

Wisniewski, Amy B., and Tom Mazur. 2009. "46,XY DSD with Female or Ambiguous External Genitalia at Birth Due to Androgen Insensitivity Syndrome, 5α-Reductase-2 Deficiency, or 17ß-Hydroxysteroid Dehydrogenase Deficiency: A Review of Quality of Life Outcomes." *International Journal of Pediatric Endocrinology* 2009 (567430): 1–7. https://doi.org/10.1155/2009/567430.

Wodda, Aimee, and Vanessa R. Panfil. 2014. "'Don't Talk to Me about Deception': The Necessary Erosion of the Trans Panic Defense." *Albany Law Review* 78: 927–71.

Wolbring, Gregor. 2012. "Paralympians Outperforming Olympians: An Increasing Challenge for Olympism and the Paralympic and Olympic Movement." *Sport, Ethics and Philosophy* 6 (2): 251–66. https://doi.org/10.1080/17511321.2012.667828.

Womack, Ytasha. 2013. *Afrofuturism: The World of Black Sci-Fi and Fantasy Culture.* Chicago: Chicago Review Press.

Woodgate, Roberta L., et al. 2016. "Childhood Brain Cancer and Its Psychosocial Impact on Survivors and Their Parents: A Qualitative Thematic Synthesis." *European Journal of Oncology Nursing* 20: 140–49. https://doi.org/10.1016/j.ejon.2015.07.004.

World Health Organization. 2003. *World Atlas of Birth Defects.* 2nd ed. Geneva: World Health Organization.

World Medical Association. 2019. "WMA Urges Physicians Not to Implement IAAF Rule on Classifying Women Athletes." April 25. https://www.wma.net/news-post/wma-urges-physicians-not-to-implement-iaaf-rules-on-classifying-women-athletes/.

Wormsley, Alisha B. n.d. "There Are Black People in the Future." https://alishabwormsley.com/there-are-black-people-in-the-future.

Xuetong, Yan. 2006. "The Rise of China and Its Power Status." *Chinese Journal of International Politics* 1 (1): 5–33. https://doi.org/10.1093/cjip/pol002.

Yaniv, Oren. 2009. "Semenya, Forced to Take Gender Test, Is a Woman ... and a Man." *Daily News* (New York), September 10. https://www.nydailynews.com/news/world/semenya-forced-gender-test-woman-man-article-1.176427.

Yaszek, Lisa. 2006. "Afrofuturism, Science Fiction, and the History of the Future." *Socialism and Democracy* 20 (3): 41–60. https://doi.org/10.1080/08854300600950236.

Young, Cathy. 2019. "The Future Is Female. And She's Furious." *Reason,* February. https://reason.com/2019/01/28/the-future-is-female-and-shes/.

Young, Stella. 2012. "We're Not Here for Your Inspiration." *ABC News,* July 2. https://www.abc.net.au/news/2012-07-03/young-inspiration-porn/4107006.

–. 2014. "I'm Not Your Inspiration, Thank You Very Much." *TED,* April. https://www.ted.com/talks/stella_young_i_m_not_your_inspiration_thank_you_very_much?language=en.

Zaccone, Laura A. 2010. "Policing the Policing of Intersex Bodies: Softening the Lines of Title IX Athletic Programs." *Brooklyn Law Review* 76 (1): 385–438.

Zamalin, Alex. 2019. *Black Utopia: The History of an Idea from Black Nationalism to Afrofuturism.* New York: Columbia University Press.

Zeigler, Cyd. 2016a. "Dutee Chand's Early 100-Meter Exit Says a Lot about Caster Semenya." *Outsports,* August 14. http://www.outsports.com/2016/8/14/12475190/caster-semenya-dutee-chand-intersex-olympics.

–. 2016b. "Exclusive: Read the Olympics' New Transgender Guidelines That Will Not Mandate Surgery." *Outsports,* January 12. http://www.outsports.com/2016/1/21/10812404/transgender-ioc-policy-new-olympics.

Zeiler, Kristin, and Anette Wickström. 2009. "Why Do 'We' Perform Surgery on Newborn Intersexed Children? The Phenomenology of the Parental Experience of Having a Child with Intersex Anatomies." *Feminist Theory* 10 (3): 359–77. https://doi.org/10.1177/1464700109343258.

Zhang, Heng, et al. 2013. "Long-Term Evaluation of Patients Undergoing Genitoplasty Due to Disorders of Sex Development: Results from a 14-Year Follow-Up." *Scientific World Journal* 2013: 1–7. https://doi.org/10.1155/2013/298015.

Zieselman, Kimberly. 2015. "Invisible Harm." *Narrative Inquiry in Bioethics* 5 (2): 122–25. doi:10.1353/nib.2015.0056.

Zucker, Kenneth J. 2012. "Born This Way: Comment on Factitious Intersex Conditions." *International Journal of Sexual Health* 24 (2): 97–98. https://doi.org/10.1080/19317611.2012.685024.

Index

Note: "AIS" refers to androgen insensitivity syndrome; "CAH" to congenital adrenal hyperplasia; "CAIS" to complete androgen insensitivity syndrome; "DSD" to disorders of sex development; "HRT" to hormone replacement therapy; "PGD" to preimplantation genetic diagnosis.

of disability, 16–19; disease as metaphor, 254; DSD terminology, 8–9, 10; identity nomenclature, 20–25; in medical discourse, 240; for medical interventions, 28; pro-consent rhetoric, 159–60; of queering, 64–65. *See also* haunting and hauntology

Laqueur, Thomas: on sex dimorphism, 275n6

Latham, Rachael, 185

Laurent, Bo (Cheryl Chase): on curative medical practices, 62; on female assignment, 59; on surgeries, 79–80

Law, Alvin, 187

Layden, Tim, 167–68, 176

Lee, Peter A., 75

Leite, Renato, 185

lesbian politics and sexuality, 167, 263–64

Levant, Ronald F., 206

LGBTQIA2 people: asked to "prove" identity, 128; "I" (intersex) in, 4

Long, Christopher J., 97

Long, Lynnell Stephani, 82–83, 122

lower urinary tract symptoms (LUTS), 38, 39

Luk, Small, 59

lying, 85–91; about intersex identity, 132–33; vs deceiving, 86; by medical professionals, 114

Magubane, Zine, 118–19, 120–21

Maheshwari, Abha, 51, 240

male privilege: and trans men, 131

males (assigned): fertility of, 53

Mansfield, Caroline, 284n8

Mäntyranta, Eero, 152

Marquez, Anunnaki Ray, 136

marriage. *See* same-sex/different-sex marriage

masculinity: failure of, 99; hetero-masculinity, 100; and hormones, 67, 70

masculinization: of (assigned) females, 40; psychological, 40–41; of sports, 208; surgeries, 60–61

masculinizing corrections, 95. *See also* hypospadias and hypospadias cripple

Mastenbroek, Sebastiaan, 285n9

MaterniT21, 212, 284n5

Matrau, Theresa M., 284n8

Mayer-Rokitansky-Küster-Hauser syndrome (MRKH), 123, 127

Mazur, Tom, 53–54, 276n3

M.C. (pseud., intersex child), 16–17

McDermott, Nick, 116

McRuer, Robert, 6, 129; ableism of same-sex marriage discourse, 265. *See also* crip theory

medical discourse, 98, 240

medical examinations. *See* genitals, examinations and displays

medical interventions: body-mind disabilities from, 65; consequences of, 64; dyadic views of, 55; and medical education, 35; and reproductive capacity, 51. *See also* gender affirmation

medical malpractice: errors, 93–94; and intersex activism, 107; long-term consequences of, 108; as "mistakes," 107; as part of medical practice, 93–94; practices constituting, 104–5; "treatments" as, 104

medical photography, 82

medical professionals: communication from, 44–45, 236, 249, 257; creation of disabled subjects, 14, 29; education of, 268–70; gender/sex identity of intersex people, 57; intentions of, 28, 35, 61; intersex as medical emergency, 3, 4–5; and misinformation, 85; mis/recognition of trauma, 95, 106; perceptions of, 100–1; power over intersex, 252; quoted (on surgeries), 74; and sex dyad, 5; status of, 62, 92, 105, 108; on surgeries, 79; on women in sports, 151. *See also* genitals, examinations and displays; hormone replacement therapy (HRT); surgeries

medication: use of term, 58, 160